Anxiety Disorders

Guest Editors

HANS-ULRICH WITTCHEN, PhD
ANDREW T. GLOSTER, PhD

PSYCHIATRIC CLINICS OF NORTH AMERICA

www.psych.theclinics.com

September 2009 • Volume 32 • Number 3

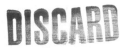
SAUNDERS an imprint of ELSEVIER, Inc.

W.B. SAUNDERS COMPANY
A Division of Elsevier Inc.

1600 John F. Kennedy Boulevard ● Suite 1800 ● Philadelphia, PA 19103-2899

http://www.theclinics.com

PSYCHIATRIC CLINICS OF NORTH AMERICA Volume 32, Number 3
September 2009 ISSN 0193-953X, ISBN-13: 978-1-4377-1270-4, ISBN-10: 1-4377-1270-3
Editor: Sarah E. Barth
Developmental Editor: Donald Mumford

Psychiatric Clinics of North America (ISSN 0193-953X) is published quarterly by Elsevier Inc., 360 Park Avenue South, New York, NY 10010-1710. Months of issue are March, June, September, and December. Business and Editorial Offices: 1600 John F. Kennedy Blvd., Suite 1800, Philadelphia, PA 19103-2899. Periodicals postage paid at New York, NY and additional mailing offices. Subscription prices are $230.00 per year (US individuals), $398.00 per year (US institutions), $116.00 per year (US students/residents), $275.00 per year (Canadian individuals), $495.00 per year (Canadian Institutions), $342.00 per year (foreign individuals), $495.00 per year (foreign institutions), and $171.00 per year (international & Canadian students/residents). Foreign air speed delivery is included in all Clinics' subscription prices. All prices are subject to change without notice. **POSTMASTER:** Send address changes to Psychiatric Clinics of North America, Elsevier Health Sciences Division, Subscription Customer Service, 3251 Riverport Lane, Maryland Heights, MO 63043. Customer Service: 1-800-654-2452 (US). From outside the United States, call 1-314-447-8871. Fax: 1-314-447-8029. E-mail: journalscustomerservice-usa@elsevier.com (for print support) and journalsonlinesupport-usa@elsevier.com (for online support).

Reprints. For copies of 100 or more, of articles in this publication, please contact the Commercial Reprints Department, Elsevier Inc., 360 Park Avenue South, New York, New York 10010-1710. Tel.: (212) 633-3813, Fax: (212) 462-1935, E-mail: reprints@elsevier.com.

Psychiatric Clinics of North America is covered in MEDLINE/PubMed (Index Medicus), Current Contents/Social and Behavioral Sciences, Social Science Citation Index, Embase/Excerpta Medica, and PsycINFO.

Printed in the United States of America.

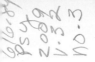

Contributors

GUEST EDITORS

HANS-ULRICH WITTCHEN, PhD
Institute of Clinical Psychology & Psychotherapy, Department of Psychology, Technische Universität Dresden, Dresden, Germany

ANDREW T. GLOSTER, PhD
Institute of Clinical Psychology & Psychotherapy, Department of Psychology, Technische Universität Dresden, Dresden, Germany

AUTHORS

CHRISTER ALLGULANDER, MD, PhD
Senior Lecturer and Associate Professor, Department of Clinical Euroscience, Karolinska Institutet, Section of Psychiatry at Karolinska University Hospital, Huddinge, Sweden

JOANNA J. ARCH, PhD
Post-Doctoral Fellow, Department of Psychology, University of California Los Angeles, Los Angeles, California

KATJA BEESDO, PhD
Academic Assistant, Institute of Clinical Psychology & Psychotherapy, Department of Psychology, Technische Universität Dresden, Dresden, Germany

ELISABETH BINDER, MD, PhD
Research Group Leader, Max-Planck Institute of Psychiatry, Munich, Germany; Assistant Professor, Department of Psychiatry and Behavioral Sciences; and Assistant Professor, Department of Human Genetics, Emory University School of Medicine, Atlanta, Georgia

MICHELLE G. CRASKE, PhD
Professor, Department of Psychology; and Department of Psychiatry and Biobehavioral Sciences, University of California Los Angeles, Los Angeles, California

DAMIAAN DENYS, MD, PhD
Department of Psychiatry, Academic Medical Center, University of Amsterdam; and the Institute for Neuroscience of the Royal Netherlands Academy of Arts and Sciences, Amsterdam, The Netherlands

ANDREW T. GLOSTER, PhD
Institute of Clinical Psychology & Psychotherapy, Department of Psychology, Technische Universität Dresden, Dresden, Germany

ALFONS O. HAMM, PhD
Professor, Department of Clinical Psychology, University of Greifswald, Greifswald, Germany

RICHARD G. HEIMBERG, PhD
Professor and Distinguished Faculty Fellow in Psychology; and Director, Adult Anxiety
Clinic of Temple, Department of Psychology, Temple University, Philadelphia,
Pennsylvania

ERIC HOLLANDER, MD
Department of Pyschiatry, Montefiore Medical Center, University Hospital of Albert
Einstein College of Medicine, Bronx, New York

JUERGEN HOYER, PhD
Professor, Institute of Clinical Psychology & Psychotherapy, Department of Psychology,
Technische Universität Dresden, Dresden, Germany

ELLEN C. JØRSTAD-STEIN, MSc
Doctoral Student in Clinical Psychology, Adult Anxiety Clinic of Temple, Department
of Psychology, Temple University, Philadelphia, Pennsylvania

SUSANNE KNAPPE, Dipl-Psych
Research Assistant, Institute of Clinical Psychology & Psychotherapy; and Faculty
of Science, Technische Universität Dresden, Dresden, Germany

JAMES F. LECKMAN, MD
Professor of Child Psychiatry, Pediatrics, and Psychology, Child Study Center, Yale
University, New Haven, Connecticut

ELIZABETH I. MARTIN, PhD
Laboratory of Neuropsychopharmacology, Department of Psychiatry and Behavioral
Sciences, Emory University, Atlanta, Georgia

R. KATHRYN McHUGH, MA
Graduate Student, Department of Psychology, Boston University, Boston,
Massachusetts

CHARLES B. NEMEROFF, MD, PhD
Reunette W. Harris Professor, Laboratory of Neuropsychopharmacology, Department
of Psychiatry and Behavioral Sciences, Emory University, Atlanta, Georgia

MICHAEL W. OTTO, PhD
Professor, Department of Psychology, Boston University, Boston, Massachusetts

KATHARINE A. PHILLIPS, MD
Department of Psychiatry and Human Behavior, Brown University, Providence, Rhode
Island

DANIEL S. PINE, MD
Director, Section on Development and Affective Neuroscience, Department of Health
and Human Services, National Institute of Mental Health, National Institutes of Health,
Bethesda, Maryland

SCOTT L. RAUCH, MD
Professor of Psychiatry, Harvard Medical School; and President and Psychiatrist in Chief,
McLean Hospital, Belmont, Massachusetts

KERRY J. RESSLER, MD, PhD
Investigator, Howard Hughes Medical Institute, Chevy Chase, Maryland; and Associate Professor, Department of Psychiatry and Behavioral Sciences, Yerkes Research Center, Emory University, Atlanta, Georgia

ARIEH Y. SHALEV, MD
Professor and Chair, Department of Psychiatry, Hadassah University Hospital, Jerusalem, Israel

JASPER A.J. SMITS, PhD
Assistant Professor, Department of Psychology, Southern Methodist University, Dallas, Texas

DAN J. STEIN, MD, PhD
Deparment of Psychiatry and Mental Health, University of Cape Town, Cape Town, South Africa

HANS-ULRICH WITTCHEN, PhD
Institute of Clinical Psychology & Psychotherapy, Department of Psychology, Technische Universität Dresden, Dresden, Germany

Contents

predictors for onset, course, and outcome will require prospective designs that assess a wide range of putative vulnerability and risk factors. This type of information is important for improved early recognition and differential diagnosis as well as prevention and treatment in this age span.

In this article, the authors assess the successes, remaining challenges, and new developments in cognitive behavioral therapy (CBT) for anxiety disorders. They define CBT, examine treatment components, review treatment efficacy, and discuss the challenges of attrition, long-term follow-up, co-occurring/comorbid disorders, limited treatment comparisons, treatment mediators, and broader implementation. In addition, they present recent developments in cognitive behavioral therapy for anxiety disorders, including linking exposure therapy to basic science, mindfulness and acceptance-based treatments, and unified or transdiagnostic treatment protocols.

Anxiety disorders are highly comorbid with each other and with major depressive disorder. As syndromes, anxiety and mood disorders share many symptoms, and several treatments are effective for both. Despite this overlap, there exist many distinguishing features that support the continued classification of individual anxiety disorders that are distinct from each other and from major depression. The goal of this article is to describe the key biological similarities and differences between anxiety disorders.

Exposure based treatments in which patients are systematically confronted with their feared objects of situations are highly effective in the treatment of specific phobias and produce stable improvement both in reported fear and behavioral avoidance. Exposure in reality is more effective in most cases than exposure in sensu. For situations that are difficult to realize, exposure in virtual environments has become increasingly valuable. Exposure in vivo is clearly superior to pharmacotherapy, although cognitive enhancers have been successfully used recently to increase the effect of exposure therapy. The induction of relaxation is not a necessary precondition for exposure therapy. Rather the current mechanisms of change focus on extinction learning as being the central mechanism both on a cognitive level namely that the feared object is no longer associated with severely threatening consequence but also on an affective level, meaning that feared cue is no longer capable to activate the fear circuit in the brain. Accordingly future diagnostic categorizations of phobic disorders in the DSM-V should rather focus on the pattern of the fear response that needs to be changed than on the eliciting cues or situations that are avoided.

This article provides an empirical review of the elements and efficacy of both pharmacologic and psychosocial treatments for panic disorder. Both monotherapies and combination treatment strategies are considered. The available evidence suggests that both cognitive behavioral therapy (CBT) and pharmacotherapy (prominently, selective serotonin reuptake inhibitors or serotonin-norepinephrine reuptake inhibitors) are effective first-line agents and that CBT offers particular cost efficacy relative to both pharmacotherapy alone and combined pharmacotherapy and CBT. Predictors of non-response and mechanisms of action are considered, as are novel treatment strategies, including the use of memory enhancers to improve CBT outcome.

This article presents the current evidence base for pharmacotherapy of generalized anxiety disorder (GAD) and an update on the phenomenology of GAD and its association with other psychiatric and somatic conditions. It discusses nosological issues and suggests ways to improve recognition, treatment, and care for patients who have GAD.

Generalized anxiety disorder (GAD) differs from other anxiety disorders. Patients do not fear a specific external object or situation; there is no distinct symptomatic reaction pattern; and the feared scenarios are not bizarre, improbable, or inflexible. Avoidance, although central, is less obvious and often is prominent only on the cognitive-emotional level. The key component of GAD, uncontrollable and persistent worrying, is easily confused with the lay concept of worry, and comorbid disorders often make the recognition of GAD difficult. This article discusses the challenges and the innovative, promising, and specific new developments in treating GAD.

THE CLINICS ARE NOW AVAILABLE ONLINE!
Access your subscription at:
www.theclinics.com

Developments in the Treatment and Diagnosis of Anxiety Disorders

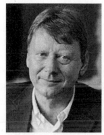 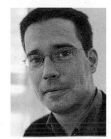

Hans-Ulrich Wittchen, PhD   Andrew T. Gloster, PhD
Guest Editors

A wide range of epidemiological community studies worldwide converge on several incontrovertible facts regarding anxiety disorders: they occur frequently, begin at an early age, significantly impair multiple areas of development and life, and are associated with numerous adverse correlates and consequences. Furthermore, evidence clearly points to the fact that the majority of patients who have anxiety disorders still go undetected and undertreated, despite considerable efforts over the last two decades to improve this situation.[1] Less than half receive any treatment at all and only a fraction of those receive what can be considered even "minimally adequate treatment."[2,3]

In addition to personal hardship resulting from anxiety disorders, increasing convergent evidence clearly points to an immense societal burden. Factors such as school failure, unemployment and underemployment, academic underachievement, interactional and marital problems, and excessive use of health care facilities insidiously combine so that the overall costs and burden to society are immense, with estimates of approximately $42 billion per year in the United States[4] and comparable rates in Europe.[2,5] Above and beyond monetary estimates, the costs extend outward from the patient and affect family and friends,[6] and multiple sources of evidence suggest that these costs are passed on to the next generation via an increased risk for mental health complications.[7,8]

Research over the past two decades ranging from cross-sectional and longitudinal epidemiological studies to clinical trials consistently documents the fact that mental disorders seldom occur in isolation.[2,9,10–13] Recent studies have contributed to a better understanding of the high rates of comorbidity, its implications, and, in some cases, the putative causes. Substantially increased rates of depressive disorders and, to a lesser degree, substance use disorders predominantly develop in the years after the onset of an anxiety disorder[14] (see article by Beesdo, Knappe, & Pine, in this issue). This has led many researchers to consider anxiety disorders as powerful—in fact, the

Psychiatr Clin N Am 32 (2009) xiii–xix
doi:10.1016/j.psc.2009.07.001
0193-953X/09/$ – see front matter © 2009 Elsevier Inc. All rights reserved.

most powerful—risk factor for depression.[15–18] Further evidence of this assumption lies in the fact that there is a dose–response relationship between anxiety disorders and subsequent mental disorders and that different anxiety disorders carry substantially different risks.[17,18]

Nevertheless, after many years of investigation, it remains unclear which mechanisms and processes best account for the high comorbidity risk in the anxiety disorders. Some suggest direct and indirect pathways of anxiety–associated features and complications, such as neurobiological factors or persistent avoidance that in themselves contribute to anxiety patients' increased risk for depression.[15] Besides shared vulnerability factors (see articles by Beesdo, Knappe, & Pine, and by Martin, Ressler, Binder, & Nemeroff, both in this issue), likely candidates that have been considered are cognitive-behavioral factors (Arch & Craske, this issue) and neurobiological sensitization processes (Martin, Ressler, Binder, & Nemeroff, this issue), leading to an accumulation of depression-specific risk factors. Others have suggested that the high rates of comorbidity indicate the existence of an underlying shared higher-order factor or liability dimension for a range of anxiety and depressive and even somatoform disorders.[19–21] These explorations argue that all these disorders should be regarded as "internalizing" disorders, characterized by emotional dysregulation and a similar and only gradually different set of vulnerability and risk factors. This latter perspective has recently received considerable, yet controversial,[22] attention within the current revision process of DSM-V and ICD-11 (see article by Wittchen, Beesdo, & Gloster, this issue).[21–25] The allure of this model for some may be its implicit (but untested) promise of a seemingly simpler diagnostic classification system.

This special issue on anxiety disorders comes together at a time of much development in the understanding, treatment, and diagnosis of anxiety disorders and particularly the revision processes of DSM-V and ICD-11, both expected to come into effect in 2012. We therefore decided not only to invite our colleagues to review the latest evidence in their respective fields, but also to comment on and share their thoughts with regard to the need of changes in our future diagnostic classification manual.

The reader will notice a particular emphasis on cognitive-behavioral treatments (CBT) relative to psychopharmacology in this special issue. This is due to several factors. First, although some new substances for some anxiety disorders have been marketed since the last time this journal reviewed the field of anxiety disorders (December 1995; Vol. 18, No. 4) and despite the existence of some new compounds and treatment principles in development (Martin, Ressler, Binder, & Nemeroff, this issue), there is currently little news about pharmacological approaches that are likely to affect practice in the next few years. Thus, the diagnostic specific articles in this issue (McHugh, Smits, & Otto; Allgulander; Hoyer & Gloster; Jørstad-Stein & Heimberg; Hamm; Shalev; and Stein, Denys, Gloster, Holander, Leckman, Rauch, & Phillips) highlight primarily the evidence for efficacy of established pharmacological approaches in short- and long-term outcomes as well as combination treatments with some form of CBT.

Second, relative to pharmacology, CBT is widely misunderstood, in part due to the definitions—or lack thereof—used to describe the techniques, processes, and strategies implemented by CBT practitioners and the mental health field in general. As CBT has grown to become the treatment of choice for various disorders and all anxiety disorders in particular, it is increasingly unlikely that the interventions used by practitioners are consistent with state-of-the-art CBT and many others may even run counter to the principles underlying CBT. This state of affairs is no wonder given the fact that "CBT" has become a catch-all phrase to describe nearly anything and seems to have replaced the word psychotherapy in some circles. Further, some practitioners not specifically trained in this modality nevertheless claim to deliver such treatments, motivated presumably by the desire to meet reimbursement requirements. Further complicating matters is that, unlike psychotropic medication, CBT's development and prescription are not strictly regulated. Thus, by focusing on CBT we hope to sensitize the practitioner to the fact that CBT as currently practiced might have little to do with CBT as derived from stringent research, or CBT as tested in randomized clinical trials.

Equally important, researchers also lack a clear understanding of the active and necessary treatment ingredients of what constitutes CBT. This is a core problem of the current CBT research field and represents a challenge for future research. Precise definitions are a prerequisite for any such attempt. What are the specific "cognitive" elements; what are the specific "behavioral" elements? What is their specific effect on dysfunctions of the "fear circuitry" in the brain and associated neurobiologic variables.[26,27] What therapeutic elements do unspecific elements constitute in relation to unspecific general factors of improvements, and which elements are unique? Is exposure in vivo a CBT variant? Which elements are unique for one versus another disorder? How does CBT in social phobia differ from CBT in PTSD and GAD? These are just a few examples of core research questions that need to be resolved if CBT wants to maintain the original claim that the method is scientifically sound and based on proper research. Only after this is established can mental health practitioners accurately examine their own skills to determine whether they posses the competences necessary to optimally treat the individual anxiety disorders.

The time has come to challenge the idea that CBT is simply a group of heterogeneous interventions, with the only prerequisite to be considered "CBT" is that they be loosely tied to a cognitive or behavioral conceptual model or be part of an empirically supported treatment *package*. Instead, a new generation of research needs to be initiated that investigates the modes, processes, and mechanisms of therapeutic action. This is the reason why we emphasized the use of precise definitions throughout the articles. When an accurate understanding of the active treatment ingredients is combined with an accurate self-assessment from the practitioner of his/her competencies in these mechanisms, the entire field is in a much stronger position to harness the knowledge of our state-of-the-art treatments, closely tied to basic science investigations, and in the service of our patients.

Third, we wanted to identify those components of CBT treatments that are currently believed to be active ingredients, even if the mechanisms through which they work are unclear. The reader will clearly notice that several interventions are common across disorders, both for pharmacological and psychological approaches. These include SSRI medication and, as evident in this special issue, various components of CBT such as exposure, emotional engagement, and techniques targeting reevaluation of thoughts. Indeed, research has begun to address the commonality of the disorders via treatment protocols[28,29] and explicit discussion of psychological processes extending from classical and operant conditioning and associated techniques.[30–32]

Techniques, in turn, are sometime more and sometimes less derived from basic scientific principles. Certain individual principles and techniques derived from these *do* cut across diagnoses. Chief among these are basic science principles of classical and operant conditioning and the techniques derived from them (ie, exposure, diffusion, etc.). The very nature of treatment validation, however, has limited our ability to indicate precisely which techniques and strategic maneuvers based on which exact scientific principles are at play. Therefore, identification of such dimensions vary depending on one's perspective, a troubling fact in itself. A partial list of potential dimensions ranges from learning theory (avoidance, reinforcement, fusion, etc.) to clinical cognitive theory (schemas, maladaptive cognitions, etc.), to experimental psychopathology (eg, attention biases), to emotional theory (antecedent and consequential control) to psychodynamic concepts (eg, repression, defense mechanism, etc.). In the next few years, the field must work towards a better understanding of which dimensions are the direct causal agents involved in therapeutic improvement and which are simply byproducts.

A fourth reason for the relative concentration on CBT in this issue surrounds the exciting developments that have occurred across the spectrum of anxiety disorders. Acceptance and Commitment Therapy (ACT) is one example of these developments, as is evident in most disorder-specific chapters in this issue. ACT can be seen as an example of a therapeutic stance that tries to develop interventions in close coordination with basic science. The evidence for its efficacy in anxiety disorders to date is preliminary, promising, and growing. In part, these and other similar developments arose in response to the recognition that superficial definitions of CBT and its requisite components would not lead to optimized outcomes.

Finally, we wish to acknowledge something that is seldom discussed in science, namely our own bias. In this case, our bias towards psychological treatments—in particular, variations of CBT—in our daily practice and research make us more keenly aware of the critical and crucial elements involved in this form of treatment.

Some readers might note a number of important topics that are missing, for example a chapter on translational research and service provision or on prevention. Certainly there is a range of remarkable and promising developments in the field that would have deserved close scrutiny, which were, however, impossible to cover because of page restrictions, although they were addressed to some degree in most disorder-specific chapters.

Nevertheless, we wish to emphasize the paradox that effective treatments are available, yet they reach only a minority of people affected. This situation remains a core concern that is evidently specific to many anxiety disorders. It differs from depression, where increasing treatment rates have been monitored. The paradox that CBT, the preferred method for many anxiety disorders, is still not widely available signals the need for further, more targeted action. We believe it is unlikely that recent attempts to make CBT shorter and simpler or to make it available by electronic media and telephone[33] so that it can be delivered by all health care professions or, in its extreme, without them will in and of themselves be an adequate solution. Unless we better understand how, why, and when CBT is effective in which disorder and with what type of patients, such demonstrations are not likely to be promising and might in fact lead to a corruption of CBT's scientific base and a devaluation of this method as a whole. Thus, we hope to stimulate a rethinking of the term CBT and a reorientation to its scientific foundations with the goal of specification and improvement.

Similar concerns can be expressed with regard to prevention. The moderately (and sometimes counterintuitive) negative effects of group-based general preventive efforts—frequently based on CBT methods—as compared with targeted high-risk approaches suggest that we need to better understand pathogenic pathways.[34,35] We believe that the uncritical group-based preventive strategies, typically showing limited efficacy in the field, suffer from a lack in anxiety-specific concepts about the core etiological pathways associated with the various anxiety disorders. Unless these pathways are better understood, it seems unlikely that we will ultimately be able to present more convergent and persuasive evidence on the efficacy of CBT.

We hope that this special issue offers guidance to the practitioners, aids in training (especially in light of the APA regulations regarding training of CBT), stimulates research, and leads to discussions between all those involved in the treatment of patients who have anxiety disorders. The field has progressed a long way in the last several decades. We hope and trust that the some of the critical reflections found within the pages of this special issue contribute to the refinement of this mission.

Hans-Ulrich Wittchen, PhD
Andrew T. Gloster, PhD

Institute of Clinical Psychology & Psychotherapy
Department of Psychology
Technische Universität Dresden
Chemnitzer Straße 46
D-01187 Dresden, Germany

E-mail addresses:
wittchen@psychologie.tu-dresden.de (H-U. Wittchen)
gloster@psychologie.tu-dresden.de (A.T. Gloster)

REFERENCES

1. Demyttenaere K, Bruffaerts R, Posada-Villa J, et al. Prevalence, severity and unmet need for treatment of mental disorders in the World Health Organization World Mental Health (WMH) Surveys. Journal of the American Medical Association 2004;291:2581–90.
2. Wittchen H-U, Jacobi F. Size and burden of mental disorders in Europe: a critical review and appraisal of 27 studies. European Neuropsychopharmacology 2005;15(4):357–67.
3. Craske MG, Edlund MJ, Sullivan G, Roy-Byrne PP, Sherbourne CD, Bystritsky AS. M.B. Perceived unmet need for mental health and barriers to among care patients with panic disorder. Psychiatric Services 2005;56:988–94.
4. Greenberg PE, Sisitsky T, Kessler RC, et al. The economic burden of anxiety disorders in the 1990s. Journal of Clinical Psychiatry 1999;60(7):427–35.
5. Konnopka A, Leichsenring F, Leibing E, König H-H. Cost-of-illness studies and cost-effectiveness analyses in anxiety disorders: A systematic review. Journal of Affective Disorders 2009;114:14–31.
6. Chambless DL, Floyd FJ, Rodebaugh TL, Steketee G. Expressed emotion and familial interaction: A study with agoraphobic and obsessive compulsive patients and their relatives. Journal of Abnormal Psychology 2007;116:754–61.
7. Weissman MM, Wickramaratne P, Nomura Y, Warner V, Pilowsky D, Verdeli H. Offspring of depressed parents: 20 years later. American Journal of Psychiatry 2006;163:1001–8.
8. Knappe S, Lieb R, Beesdo K, et al. The role of parental psychopathology and family environment for social phobia in the first three decades of life. Depression and Anxiety 2009;26(4):363–70.
9. Kessler RC, Chiu WT, Demler O, Walters EE. Prevalence, severity, and comorbidity of 12-month DSM-IV disorders in the National Comorbidity Survey Replication. Archives of General Psychiatry 2005;62:617–27.
10. Bruce SE, Yonkers KA, Otto MW, et al. Influence of psychiatric comorbidity on recovery and recurrence in generalized anxiety disorder, social phobia, and panic disorder: A 12-year prospective study. American Journal of Psychiatry 2005;162:1179–87.
11. Jacobi F, Wittchen H-U, Hölting C, et al. Prevalence, comorbidity and correlates of mental disorders in the general population: results from the German Health

Interview and Examination Survey (GHS). Psychological Medicine 2004;34(4): 597–611.

12. de Graaf R, Bijl RV, ten Have M, Beekman ATF, Vollebergh WAM. Pathways to co-morbidity: the transition of pure mood, anxiety and substance use disorders into comorbid conditions in a longitudinal population-based study. Journal of Affective Disorders 2004;82:461–7.

13. Newman DL, Moffitt TE, Caspi A, Magdol L, Silva PA. Psychiatric disorder in a birth cohort of young adults: prevalence, comorbidity, clinical significance, and new case incidence from age 11 to 21. Journal of Consulting and Clinical Psychology 1996;64(3):552–62.

14. Beesdo K, Pine DS, Lieb R, Wittchen HU. Similarities and differences in incidence and risk patterns of anxiety and depressive disorders: The position of Generalized Anxiety Disorder. Archives of General Psychiatry. In press.

15. Wittchen H-U, Kessler RC, Pfister H, Lieb R. Why do people with anxiety disorders become depressed? A prospective-longitudinal community study. Acta Psychiatrica Scandinavica 2000;102(Suppl. 406):14–23.

16. Merikangas KR, Zhang H, Avenevoli S, Acharyya S, Neuenschwander M, Angst J. Longitudinal trajectories of depression and anxiety in a prospective community study. Archives of General Psychiatry 2003;60:993–1000.

17. Bittner A, Goodwin RD, Wittchen H-U, Beesdo K, Höfler M, Lieb R. What characteristics of primary anxiety disorders predict subsequent major depressive disorder? Journal of Clinical Psychiatry 2004;65(5):618–26.

18. Kessler RC, Nelson CB, McGonagle KA, Liu J, Schwartz M, Blazer DG. Comorbidity of DSM-III-R major depressive disorder in the general population: results from the US National Comorbidity Survey. British Journal of Psychiatry 1996;168:17–30.

19. Krueger RF. The structure of common mental disorders. Archives of General Psychiatry 1999;56:921–6.

20. Watson D. Rethinking the mood and anxiety disorders: a quantitative hierarchical model for DSM-V. Journal of Abnormal Psychology 2005;114(4):522–36.

21. Andrews G, Pine DS, Hobbs MJ, Anderson TM, Sunderland M. Neurodevelopmental disorders: Cluster 2 of the proposed meta-structure for DSM-V and ICD-11. Psychological Medicine. In press.

22. Wittchen H-U, Beesdo K, Gloster AT. A New Metastructure of Mental Disorders: Helpful Step Into the Future or a Harmful Step Back to the Past? (Commentary). Psychological Medicine. In press.

23. Andrews G, Goldberg DP, Krueger RF, et al. Exploring the feasibility of a meta-structure for DSM-V and ICD-11: Could it improve utility and validity? Psychological Medicine. In press.

24. Beesdo K, Höfler M, Gloster AT, et al. The structure of common mental disorders: A replication study in a community sample of adolescents and young adults. In preparation.

25. Wittchen H-U, Beesdo K, Gloster A, Höfler M, Klotsche J, et al. The structure of mental disorders reexamined: Is it developmentally stable and robust against additions? International Journal of Methods in Psychiatric Research. In press.

26. Gloster AT, Wittchen H-U, Einsle F, Höfler M, Lang T, et al. Mechanism of Action in CBT (MAC): Methods of a Multi-Center Randomized Controlled Trial in 369 Patients with Panic Disorder and Agoraphobia. European Archives of Psychiatry and Clinical Neuroscience. In press.

27. Andrews G, Charney DS, Sirovatka PJ, Regier DA, editors. Stress-Induced and Fear Circuitry Disorders: Refining the Research Agenda for DSM-V. Arlington, VA: APA; 2009.

28. Allen LB, McHugh RK, Barlow DH. Emotional disorders: A unified protocol. In: Barlow DH, editor. Clinical Handbook of Psychological Disorders. 4 edition. New York: The Guilford Press; 2008.
29. Norton PJ, Hope DA. Preliminary evaluation of a broad-spectrum cognitive-behavioral group therapy for anxiety. Journal of Behavior Therapy and Experimental Psychiatry 2005;36:79–97.
30. Wilson KG. Science and Treatment Development: Lessons from the history of behavior therapy. Behavior Therapy 1997;28:547–58.
31. Hayes SC, Barnes-Holmes D, Roche B, editors. Relational Frame Theory: A Post-Skinnerian Account of Human Language and Cognition. New York: Kluwer Academic/Plenum Publishers; 2001.
32. Kohlenberg RJ, Tsai M. Functional Analytic Psychotherapy: A guide for creating intense and curative therapeutic relationships. New York: Plenum; 1991.
33. Perini S, Titov N, Andrews G. Clinician-assisted internet-based treatment is effective for depression: randomized controlled trial. Aust N Z J Psychiatry 2009;43: 571–8.
34. Gs G. The Child Anxiety Prevention Study: intervention model and primary outcomes. Journal of Consulting and Clinical Psychology 2009;77(3):580–7.
35. Merry S, McDowell H, Hetrick S, Bir J, Muller N. Psychological and/or educational interventions for the prevention of depression in children and adolescents. Cochrane Database Syst Rev 2004:CD003380.

The Position of Anxiety Disorders in Structural Models of Mental Disorders

Hans-Ulrich Wittchen, PhD*, Katja Beesdo, PhD, Andrew T. Gloster, PhD

KEYWORDS

• Diagnostic classification • Structural models
• Internalizing • Externalizing • Anxiety disorders

"Comorbidity" among mental disorders is commonly observed in both clinical and epidemiological samples. The robustness of this observation is rarely questioned; however, what is at issue is its meaning. Is comorbidity "noise"—nuisance covariance that researchers should eliminate by seeking "pure" cases for their studies—or a "signal"—an indication that current diagnostic systems are lacking in parsimony and are not "carving nature at its joints?"

(Krueger, p. 921).[1]

With these words, Krueger[1] started a discussion on the structure of mental disorders, which suggested that a 3-factor model of common mental disorders existed in the community. These common factors were labeled "anxious-misery," "fear" (constituting facets of a higher-order internalizing factor), and "externalizing." Along with similar evidence from personality research and psychometric explorations[2–4] and selective evidence from genetic and psychopharmacologic studies,[5–10] Krueger[1] suggested that this model might not only be phenotypically relevant, but might actually improve our understanding of core processes underlying psychopathology. Since then, this suggestion has become an influential, yet also controversial topic in the scientific community, and has received attention particularly in the context of the current revision process of the Manual of Mental Disorders (Fifth Edition) (DSM-V) and the International Classification of Diseases, 11th Revision (ICD-11).[11,12]

Focusing on anxiety disorders, this article critically discusses the methods and findings of this work, calls into question the model's developmental stability and utility for

Institute of Clinical Psychology and Psychotherapy, Department of Psychology, Technische Universität Dresden, Chemnitzer Straße 46, D-01187 Dresden, Germany
* Corresponding author.
E-mail address: wittchen@psychologie.tu-dresden.de (H-U. Wittchen).

Psychiatr Clin N Am 32 (2009) 465–481
doi:10.1016/j.psc.2009.06.004
0193-953X/09/$ – see front matter © 2009 Elsevier Inc. All rights reserved.

clinical use and clinical research, and challenges the wide-ranging implications that have been linked to the findings of this type of exploration. This critical appraisal is intended to flag several significant concerns about the method. In particular, the concerns center around the tendency to attach wide-ranging implications (eg, in terms of clinical research, clinical practice, public health, diagnostic nomenclature) to the undoubtedly interesting statistical explorations.[11–13]

INTERNALIZING AND EXTERNALIZING AS CORE DIMENSIONS OF THE STRUCTURE OF MENTAL DISORDERS
The Approach

Krueger[1] used the epidemiological diagnostic data from the US National Comorbidity Survey (NCS)[14] to analyze patterns of comorbidity among DSM-III-R mental disorders. Ten diagnoses were selected for this analysis from a wider set of all diagnoses in the NCS, namely: major depressive episode (MDE), dysthymia (DYS), panic disorder (PD), agoraphobia (AGPH), social phobia (SOP), simple phobia (SIP), generalized anxiety disorder (GAD), alcohol dependence (AD), drug dependence (DD), and antisocial personality disorder (APD). All 10 disorders were submitted to confirmatory factor analysis (CFA), a formal statistical means of evaluating dimensional accounts of comorbidity among mental disorders. Four competing models, positing from 1 latent factor to 4 latent factors, were evaluated to determine their fit in the entire NCS sample and various subsamples (**Fig. 1**).

Krueger's[1] main findings were noteworthy. For the entire NCS sample, across sexes, and across random halves, a 3-factor model provided the best fit to the correlations among the 10 disorders. These factors were labeled "anxious-misery," "fear," and

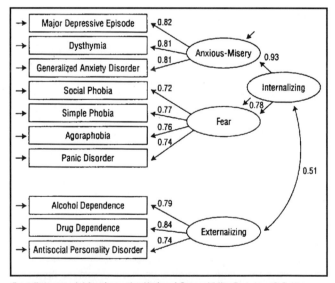

Best-fitting model for the entire National Comorbidity Survey, a 3-factor variant of the 2-factor internalizing/externalizing model. All parameter estimates are standardized and significant at P<.05.

Fig.1. Krueger's 3-factor model based on 10 lifetime disorders (NCS-Data). (*From* Krueger RF. The structure of common mental disorders. Arch General Psychiatry 1999;56:921–6; with permission.)

"externalizing." Because of the high correlation between the anxious-misery and fear factors in the 3-factor model (0.73), these factors were described as meaningful expressions of subfactors of a higher-order "internalizing" factor. Consistent with this, the 2-factor internalizing-externalizing model was also found to provide the best fit in a treatment-seeking subsample of his exploration. Thus, at the highest level of the factor hierarchy, a broad internalizing factor (with anxious-misery and fear subfactors) and a broad externalizing factor explained the pattern of correlations among mental disorders.

The Conclusion

Krueger concluded that his findings provide evidence for (a) refocusing the study of common mental disorders on their common substrates, namely broad, higher-order internalizing and externalizing dimensions, and (b) that the model helps to organize observations of psychopathology by suggesting directions for future research in psychiatric epidemiology, psychopharmacology, and psychiatric genetics in several ways (Krueger,[1] pp 925–926): First, regarding psychiatric epidemiology, it is suggested that the model would organize common psychopathological variance into psychologically sensitive patterns labeled internalizing, such as pervasive anxiety and sadness (anxious-misery) and phobic avoidance (fear), and externalizing patterns involving antisocial behaviors (APD) and lifestyles (AD, DD).

Psychologically speaking, the model suggests that maladjustment can be expressed primarily inward, as anxious misery or fear, or primarily outward, as antisocial, disruptive behavior. Second, according to the author's conclusions, the model might suggest directions for psychopharmacology because it "predicts" the observed effectiveness of similar interventions for putatively different common mental disorders. For example, the selective serotonin reuptake inhibitors (SSRIs), although initially regarded as an antidepressant, have been found to be effective in treating other internalizing conditions, such as PD and DYS. The author claims that SSRIs may be effective in treating all these conditions because they influence a core internalizing process—perhaps the personality trait of neuroticism/negative emotionality, which has also been shown to be reduced by SSRI administration. Third, the author claimed that the model is consistent with genetic findings, because internalizing disorders share a considerable degree of genetic variance. As predicted by the model, MDE and GAD are closely linked, PD and the phobias are closely linked, and MDE and the phobias, although significantly linked, are linked to a lesser degree. In addition, APD and substance use disorders share significant genetic variance. Although it is admitted that multivariate and molecular genetic research framed in terms of the model is needed to verify this possibility, existing research is interpreted to suggest that the model may organize common psychopathological variance by shared genetic etiology.

BEYOND THE INTERNALIZING-EXTERNALIZING MODEL: ADDITIONAL IMPACT AND FAR-REACHING IMPLICATIONS FOR DSM-V AND ICD-11

Since the publication of the article by Krueger[1]—and despite a range of critical concerns[15]—this approach has received considerable attention and extensions. Positive replications of the internalizing-externalizing structure clearly outnumber failures, particularly if identical or only a slightly different set of diagnoses and identical methods were used (see Refs.[12,16]). However, it should be stated up front that there were also several failures to replicate this structure for various reasons, and there are also some studies that revealed different structures, some of which suggest a considerably larger number of classes.[16,17]

In light of the seemingly attractive possibility of simplifying our current diagnostic classification structure, the DSM-V Task Force chose this approach as one of several guiding principles with which to explore the option of simplifying the classificatory structure of the future DSM and ICD.[13] By broadening the model to cover a wider range of disorders, and ultimately the whole spectrum of mental disorders currently listed in the DSM,[13,18] a new "metastructure of mental disorders" consisting of 5 "clusters" was suggested in the context of the DSM-V revision process (see special issue of *Psychological Medicine*, 2009, in press). In addition to an "externalizing" and "internalizing" (labeled "emotional") cluster, 3 further groupings were suggested as part of this proposition, labeled "Neurocognitive," "Neurodevelopmental" and "Psychotic."

At first sight, this structural grouping of a metastructure appears considerably simpler than the current diagnostic classification structures used in the DSM Fourth Edition, Text Revision (DSM-IV-TR) (17 categories)[18] and, in some parts, more convergent with the Tenth Revision of ICD (ICD-10) (10 categories).[19] Responding to some dissatisfaction expressed with the current diagnostic classification structure and its mostly descriptive principles, the authors of the proposed metastructure[11] made an impressive attempt to provide evidence for this position via a selective critical review of relevant research. In addition to extensive reference to CFA findings similar to Krueger's original exploration,[1] evidence was examined to address the question of whether current individual mental disorders sufficiently differ from each other, and whether the current more fine-graded distinction of specific mental disorders and their grouping in 10 major classes according to ICD-10 and 17 in DSM-IV-TR is justified. A priori criteria were chosen in the form of a wide range of "validators" grouped into so-called causal risk factors (ie, shared genetic risk factors, familiality, shared environmental risks, shared neural substrates, shared biomarkers, shared temperamental antecedents), and factors believed to reflect the clinical picture itself (shared abnormalities of cognitive and emotional processing, symptom similarity, rates of comorbidity, course, treatment response).[11] The outcome of this admittedly selective exploration was interpreted as proof for the proposed 5 metastructure clusters. However, there was also a fairly large residual category of disorders not yet assigned. Particularly noteworthy examples for classificatory changes associated with the proposed metastructure involve: the suggestion to group anxiety, somatoform, and depressive disorders together under the term "emotional disorders"; the allocation of bipolar disorders to the "psychotic cluster"; and the formation of a broad externalizing cluster that comprises substance use disorders, some of the personality disorders, and impulse control disorders.

Several core motivations and promises are presented by the authors of the proposed new metastructure to justify their proposal.[11]

1. *Increased utility* to the degree that the current system has been found to be overly complicated and too complex for routine care, in particular by nonspecialists like primary care physicians. From this perspective, the proposed metastructure is also expected to provide considerable simplification for research and a better adoption in routine care and public administration.
2. *Increased validity and advantages for research*, in the sense that proposed grouping would move classification of mental disorders away from one based purely on symptomatology and closer to current understanding of shared putative causal risk and clinical factors identified in research.

3. *Increased homogeneity within clusters*, in that the proposed metastructure would more appropriately highlight similarities rather than subtle differences between our current specific diagnoses.

FROM A FACTOR ANALYTIC EXPLORATION TO A CLASSIFICATORY METASTRUCTURE OF MENTAL DISORDERS?

Given this set of promises, the deeper meaning apparently ascribed to the metastructure, and the potentially far-reaching implications for research and practice, Wittchen and colleagues recently criticized and challenged these assumptions and predictions of the model in a commentary, highlighting a range of deficits and problems.[20] The commentary emphasized that the claims and promises remain largely untested and unproven, and that evidence provided was selective, "biased toward" confirming the proposition. Further, doubts were raised about how methodologically sound and valid factor analytic approaches are in deriving a classification structure that is meaningful and sensitive to clinical issues. If the intent, motivation, and claims of the authors would have been more moderate, then the proposed metastructure would be a helpful step. For example, focusing primarily on the technical aspect of reducing the number of major groups of mental disorder without overly ambitious claims of a deeper meaning and increased clinical utility would have been useful. However, the goal of this proposal is much more ambitious, namely to develop a more parsimonious metastructure based on risk factors and clinical factors with the long-term goal of improving clinical practice, administration, research, and even training and education.

Wittchen and colleagues[20] came to the conclusion that such a metastructure proposal might actually imply more risks for harm than benefits. For example, it may lead to an oversimplification of mental disorders, the deletion of disorders from the classification, premature adoption of putative common risk factors to the exclusion of other valid factors, diminished specificity with regard to recognition of established diagnoses, and the overemphasis of common treatment procedures that might in fact be very different. From a diagnostic perspective, the serious concern is that the broader, higher-order factor statistical approach might largely miss the subtle distinctions between disorders that constitute the essential difference for improved recognition and improved allocation of optimal treatment. Finally, from a technical perspective, the authors of this article are disquieted that numerous caveats and concerns regarding statistical and methodological limitations of higher-order factorial methods are not acknowledged. This disquiet also applies to concerns about the interpretation of results, the value and implications of these findings for general classificatory issues, and the propositions for a simplified metastructure of diagnostic classification systems based on these results.

A CRITICAL REAPPRAISAL OF THE "STRUCTURE OF MENTAL DISORDERS"

The new metastructure proposal[11] that is meant to inform the structure of a clinical diagnostic classification system seems to be driven by the 2- and 3-factor solutions within the "internalizing and externalizing" model. The structure is largely based on epidemiologic data collected from diagnostic instruments and self-report data, and derived using higher-order factor analytic methods. The concerns expressed earlier prompted us to conduct a critical appraisal of these methods and findings.

With support from the DSM-V Task Force, we were commissioned to reexamine the assumptions, models, and findings of this line of research. Specifically, we examined the effects of using a considerably broader scope of diagnoses than originally included, examined the stability/instability of the factors in different age groups, and explored the value and limitations for specific diagnostic areas, with a particular emphasis on anxiety. In addition, we explored models and solutions that might be potentially more sensitive to clinical, developmental, and prospective-longitudinal epidemiological data and issues, to inform about an alternative and potentially more appropriate grouping of disorders. That is, we examined which disorders and to what degree sufficiently fit the proposed 3-cluster solution and which disorders do not. Although the proposal might have implications for various other diagnostic groups, emphasis for the purpose of this article was deliberately placed on anxiety disorders.

Method

The aims and methods of this comprehensive appraisal and corresponding findings have been described elsewhere in greater detail.[21] In brief, we used 2 large epidemiological data sets: (a) the prospective-longitudinal Early Developmental Stages of Psychopathology (EDSP) study data[22,23] with 4 waves of investigation (n = 3021, age range 14–34 years) and (b) the cross-sectional German National Health Interview and Examination Survey—Mental Health Supplement (GHS-MHS) (n = 4181, age range 18–65 years)[24] to test the following 4 core aspects of the model.

1. Using CFA, we first attempted to *replicate* Krueger's cross-sectional model (ie, factor solutions and model fit) using identical methods and conventions with respect to diagnoses, diagnostic assessment, and referent time frame of the assessment.
2. We examined the *stability* of factor solutions against minor and major additions to the diagnoses included in the model by examining the effects of adding additional diagnoses. Additional diagnoses were added in stepwise, grouped, and comprehensive manner. The additional diagnoses to those used in initial analyses were: group (a) hypomanic episodes (HME), manic episodes (MNE), separation anxiety disorder, obsessive compulsive disorder (OCD), posttraumatic stress disorder (PTSD), specific phobia subtypes; group (b) pain disorders, somatoform disorders (SSI4/6); group (c) psychotic disorders; group (d) eating disorders; and group (e) childhood disorders (attention deficit hyperactivity disorder [ADHD], oppositional defiant disorder [ODD], tics, elimination disorders).
3. We also examined the *developmental stability* of the model by examining whether the solution and model fits differ substantially by age group (ie, 14–17, 18–21, 22+). These tests were conducted for Krueger's standard diagnostic set[1] as well as a broader range of diagnoses.
4. Finally, we also examined the structure of DSM-IV anxiety disorders using exploratory factor analysis (EFA) to explore the existence of similarly acceptable solutions.

Model Specifications

Irrespective of the considerable range of general and specific statistical problems inherent in factor analytic approaches (ie, violations of basic assumptions, which render all subsequent results suspect), we expected to replicate Krueger's findings[1] of 2-factor (internalizing versus externalizing) and 3-factor (anxious-misery, fear, externalizing) solutions only when using exactly the same restricted set of DSM diagnoses assessed cross-sectionally. In contrast, we did not expect to replicate the 2- and 3-factor solutions (ie, insufficient model fit) when examining the sample with restricted age groups of young and older subjects. This method provides information as to whether the model is robust against developmental and age changes.

We also did not expect that the 2- or 3-factor model provides a sufficient model fit when adding other diagnoses to the model. The latter 2 cases provide information as to whether the model is robust against even minor modifications of the diagnoses included.

It should be noted that we do not separately address the considerably more general limitations of the factor analytic approach for classificatory diagnostic purposes, which have been expressed and discussed elsewhere in greater detail.[15] However, in light of these severe limitations we emphasize that considerable caution is warranted when interpreting the implications of positive replications of the Krueger model[1] on the one hand, and any alternative structure solution on the other.

Replication: Can the 3-Factor Solution be Replicated if Exactly the Same Diagnoses are Used?

In the first step of our examination,[16] we used exactly the same conventions and diagnoses as in Krueger's original work[1] using *cross-sectional (12-month) data*. We found that, by and large, a 3-factor model fit the data in both samples (EDSP and GHS-MHS) used, separating fear, anxious-misery, and externalizing. However, Krueger[1] suggested that anxious-misery and fear constitute second-order factors of a latent "higher" dimension called "internalizing." This factoring could not be replicated consistently. Further, some of the factor loadings were much smaller than in Krueger's work,[1] which is particularly evident for the "fear" factor on specific phobia (0.43 vs 0.77). This result might indicate that "fear" is less strongly related to specific phobia in this replication sample. In general we found more heterogeneity between loadings of latent variables on diagnoses, probably due to the prospective-longitudinal nature of the EDSP data set used. However, with the factor loadings freely estimated, the Krueger[1] model fits the data well.

In the *lifetime* data set, the model once again necessitated the omission of the higher-order factor "internalizing," which resulted from the failure to differentiate the "fear" and "anxious-misery" factor as subordinate factors of internalizing. Overall, in both the EDSP and GHS-MHS samples the model fit was satisfactory only when the second-order latent factor "internalizing" was omitted (**Table 1**).

Stability: How Robust is the 3-Factor Model Against the Additional Inclusion of Disorders?

In the second step, additional disorders were assigned to the 3 assumed factors. The following diagnoses were added: group (a) HME, MNE, separation anxiety disorder, OCD, PTSD, specific phobia subtypes; group (b) pain disorders, somatoform disorders (SSI4/6); group (c) psychotic disorders; group (d) eating disorders; group (e) childhood disorders (ADHD, ODD, tics, elimination disorders). Assignment of diagnoses was explored by testing whether assignment of additional disorders to different factors led to different results. Models were tested using all diagnoses as well as sequentially adding them by group of disorders.

We found that the addition of anxiety diagnoses and HME and MNE to the Krueger[1] model could not be fitted, or only just fitted when the factor "internalizing" was omitted (**Table 1**). After adding the somatoform disorders the model fit became particularly poor. Adding psychotic disorder and childhood disorder further impaired the fit.

In conclusion, the model could not be appropriately fitted in any of the analyses when several or many additional diagnoses were added. This lack of fit suggests that the model is very sensitive to even minor changes and is thus not robust.

Table 1
Results of the CFA

Sample	Age Range	N	RMS[b]	Which Model Could be Fitted?
EDSP, 12-month diagnoses at T0, T1, T2 and T3	14–34	9,007	**0.044**	"Internalizing" omitted[a]
	14–15	1,091	0.144	"Internalizing" omitted[a]
	16–20	3,333	0.088	"Internalizing" omitted[a]
	21–25	2,878	**0.071**	"Internalizing" omitted[a]
	26–30	1,323	0.147	"Internalizing" omitted[a]
	31–34	382	0.178	"Internalizing" omitted[a]
GHS-MHS, 12-month diagnoses, one assessment	18–65	4,181	**0.019**	"Internalizing" omitted[a]
EDSP cumulative lifetime diagnoses (T0–T3)	14–34	3,021	**0.066**	"Internalizing" omitted[a]
EDSP person-year data	1–34	74,634	**0.058**	"Internalizing" omitted[a]
	1–13	38,779	0.138	"Internalizing" omitted[a]
	14–17	11,803	**0.076**	"Internalizing" omitted[a]
	18–21	10,730	**0.066**	"Internalizing" omitted[a]
	22–34	13,322	0.089	"Internalizing" omitted[a]
EDSP person-year data, subsequently added diagnoses:				
Specific phobia subtypes, other anxiety disorders, HME and MNE[c]	1–34	74,389	0.082	"Internalizing" omitted[a]
Somatoform disorders[d]	1–34	74,330	0.109	"Internalizing" omitted[a]
Psychotic disorder to "externalizing"	1–34	74,330	0.114	"Internalizing" omitted[a]
any eating disorder to "anxious-misery"	1–34	74,278	0.112	"Internalizing" omitted[a]
Repeated in the data set of 1053 persons with T1-family assessment[e]	1–28	23,046	0.122	"Internalizing" omitted[a]
Childhood disorders[f]	1–28	22,930	0.146	"Internalizing" omitted[a]

EDSP, early developmental stages of psychopathology; GHS-MHS, German Health Survey—Mental Health Supplement.
[a] Three (correlated) latent factors, "Anxious-misery," "Fear," and "Externalizing," were maintained, but the second-order factor "Internalizing" posed on "Anxious-misery" and "Fear" was omitted.
[b] RMS = Standardized root mean squared residual (**bold**: satisfactory model fit = RMS < 0.08).
[c] OCD and PTSD, HME, and MNE were assigned to "Anxious-misery," separation anxiety was added to "Fear".
[d] Pain disorder and hypochondrias were added to "Fear," SSI4/6 was added to "Anxious-misery".
[e] ADHD and ODD were added to "Externalizing," tics and elimination disorder were added to "Anxious-misery".
[f] Only among those where information on childhood disorders is present.

Developmental Stability: How Robust is the 3-Factor Model when Examined Across Different Developmental Stages?

In the third step, and based on considerable evidence that the comorbidity patterns in children and young adolescents differ considerably from those in older adults,[17,25–27] we examined whether the factor solution and model fits substantially differ across the age span (1–13, 14–17, 18–21, 22+ years). These ages are considered a proxy for developmental stages ranging from childhood through adolescence to adulthood. Using the same diagnoses as in the original Krueger[1] work, we found that the model fit was appropriate for some age groups, namely 14- to 17-year-olds and 18- to 21-year-olds, but does not fit in the younger or the older cohorts (**Table 1**). The age-related increase in comorbidity seems to yield an association structure that is neither consistent with nor in line with the 3-factor model. Where the model could be fit, its overall model fit was reasonable in some age groups only if the second-order factor "internalizing" was ignored. To conclude, the model could not be consistently replicated in different age groups, despite some evidence for acceptable fits in some age groups. Thus, overall the model seems to be developmentally unstable.

Is There a Better Factor Solution?

Given that the 3-factor CFA solutions were neither robust nor developmentally stable, we also explored whether other meaningful and stable factor models could be identified when using EFA. Separate EFA were conducted in the total sample and different age groups as well as by including and excluding various groups of disorders. The scree test combined with parallel analyses suggested different numbers of factors across age spans, with up to 8 necessary factors. Moreover, the factor structures of the different models were not nested. That is, when more factors are extracted the factors did not simply add up to subfactors. Therefore, it seems that there is no one single model that would apply to all different age spans examined.

Nevertheless, the factor solutions may offer a range of clinically meaningful groupings, with some consistency across factor solutions. For example, the fairly consistent emergence of an externalizing-like factor (ie, substance dependence, ASP/CD), the frequent emergence of a panic/agoraphobia factor, a phobia factor (specific subtypes of phobia) and, less consistently and depending on age group considered, a psychotic factor, an ADHD/ODD/CD factor, and so forth. It is also noteworthy that some disorders such as OCD, psychotic, and hypomania/mania did not consistently reveal particularly high loading on one single factor but rather displayed moderate loadings on several factors. The factor structures became even more heterogeneous when adding childhood disorders and when running the analyses only among children and adolescents. For example, among the youngest cohort subjects a 4-factor solution emerged: The first factor loads high on MDE (0.86), dysthymia (0.51), OCD (0.50), and eating disorders (0.48), the second on some specific phobias, the third on GAD, ADHD, ODD, and elimination disorders, and the fourth on panic, agoraphobia, separation anxiety, and some phobias.

An example of this exploration is presented in **Fig. 2**, namely a 6-factor solution from the total sample based on EFA with good fit values. Partly consistent with the 3-factor model, this model describes a first "externalizing" factor (alcohol and drug dependence, conduct/ASP), and second factor that resembles the "anxious-misery" factor (MDE, DYS, and GAD), albeit with the addition of OCD and eating disorders. Krueger's[1] "fear factor" is, however, reflected by 3 factors, namely panic/agoraphobia, specific phobias (animal and environmental), and specific phobias (blood injury, situational, and other type). It is noteworthy that social phobia falls somehow

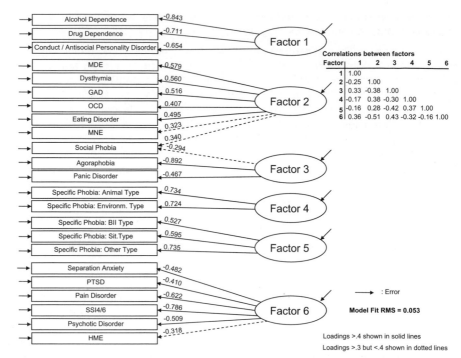

Fig. 2. Result of the exploratory factor analysis (EFA) including anxiety, mood and other disorders (EDSP, total sample, 6 factors). GAD, generalized anxiety disorder; HME, hypomanic episodes; MDE, major depressive episode; MNE, manic episodes; OCD, obsessive compulsive disorder; PTSD, posttraumatic stress disorder; RMS, root mean square; SSI4/6, somatoform disorders.

in between factors 2 (anxious-misery) and 3 (panic and agoraphobia). In addition, we found a sixth factor that describes a clinically more heterogeneous group of disorders, namely separation anxiety, PTSD, pain and somatoform disorders, and psychotic disorder.

In conclusion, this exploration suggests various clinically meaningful patterns with good fit, which go substantially beyond the original Krueger[1] structure. However, as with the Krueger structure, there is little consistency in findings when different age groups or different diagnostic groups are included or excluded. Further, it is noteworthy that a higher-order factor of "internalizing" could be substantiated in any of the explorations. This finding suggests that even when reducing the association structure to a matrix of 2-way tetrachoric correlations (although there might be higher dimensional structures), there seems to be no simplified structure that is stable over and across age groups. Instead, there is strong evidence that there might be more than 3 dimensions behind expressions of psychopathology as assessed in this data set.

Structures of DSM-IV Anxiety Disorders?

Finally, we also subjected the anxiety disorders (including separation anxiety disorder and specific phobia subtypes) to an EFA to explore whether a meaningful model could be identified within anxiety disorders. The scree plots and parallel analyses consistently indicated 3-factor solutions with acceptable model fits overall and by age group considered. Despite some differences in the loadings and the grouping of specific disorders there are common findings. (a) Agoraphobia and PD were always found in the same factor. (b) GAD and social phobia were always found in the same factor. (c) In all 3-factor solutions from age 14 on (and in the total sample) GAD, social phobia, PTSD, agoraphobia, PD, OCD and separation anxiety where assigned, with some variations, to the same factor. (d) The specific phobia subtypes animal and natural environment are always assigned to the same factor; in the age spans 14 to 17 and 18 to 21 they form a factor on their own, in the age span 1 to 13 they cluster with GAD and social phobia, and in the age span 22 to 34 with the situational subtype. (e) The blood injection injury specific phobia subtype could not be clearly assigned to one single factor.

DISCUSSION
Serious Limitation of the Internalizing-Externalizing Construct

In the decade following Krueger's initial landmark article[1] there is still insufficient evidence for a meaningful, relatively simple structure of common mental disorders. The results of this article challenge the higher-order factor of "internalizing" disorders with 2 subfactors of "anxious-misery" and "fear" conditions. Overall, our findings strongly suggest that even sophisticated factor analytic methods are too vulnerable for the type of diagnostic and comorbidity data used in such explorations. We have demonstrated that such methods lead to findings that are neither sensitive for developmental variations in the expression of psychopathology, nor sufficiently robust against even minor modifications with regard to the type and range of diagnoses covered. Despite the existence of several replications of Krueger's[1] work,[3] we and others[17] were unable to replicate the model in the majority of analyses with sufficient confidence and integrity. This failure, along with further methodological constraints discussed later in this article, strongly suggests that it is unwise and inappropriate to draw strong conclusions based on such findings. This reservation applies in particular to diagnostic classificatory issues and the extension of this model in the context of a metastructure proposition for DSM-V and ICD-11 recently presented.[11,12] These concerns further extend to the wide-ranging implications attached to the model, for example in terms of future research needs in psychiatric epidemiology, genetics, pharmacology, and intervention research. In particular, there is little evidence for the claim that this approach and the available explorative data justify the decision to refocus the study of common disorders on their common substrates, namely broad, higher-order internalizing and externalizing dimensions, simply because they might reflect "core psychopathological processes."[1]

It is difficult to dispute that the internalizing-externalizing distinction is and has been a fertile phenotypic construct to study personality, temperament, and cross-sectional self-report on symptoms within a dimensional questionnaire assessment of patients from a psychometric and quantitative psychological perspective. As compared with categorical clinical diagnoses, the dimensional nature of latent constructs has also been shown to be advantageous with regard to identifying associations with validators, such as neurobiological and genetic variables. We also do not dispute that identifying dimensions that are common across disorders can be helpful in understanding some of the mechanisms involved in etiology, maintenance, and treatment of mental disorders.[28]

One should be seriously concerned, however, when this model and its findings are used as a basis for designing the structure of diagnostic classification, the development of diagnostic interviews, clinical decision making, and public health decisions.

More generally speaking, one should be concerned about making far-reaching implications beyond the fact that this work represents a potentially useful phenotypic exploration. These concerns have been previously discussed in greater detail elsewhere[15,20] and will not be presented here again. In brief, in terms of the data used the significant limitations refer to the use of categorical (instead of dimensional), threshold (instead of subthreshold and threshold) disorders based on structured diagnostic interviews, the very limited range of diagnoses covered, the lack of consideration to temporal and developmental issues, and the lack of data beyond subjective-verbal information from the respondent. In terms of the statistical method, limitations lie in the fact that confirmatory factor analytic methods typically allow for the derivation of quite different models, all of which might be justified by the data. There are simply too many unknown parameters (factor loadings, variances and covariances of residuals) in the presence of an insufficient number of equations. Basic problems (eg, the use of tetrachoric correlations, see Ref.[29]) of this sort force almost invariably a relatively arbitrary choice of models, most likely those that are easy to interpret or those that fit the researchers' intention best. Therefore, as replication alone is insufficient and misleading, CFA may be used to reject or support a model but never to prove that a theory holds. In this respect, Krueger[1] has provided some evidence that the model might hold for his restricted set of diagnoses and his particular set of analyses. Replications to date have also used a similar set and range of diagnoses.[3] However, as shown in the data exploration of this article, the model evidently does not hold in general when other (even similar) diagnoses are taken into account, or even minor variations by age group are introduced. It is unlikely that the 2- and 3-factor models can be invalidated, but our exploration within the same limitations as in Krueger[1] shows that there is a wide range of alternative, clinically meaningful solutions or typologies that might be regarded as equally well supported as the Krueger model. In particular, the "internalizing" concept seems to be highly problematic, and only poorly reflects the structure of mental disorders and the structure of anxiety disorders in particular.

Of course, these restrictions should drastically limit the level of speculation attached to this type of exploration and the models derived. Yet, it is concerning to what degree the model continues to generate even further speculation and considerable extension not appropriately supported by data. Thus, beyond the possibility of identifying shared phenotypic expressions, extreme caution is warranted with regard to the potential clinical, cognitive-behavioral, genetic, and other neurobiological considerations, as well as with regard to suggested implications[11,12] for interventions research, clinical practice and public health.

Is There an Alternative?

Having summarized the severe restrictions of the factor analytic approach for diagnostic classificatory issues and this type of investigations in general, the question of whether there is a better or alternative solution possible within such an approach has to be denied. These types of methods are not suitable for the definitive detection of latent dimensions, or the relationships between latent factors and their observed variables. This nonsuitability applies to the structure of anxiety disorders as well as the structure of mental disorders in general. In this respect, the presentation of our more comprehensive structural model (see **Fig. 2**) was meant only as an example that there are other possible structural models that can be justified with similar or even better values, and that may or may not be much more useful clinically. These models should in no way, however, be interpreted as proof of a better or even alternative model. Factor analytic models should simply not be used for this purpose.

Yet, overall, we have little doubt that the data presented in our article suggest clearly that the assumption of the existence of more than 3 dimensions is much more likely to reflect expressions of psychopathology as the Krueger[1] model.

The Metastructure and Implications for DSM-V and ICD-11?

Even though somewhat repetitious in argumentation, we now comment on the use or misuse of this model for the clinical classification of mental disorders in general. The fact that such factor analytic findings are currently seriously being considered to provide guidance for a DSM-V diagnostic classificatory metastructure[11,12] is concerning.[20] Within the metastructure proposal,[11] the emotional cluster (almost identical to internalizing) lumps together all anxiety disorders along with depression and somatoform disorders under one umbrella. It is fair to state that such a proposition is actually not new and has in fact a long history. From the perspective of diagnostic classification, with its neurosis concept it resembles the ICD sixth to eighth revision, and is consistent with the old neurotic versus endogenous distinction as well as "disorders of temperament and personality" in the case of the externalizing dimension. It is also largely consistent with quantitative psychology and psychometric evaluations of cross-sectional questionnaires and scales based on self-report, and the psychological tradition of trait and personality research. These approaches have always opted for restricted 1-factor (general distress), 2-dimensional (eg, positive and negative affect), or 3-dimensional structures (og, tripartite model).[30–35] It is further noteworthy that scales that have claimed to have more factors (SCL-90) have been shown to load strongly on one factor with little discriminate value among the subscales.[36] Thus, it seems fair to state that the level of differentiation that is reliably achievable by self-report measures is limited; its value lies in the dimensional description of facets of self reported behavior, cognitive-emotional and circumscribed symptom elements, and in the dimensional characterization of perceived distress of a person.

Yet is this sufficient basis for revising diagnostic classification or even suggesting a new metastructure? Is correlational evidence that the assumed dimensions are more consistent with selected evidence from neurobiological, genetic, and treatment research than single categorical diagnosis a sufficient justification? Taking into account the serious limitations of the factor analytic approach, and if examined against the criteria for establishing diagnostic entities by Robins and Guze[37] or its extensions (Hyman and colleagues, citod in Ref.[11]), these questions must be denied. So what might be the additional benefit?

Could it help to decide on the deletion of groups of disorders or specific diagnoses from our research and clinical practice agenda? Would it help to improve current diagnostic practice by allowing the cluster labels to be used as a sufficient global diagnostic substitute, thus easing the burden of careful differential diagnostic workups? Will it reduce spurious comorbidity, by assuming that "relevant" comorbidity only exists between the 5 clusters? All these claims have been recently stated by promoters of the new metastructure with more or less pronounced limitations. Given the very limited exploratory evidence for the clusters, its adoption seems premature. It is therefore disconcerting that Andrews and colleagues[11] and others suggest the proposed metastructure as a basis for research on treatment, prognosis, and even practice. Yet there is neither explanation nor proof as to why one would expect the proposition to have greater utility and validity compared with the current DSM grouping.

Harmful Effects?

Leaving aside the substantial gaps regarding supporting data, might the lumping of anxiety, somatoform, and depressive disorders under the broad umbrella of "emotional cluster" revive the stigmatizing and otherwise controversial concept of neurosis? The initial beauty and simplicity of grouping mental disorders into conditions that could be mainly characterized by constructs like "emotional dysregulation" as in the emotional cluster, and "disinhibition" as in the externalizing cluster, does not protect against the revival of potentially stigmatizing diagnostic group labels. Even worse, such an organization carries an increased risk of losing sight of research-based distinctions and considerably different intervention needs of the specific anxiety, depressive, somatoform, and other "emotional cluster" disorders. It took 2 decades to communicate—albeit sometimes too subtly—that diagnosing specific mental disorder matters. For example, it is certainly true that the cross-sectional picture of a person with PD with past uncued panic attacks might not be that different from agoraphobia, severe specific phobia, GAD, or even depression with anxiety features when considering presenting symptoms, distress, and associated neurobiological and behavioral correlates. However doesn't the occurrence of initial spontaneous panic attacks tell us something extremely useful with regard to prognosis[38] as well as treatment[39]? Isn't there persuasive evidence that PD *without* agoraphobia is a quite different "animal" from panic disorder *with* agoraphobia[39]? How damaging will a broad cluster proposition be in this respect if a "deeper" meaning is involved? One might also ask what progress might be impeded if these factors, or dimension, or proposed metastructures are incomplete or incorrect. Intended or not, the diagnostic system will always influence the field's thinking about psychopathology and treatment. Is it therefore wise to adopt such a structural system with a "deeper meaning" that has not been adequately tested? (**Fig. 3**)

	Specific and shared evaluation domains* according to diagnostic criteria						
DSM-IV anxiety diagnoses	Diagnosis-specific features	Anxiety reaction/panic	anticipatory anxiety	Avoidance behavior	Impairment, disability	Distress/ neg. affect	Duration, persistence
Panic disorder. w/o Agoraphobia							
Panic disorder with Agoraphobia							
Agoraphobia w/o history of panic							
GAD							
Specific phobias							
Social phobia							
OCD							
PTSD							
Acute stress disorder							
Separation anxiety disorder							

By Anxiety Diagnosis

Across diagnoses by domain

* Each domain can be rated continously by severity, frequency, etc, Other possible domains may include etiological factors (neurobiological, developmental, etc.)

Fig. 3. Diagnosis-specific and cross-cutting assessment domains of anxiety disorders. (*From* Shear MK, Bjelland I, Beesdo K, Gloster AT, Wittchen H-U. Supplementary dimensional assessment in anxiety disorders. Int J Methods Psychiatr Res 2007;16(suppl 1):S54; with permission.)

To conclude, we currently see no solid evidence to adopt a new structure of mental disorders along the lines of factor analytic explorations and other statistical methods. In particular, we have deep concerns about adopting the 2-factor model of "internalizing" and "externalizing" or the 3-factor model of "anxious-misery," "fear," and "externalizing," or similar extensions of this sort. We do not see evidence of immediate or long-term advantages but have significant concerns about potentially critically harmful effects for basic and clinical research as well as treatment practice and public health issues. However, we share the strong feeling that a wider inclusion of dimensional measures for diagnosis and syndrome-specific core features of mental disorders may be fruitful. These measures could be conceptualized for single diagnoses as well as for cross-cutting diagnostics. Such alternative propositions to revising DSM-V have been recently elaborated[28,40] (see **Fig. 3** for an example), and seem to address the current needs in research and practice much more appropriately and straightforwardly.

REFERENCES

1. Krueger RF. The structure of common mental disorders. Arch Gen Psychiatry 1999;56:921–6.
2. Achenbach T, Edelbrock C. Psychopathology of childhood. Annu Rev Psychol 1984;35:227–56.
3. Krueger RF, Markon KE. Reinterpreting comorbidity: a model-based approach to understanding and classifying psychopathology. Annu Rev Clin Psychol 2006;2: 111–33.
4. Markon K, Krueger R, Watson D. Delineating the structure of normal and abnormal personality: an integrative hierarchical approach. J Pers Soc Psychol 2005;88(1):139–57.
5. Kendler KS. Major depression and generalised anxiety disorder. Same genes, (partly) different environments—revisited. Br J Psychiatry 1996;168(Suppl 30): 68–75.
6. Kendler KS, Walters EE, Neale MC, et al. The structure of the genetic and environmental risk factors for six major psychiatric disorders in women. Arch Gen Psychiatry 1995;52(5):374–83.
7. Kendler KS, Prescott CA, Myers J, et al. The structure of genetic and environmental risk factors for common psychiatric and substance use disorders in men and women. Arch Gen Psychiatry 2003;60:929–37.
8. Hettema JM, Neale MC, Myers JM, et al. A population-based twin study of the relationship between neuroticism and internalizing disorders. Am J Psychiatry 2006;163:857–64.
9. Morilak D, Frazer A. Antidepressants and brain monoaminergic systems: a dimensional approach to understanding their behavioural effects in depression and anxiety disorders. Int J Neuropsychopharmacol 2004;7(2):193–218.
10. Andrews W, Parker G, Barrett E. The SSRI antidepressants: exploring their "other" possible properties. J Affect Disord 1998;49(2):141–4.
11. Andrews G, Goldberg DP, Krueger RF, et al. Exploring the feasibility of a meta-structure for DSM-V and ICD-11: Could it improve utility and validity? Psychol Med, in press.
12. Goldberg DP, Krueger RF, Andrews G, et al. Emotional disorders: cluster 4 of the proposed meta-structure for DSM-V and ICD-11. Psychol Med, in press.
13. Regier DA, Narrow WE, Kuhl EA, et al. The conceptual development of DSM-V. Am J Psychiatry 2009;166(6):645–50.

14. Kessler RC, McGonagle KA, Zhao S, et al. Lifetime and 12-month prevalence of DSM-III-R psychiatric disorders in the United States: results from the National Comorbidity Survey. Arch Gen Psychiatry 1994;51:8–19.

15. Wittchen H-U, Höfler M, Merikangas KR. Towards the identification of core psychopathological processes? Arch Gen Psychiatry 1999;56(10):929–31.

16. Beesdo K, Höfler M, Gloster AT, et al. The structure of common mental disorders: a replication study in a community sample of adolescents and young adults. Submitted.

17. Kessler RC, Chiu WT, Demler O, et al. Prevalence, severity, and comorbidity of 12-month DSM-IV disorders in the National Comorbidity Survey Replication. Arch Gen Psychiatry 2005;62:617–27.

18. APA. Diagnostic and statistical manual of mental disorders. text revision. 4th edition. Washington, DC: American Psychiatric Press; 2000.

19. WHO. The ICD-10 classification of mental and behavioural disorders: diagnostic criteria for research. Geneva (Switzerland): World Health Organization; 1993.

20. Wittchen H-U, Beesdo K, Gloster AT. A new metastructure of mental disorders: helpful step into the future or a harmful step back to the past? (Commentary). Psychol Med, in press.

21. Wittchen H-U, Beesdo K, Gloster A, et al. The structure of mental disorders reexamined: is it developmentally stable and robust against additions? Int J Methods Psychiatr Res, in press.

22. Wittchen H-U, Perkonigg A, Lachner G, et al. Early developmental stages of psychopathology study (EDSP)—objectives and design. Eur Addict Res 1998; 4(1–2):18–27.

23. Lieb R, Isensee B, von Sydow K, et al. The Early Developmental Stages of Psychopathology Study (EDSP): a methodological update. Eur Addict Res 2000;6:170–82.

24. Jacobi F, Wittchen H-U, Hölting C, et al. Estimating the prevalence of mental and somatic disorders in the community: aims and methods of the German National Health Interview and Examination Survey. Int J Methods Psychiatr Res 2002; 11(1):1–18.

25. Wittchen H-U, Lieb R, Schuster P, et al. When is onset? Investigations into early developmental stages of anxiety and depressive disorders. In: Rapoport JL, editor. Childhood onset of "adult" psychopathology, clinical and research advances. Washington: American Psychiatric Press; 1999. p. 259–302.

26. Wittchen H-U, Kessler RC, Pfister H, et al. Why do people with anxiety disorders become depressed? A prospective-longitudinal community study. Acta Psychiatr Scand 2000;102(Suppl 406):14–23.

27. Newman DL, Moffitt TE, Caspi A, et al. Psychiatric disorder in a birth cohort of young adults: prevalence, comorbidity, clinical significance, and new case incidence from age 11 to 21. J Consult Clin Psychol 1996;64(3):552–62.

28. Shear MK, Bjelland I, Beesdo K, et al. Supplementary dimensional assessment in anxiety disorders. Int J Methods Psychiatr Res 2007;16(suppl 1):S52–64.

29. Kraemer HC. What is the 'right' statistical measure of twin concordance (or diagnostic reliability and validity)? Arch Gen Psychiatry 1997;54(12):1121–4.

30. Clark LA, Watson D. Tripartite model of anxiety and depression: psychometric evidence and taxonomic implications. J Abnorm Psychol 1991;100(3):316–36.

31. Brown TA, Chorpita BF, Barlow DH. Structural relationships among dimensions of the DSM-IV anxiety and mood disorders and dimensions of negative affect, positive affect, and autonomic arousal. J Abnorm Psychol 1998;107(2):179–92.

32. Mineka S, Watson D, Clark LA. Comorbidity of anxiety and unipolar mood disorders. Annu Rev Psychol 1998;49:377–412.
33. Clark LA, Watson D, Mineka S. Temperament, personality, and the mood and anxiety disorders. J Abnorm Psychol 1994;103(1):103–16.
34. Zinbarg RE, Barlow DH. Structure of anxiety and the anxiety disorders: a hierarchical model. J Abnorm Psychol 1996;105(2):181–93.
35. Goldberg D. A dimensional model for common mental disorders. Br J Psychiatry 1996;168(Suppl 30):44–9.
36. Schmitz N, Hartkamp N, Kiuse J, et al. The symptom check-list-90-R (SCL-90-R): a German validation study. Qual Life Res 2000;9:185–93.
37. Robins E, Guze SB. Establishment of diagnostic validity in psychiatric illness: its application to schizophrenia. Am J Psychiatry 1970;126(7):983–7.
38. Wittchen H-U, Höfler M, Gloster AT, et al. Options and dilemmas of dimensional measures for DSM-V: which type of measures fair best in predicting course and outcome? APPA monograph: APA; in press.
39. Craske MG, Kircanski K, Epstein A, et al. Panic disorder literature review. DSM V Anxiety, OC Spectrum, Posttraumatic, and Dissociative Disorder Work Group. Depress Anxiety, in press.
40. Special Issue: Dimensional approaches to psychiatric classification. refining the research agenda for DSM-V. Int J Methods Psychiatr Res 2007;16(Suppl 1).

Anxiety and Anxiety Disorders in Children and Adolescents: Developmental Issues and Implications for DSM-V

Katja Beesdo, PhD[a],*, Susanne Knappe, Dipl-Psych[a], Daniel S. Pine, MD[b]

KEYWORDS

- Anxiety • Assessment • Diagnosis • Boundaries
- Onset • Course • Outcome

ANXIETY AND ANXIETY DISORDERS IN CHILDREN AND ADOLESCENTS AND ITS ASSESSMENT

Childhood and adolescence Is the core risk phase for the development of symptoms and syndromes of anxiety that may range from transient mild symptoms to full-blown anxiety disorders. Challenges from a research perspective include its reliable and clinically valid assessment to determine its prevalence and patterns of Incidence, and the longitudinal characterization of its natural course to better understand what characteristics are solid predictors for more malignant courses as well as which are likely to be associated with benign patterns of course and outcome. This type of information is particularly needed from a clinical perspective to inform about improved early recognition and differential diagnosis as well as preventions and treatment in this age span.

Anxiety refers to the brain response to danger, stimuli that an organism will actively attempt to avoid. This brain response is a basic emotion already present in infancy and childhood, with expressions falling on a continuum from mild to severe. Anxiety is not typically pathological as it is adaptive in many scenarios when it facilitates avoidance of danger. Strong cross-species parallels—both in organisms' responses to danger and in the underlying brain circuitry engaged by threats—likely reflect these adaptive aspects of anxiety.[1] One frequent and established conceptualization is that anxiety

[a] Institute of Clinical Psychology and Psychotherapy, Department of Psychology, Faculty of Science, Technische Universität Dresden, Chemnitzer Str. 46, 01187 Dresden, Germany
[b] Section on Development and Affective Neuroscience, Department of Health and Human Services, National Institute of Mental Health, National Institutes of Health, Bethesda, MD 20892-1381, USA
* Corresponding author.
E-mail address: Katja.Beesdo@tu-dresden.de (K. Beesdo).

Psychiatr Clin N Am 32 (2009) 483–524
doi:10.1016/j.psc.2009.06.002
0193-953X/09/$ – see front matter © 2009 Elsevier Inc. All rights reserved.

psych.theclinics.com

becomes maladaptive when it interferes with functioning, for example when associated with avoidance behavior, most likely to occur when anxiety becomes overly frequent, severe, and persistent.[2] Thus, pathological anxiety at any age can be characterized by persisting or extensive degrees of anxiety and avoidance associated with subjective distress or impairment. The differentiation between normal and pathological anxiety, however, can be particularly difficult in children because children manifest many fears and anxieties as part of typical development[3,4] (**Table 1**). Although these phenomena might be acutely distressing, they occur in most children and are typically transient. For example, separation anxiety normatively occurs at 12 to 18 months, fears of thunder or lightning at 2 to 4 years, and so forth. Thus, given that such anxiety occurs in most children and typically does not persist, distress, in and of itself, represents an inadequate criterion for distinguishing among normal and pathological anxiety states in children. This problem creates unique challenges when trying to distinguish among normal, subclinical, and pathological anxiety states in children. Other challenges in the assessment of childhood fears and anxiety are that children at younger ages may have difficulties in communicating cognition, emotions, and avoidance, as well as the associated distress and impairments, to the diagnostician[5] because they might lack the cognitive capabilities used to communicate information vital to the application of the diagnostic classification system. Thus, developmental differences (eg, cognition, language skills, emotional understanding) must be carefully considered when assessing anxiety in young people to make a diagnostic decision.[6]

Anxiety disorders are described and classified in diagnostic systems such as the Diagnostic and Statistical Manual of Mental Disorders (DSM, currently version IV-TR, American Psychiatric Association)[2] or the International Classification of Diseases (ICD, currently version 10, World Health Organization)[7] (**Table 2**). Across these systems, many anxiety disorders share common clinical features such as extensive anxiety, physiological anxiety symptoms, behavioral disturbances such as extreme avoidance of feared objects, and associated distress or impairment. Nonetheless, differences exist and it should be noted that narrowly categorized anxiety disorders such as panic disorder, agoraphobia, and subtypes of specific phobias also exhibit a substantial degree of phenotypical diversity or heterogeneity.

In the assessment of anxiety features in children one has to recognize that the core diagnostic criteria might present differently in the young, requiring special assessment strategies and the recognition of special features that are unique to or characteristic for this age group. DSM-IV acknowledges this by adding for some disorders, though not consistently, some of the features that might present differently in children and adolescents. With the exception of separation anxiety disorder, all of the anxiety disorders in DSM-IV are grouped together irrespective of the age at which the disorder manifests; separation anxiety disorder, in contrast, is defined as manifesting before adulthood. Thus for most of the anxiety disorders, differences between diagnostic criteria for children and adults, if any, are provided within the same criteria set. Examples include duration commentaries, differences in symptom type or count, or insights into the excessiveness/inadequacy of fear (**Table 2**). More specifically, for example, the threshold in DSM-IV for diagnosing generalized anxiety disorder is lower in children than adults (1 instead of 3 out of 6 symptoms); in phobias, children are not required to judge their anxiety as excessive or unreasonable, yet duration must be at least 6 months among individuals under the age of 18 years. For ICD-10, in contrast to DSM-IV, children receive other diagnostic codings, separate from adults, for anxiety disorders that reflect exaggerations of normal developmental trends. The specific differences in diagnosis and diagnostic criteria between children and adults for DSM-IV and ICD-10 are listed in **Table 2**.

It should be noted that it remains unspecified as to what age range the *child-specific* diagnostic criteria refer. Given cognitive and language development, the increasing importance of peer relationships, and the seeking of autonomy from parents, it is crucial to specify similarities and differences in anxiety expressions for different ages (eg, childhood up to 12 years, adolescence 13 to 17 years). This important issue is rarely acknowledged in the current diagnostic criteria, and not even in the text portions of the DSM that generally contain important additional information for diagnosticians and clinicians (see **Table 2**).

There is also little guidance in the diagnostic systems on developmentally appropriate *assessment* of anxiety disorders to identify those in need of treatment. Although the development of explicit descriptive diagnostic criteria has facilitated the development of diagnostic instruments for the assessment of anxiety disorders, diagnosticians and clinicians should be aware of their limitations, particularly related to developmental issues in obtaining self-reports from children and adolescents.[6,8,9]

Table 3 provides a selection of the most commonly used diagnostic tools for assessment of anxiety symptoms and anxiety disorders in children and adolescents. In children, applications of these tools to younger children might be more problematic than to older children, as reflected in poorer psychometric data. This problem undoubtedly at least partly reflects the difficulty young children face when trying to communicate information about internally experienced affective states.[5] Therefore, assessments in young children often require solicitation of information from multiple sources beyond the child to reliably and validly distinguish among normal anxiety, subclinical, and pathological anxiety syndromes and disorders. This assessment includes parent or teacher reports. In older children and adolescents, in contrast, diagnostic decisions can rely heavily on information provided directly by the patient, although even in this age group parallel informants can also be helpful.

Beyond these problems, unclear rules for applying diagnostic thresholds and variations in the methods used to aggregate information from different sources may drastically influence prevalence estimates (see later discussion) and might also impact findings from basic and epidemiological research. Thus, anxiety disorders in children and adolescents cannot be easily assessed with standard questionnaires or interviews that have been derived from adult instruments. In fact, the use of structured and standardized interviews for children and adolescents has much improved the reliability and validity of anxiety diagnoses in children and adolescents in the last 2 decades. Such instruments also have an advantage over symptom scales in that they allow a better delineation of transient subclinical manifestations of anxiety from anxiety disorders that were shown to have predictive validity and even concrete implications for prevention early intervention, and treatment.

The next section highlights developmental issues in anxiety, with focus on anxiety disorders (1) by critically reviewing recent data on the prevalence, incidence, age of onset, natural course, and longitudinal outcome of anxiety disorders, including comorbidity and psychosocial impairments and disabilities, and (2) by addressing important correlates and potential risk factors. The review focuses on the following categorically defined anxiety disorders: separation anxiety disorder, specific phobias, social phobia, agoraphobia, panic disorder, and generalized anxiety disorder (GAD). Obsessive-compulsive disorder and posttraumatic stress disorder are not covered in this article because of additional complicating issues involved with these diagnoses, for example, controversy in regard to their grouping with the other anxiety disorders.[10] As an attempt is made to provide information on development, the authors focus on children (defined here as up to age 12), adolescence (defined here as ages 13 to 17), and young adults (defined here as ages 18 to 35 years).

Table 1
Normative anxiety and fears in childhood and adolescence

Age		Development Conditioned Periods of Fear and Anxiety	Psychopathological Relevant Symptoms	Corresponding DSM-IV Anxiety Disorder
Early infancy	Within first weeks	Fear of loss, eg, physical contact to caregivers	—	—
	0–6 months	Salient sensoric stimuli	—	—
Late infancy	6–8 months	Shyness/anxiety with stranger		Separation anxiety disorder
Toddlerhood	12–18 months	Separation anxiety	Sleep disturbances, nocturnal panic attacks, oppositional deviant behavior	Separation anxiety disorder, panic attacks
	2–3 years	Fears of thunder and lightening, fire, water, darkness, nightmares	Crying, clinging, withdrawal, freezing, eloping seek for security and physical contact, avoidance of salient stimuli (eg, turning the light on), pavor nocturnus, enuresis	Specific phobias (environmental subtype), panic disorder
		Fears of animals	—	Specific phobias (animal subtype)
Early childhood	4–5 years	Fear of death or dead people	—	Generalized anxiety disorder, panic attacks
Primary/elementary school age	5–7 years	Fear of specific objects (animals, monsters, ghosts)	—	Specific phobias
		Fear of germs or getting a serious illness	—	Obsessive compulsive disorder
		Fear of natural disasters, fear of traumatic events (eg, getting burned, being hit by a car or truck)	—	Specific phobias (environmental subtype), acute stress disorder, posttraumatic stress disorder, generalized anxiety disorder
		School anxiety, performance anxiety	Withdrawal, timidity, extreme shyness to unfamiliar people and peers, feelings of shame	Social anxiety disorder
Adolescence	12–18 years	Rejection from peers	Fear of negative evaluation	Social anxiety disorder

Data from Morris RJ, Kratochwill TR. Childhood fears and phobias. In: Kratochwill TR, Morris RJ, editors. The practice of child therapy. 2nd ed. New York: Pergamon; 1991. p. 76–114; and Muris P, Merckelbach H, Mayer B, et al. Common fears and their relationship to anxiety disorders symptomatology in normal children. Pers Individ Diff 1998;24(4):575–8.

EPIDEMIOLOGY OF ANXIETY DISORDERS IN CHILDHOOD AND ADOLESCENCE
Prevalence and Onset

There is persuasive evidence from a range of studies that anxiety disorders are the most frequent mental disorders in children and adolescents, and thus seem to be the earliest of all forms of psychopathology. The *onset of anxiety disorders* (or symptoms/syndromes of anxiety) has been assessed in youth and adult samples, in cross-sectional and longitudinal surveys, most frequently by using the answers of the respondents to questions like "When was the first time you experienced..." (**Fig. 1**). Of note, such reports may be subject to recall bias,[11] particularly in studies among older adults or in studies that retrospectively cover long time periods. As a consequence, reports of mean ages of onset are likely to be heavily influenced by the age range of the studied population (higher mean estimates in adult studies). Thus, age of onset distribution curves that cumulate recently assessed new cases across age (**Fig. 2**) are more informative and reliable with regard to actual onset patterns and core incidence periods (ie, high-risk phases for first onset of disorders).

Findings suggest that onset of the first or any anxiety disorder is clearly in childhood (eg, Refs.[12,13,14]). Yet, leaving aside that some anxiety disorders might be preceded in their onset by other earlier comorbid anxiety disorders, there is some noteworthy heterogeneity between the specific anxiety disorders that reveals a temporal sequence of core risk periods for first onset of anxiety disorders in childhood and adolescence. In terms of validation these differences in age of onset provide one important indicator for separating different types of anxiety disorders.[15] The earliest age of onset has been consistently found for separation anxiety disorder and some types of specific phobias (particularly the animal, blood injection injury, and environmental type), with most cases emerging in childhood before the age of 12 years,[12,16,17] followed by the onset of social phobia with incidences in late childhood and throughout adolescence, with very few cases emerging after the age of 25.[12,18,19] Panic disorder, agoraphobia, and GAD, in contrast, have their core periods for first onset in later adolescence with further first incidences in early adulthood,[12,14,20] despite the fact that some cases, especially with panic attacks, might occur as early as age 12 years or before.[21] Particularly for GAD as defined by the 6-month duration criterion, new cases also emerge throughout middle and late adulthood.[12,20,22] It should be noted, however, that some doubts have been expressed about whether the 6-month duration criterion for GAD is appropriate in general[23,24] and useful in children and adolescents in particular.[25] Indirect evidence for GAD of shorter duration comes from studies using the former diagnosis of overanxious disorder (OAD), for which considerably earlier onsets and higher prevalence rates have been found among children (**Table 4**). Although the lack of specific diagnostic continuity for OAD into adulthood[26] might speak against the definition of GAD by using a shorter duration, an accordant change of diagnostic criteria of GAD for children in DSM-V is currently under investigation.

Fig. 2 graphs for males and females the age of onset distribution of anxiety disorders assessed in a prospective-longitudinal community study (Early Developmental Stages of Psychopathology, EDSP) among adolescents and young adults up to age 34 years. No remarkable gender differences in onset patterns occur with 2 exceptions: compared with females, males exhibit a somewhat earlier onset of specific phobia of natural environmental type, and a later onset of GAD.

Prevalence estimates in aggregated age groups (see **Fig. 1**) also give some convergent, though crude indications for the early onset of a disorder. Prevalence estimates (**Table 4**) tend to further increase with age among children and adolescents for GAD,

Table 2
Classification of anxiety disorders according to ICD-10 and DSM-IV

ICD-10	DSM-IV	Different criteria in children (vs adults)
Neurotic, somatoform, and stress-related disorders	Anxiety disorders	*Information on childhood anxieties as highlighted in DSM text portion*
F40 Phobic disorder		
F40.0 Agoraphobia		
F40.00 Agoraphobia without panic disorder	300.22 Agoraphobia without history of panic disorder	—
F40.01 Agoraphobia with panic disorder	300.21 Panic disorder with agoraphobia	—
F40.1 Social phobia	300.23 Social phobia	A: In children, there must be evidence of the capacity for age-appropriate social relationships with familiar people and the social anxiety must occur in peer settings, not just in interactions with adults
		B: In children, the anxiety may be expressed by crying, tantrums, freezing, shrinking from social situations with unfamiliar people
		C: In children, the C criterion (recognizes that fear is excessive/unreasonable) may be absent.
		F: In individuals < 18 years, duration is at least 6 months
		Fears of being embarrassed in social situations are common, but usually the degree of distress or impairment is insufficient to warrant a diagnosis Transient social anxiety or avoidance is especially common in childhood and adolescence (eg, an adolescent girl may avoid eating in front of boys for a short time, then resume usual behavior). Unlike adults, children may not have the option of avoiding feared situations altogether, and may be unable to identify the nature of their anxiety.
F40.2 Specific (isolated) phobia	300.29 Specific phobia	B: In children, the anxiety may be expressed by crying, tantrums, freezing, or clinging
		C: In children, the C criterion (recognizes that fear is excessive/unreasonable) may be absent
		F: In individuals < 18 years, duration is at least 6 months

Fear of animals and other objects in the natural environment are particularly common and are usually transitory in childhood. A diagnosis is not warranted unless the fears lead to clinically significant impairment (eg, unwillingness to got to school for fear of encountering a dog on the street)

F40.8	Other	—	—
F40.9	Not specified	300.00 Anxiety disorders NOS	—
F41	**Other anxiety disorders**		
F41.0	Panic disorder (episodic paroxysmal anxiety)	300.01 Panic disorder without agoraphobia	—
F41.1	Generalized anxiety disorder	300.02 Generalized anxiety disorder	C: In children, 1 instead of 3 out of 6 symptoms is required In children and adolescents the anxieties and worries often concern the quality of their performance or competence at school or in sporting events, even when their performance is not being evaluated by others. There may be excessive concerns about punctuality. They may also worry about catastrophic events such as earthquakes or nuclear war. Children may be overly conforming, perfectionist, and unsure of themselves and tend to redo tasks because of excessive dissatisfaction with less-than-perfect performance. They are typically overzealous in seeking approval and require excessive reassurance about their performance and their worries. The disorder may be overdiagnosed in children, thus a thorough evaluation of presence of other childhood anxiety disorders should be done to determine whether the worries may be better explained by one of these disorders.
F41.2	Mixed anxiety and depressive disorder	—	—
F41.3	Other mixed anxiety disorders	—	—
F41.8	Other	—	—
F41.9	Not specified	300.00 Anxiety disorders NOS	—

(continued on next page)

Table 2
(continued)

ICD-10		DSM-IV		Different criteria in children (vs adults) Information on childhood anxieties as highlighted in DSM text portion
Neurotic, somatoform, and stress-related disorders		**Anxiety disorders**		
F42	**Obsessive compulsive disorder**	300.3	Obsessive-compulsive disorder	B criterion does not apply to children *Presentations in children are generally similar to those in adulthood. Washing, checking, and ordering rituals are particularly common in children. Children generally do not request help, and the symptoms may not be ego-dystonic. More often the problem is identified by parents. Gradual declines in schoolwork secondary to impaired ability to concentrate have been reported. Like adults, children are more prone to engage in rituals than in front of peers, teachers, or strangers. For a small subset of children, the disorder may be associated with Group A beta-hemolytic streptococcal infection. This form is characterized by prepubertal onset, associated neurological abnormalities, and an abrupt onset of symptoms or an episodic course in which exacerbations are temporally related to the streptococcal infections.*
F42.0	Predominantly obsessional thoughts or ruminations			
F42.1	Predominantly compulsive acts (obsessional rituals)			
F42.2	Mixed obsessional thoughts and acts			
F42.8	Other			
F42.9	Not specified			
F43	**Reaction to severe stress and adjustment disorder**			
F43.0	Acute stress reaction	308.3	Acute stress disorder	—

F43.1	Posttraumatic stress disorder	309.81	Posttraumatic stress disorder	A(2): In children, the criterion may be expressed by disorganized or agitated behavior B(1): In young children, repetitive play may occur in which themes or aspects of the trauma are expressed B(2): In children, there may be frightening dreams without recognizable content B(3): In young children, trauma-specific reenactment may occur *Because it may be difficult for children to report diminished interest in significant activities and constrictions of affect, these symptoms should be carefully evaluated with reports from parents, teachers, and other observers. In children, the sense of foreshortened future may be evidenced by the belief that life will be too short to include becoming an adult. There may also be "omen formation," that is, belief in an ability to foresee future untoward events. Children may also exhibit various physical symptoms, such as stomachaches and headaches.*
F43.2	Adjustment disorders[a]			
F43.8	Other			
F43.9	Not specified			
F93	**Emotional disorders with onset specific to childhood**		Disorders usually first diagnosed in infancy, childhood or adolescence	
F93.0	Separation anxiety disorder of childhood	309.21	Separation Anxiety Disorder	
F93.1	Phobic anxiety disorder of childhood	—	—	
F93.2	Social anxiety disorder of childhood	—	—	
F93.8	Other childhood emotional disorders	—	—	
F93.9	Childhood emotional disorder, unspecified	—	—	

[a] Different criteria in children versus adults: In children, symptoms may also manifest as regressive behaviors such as enuresis, thumb-sucking, or baby talk. Conduct disorders may be associated feature, particularly in adolescents.
Data from ICD-10[7] (WHO) and DSM-IV[2] (APA).

Table 3
Assessment in children and adolescents

Instruments	Description	Information Level	Age	Reference
Inventories on symptom levels				
Anxiety				
CASI Child Anxiety Sensitivity Index	18-items to evaluate separation anxiety, panic attacks and agoraphobic fears and children's belief that anxiety symptoms have aversive consequences	Self-report	–	Silverman et al (1991)
MASC Multidimensional Anxiety Scale for Children	39 items, 4 scales: physical symptoms, social anxiety, harm avoidance, separation/panic anxiety	Self-report, parent report	8–16	March, Parker Sullivan, Stallings & Comers (1997)
RCMAS Revised Children's Manifest Anxiety Scale	37 items, 3 factors: physiological manifestations of anxiety, worry and oversensitivity, fear/concentration	Self-report	6–19	Reynolds & Richmond (1978)
FSS-C Fear Survey Schedule for Children—Revised	80 items describing fears, loading on 5 factors fear of failure and criticism, fear of the unknown, fear of injury and small animals, fear of danger and death, medical fears	–	7–18	Ollendick (1983)
PARS Pediatric Anxiety Rating Scale	Anxiety severity scale specifically addressing the separation anxiety, social phobia and GAD symptoms	Clinical rating	6–17	RUPP Anxiety Study Group (2002)
CBCL, YSR, TRF Child Behavior Checklist, Youth Self-Report, Teacher Report Form	Behavior inventory including a broad subscale of internalizing symptomatology, a specific depression/ anxiety scale	–	4–18; 11+ (YSR)	Achenbach (1991)
HARS Hamilton Anxiety Rating Scale	Developed according to Hamilton Anxiety Rating Scale for use in children	–		Clark & Donovan (1994)
STAIC State-Trait Anxiety Inventory for Children	2 independent 20-item inventories to assess state and trait anxiety	–	8–12	Spielberger (1973)
Social phobia				
LSAS Liebowitz Social Anxiety Scale	Evaluation of severity of fear and avoidance symptoms for social and performance-related situations; 4 subscales and total fear and total avoidance scores	Self-report	–	Liebowitz (1987)

BSPS	Brief Social Phobia Scale	Rating of fear, avoidance, severity, and somatic symptoms of social situations	Self-report	18+, adolescents	Davidson et al (1991, 1997)
SPAI-C	Social Phobia and Anxiety Inventory for Children	39 items to assess somatic, cognitive and behavioral responses to a variety of social and performance situations	Self-report	8–18	Turner et al (1989); Beidel et al (1995, 2000)
SAS-C, SAS-A	Social Anxiety Scale for Children—Revised, Social Anxiety Scale for Adolescents	22-item inventory with 3 factors: fear of negative evaluation, social avoidance and distress specific to new situations, generalized social avoidance and distress	Self-report, parent report	–	La Greca & Stone (1993)
SIAS	Social Interaction Anxiety Scale	Assesses fear of interacting in dyads and groups and fear of scrutiny	Self-report	–	Mattick & Clarke (1998)
Specific phobias					
FSS-C	Fear Survey Schedule for Children—Revised	80 items describing fears, loading on 5 factors fear of failure and criticism, fear of the unknown, fear of injury and small animals, fear of danger and death, medical fears	–	7–18	Ollendick (1983)
Generalized anxiety					
PSWQ-C	Penn State Worry Questionnaire—Children and Adolescents	Adaptation of the Penn state worry questionnaire for use with children and adolescents to assess intensity and inability to control pathological worrying with 16 items (PSWQ-C). The PSWQ-C demonstrated good convergent and discriminant validity, and excellent reliability	Self-report	6–18	Chorpita et al (1997)
Categorical diagnostic inventories					
SCARED	Screen for Child Anxiety Related Emotional Disorders	41 items assesses DSM symptoms of panic, separation anxiety, social phobia, GAD, and school phobia	Self-report, parent report	–	Birmaher et al (1997, 1999)

(continued on next page)

Table 3
(continued)

Instruments		Description	Information Level	Age	Reference
ADIS-C/P	Anxiety Disorders Interview Schedule for DSM-IV—Child and Parent Version	Semistructured, interviewer-observer format, diagnoses of lifetime and current anxiety, mood, externalizing disorders and screening for other disorders	Self-report, parent report		DiNardo, O'Brien, Barlow, Waddell & Blanchard (1983)
K-SADS	Schedule for Affective Disorders and Schizophrenia for School-age Children—Present and Lifetime Version (Kiddie-SADS)	Semistructured diagnostic interview to derive DSM diagnoses, including severity ratings	Self-report, parent report	6–17	Kaufman, Birmaher, Brent, Rao & Ryan (1997)
NIMHDISC-IV	NIHM Diagnostic Interview Schedule for Children Version IV	Highly structured interview, follows a symptom-orientated structure and covers most axis-I disorders	Self-report	6–17	Shaffer, Fisher, Lucas, Dulcan & Schwab-Stone (2000)
DICA	Diagnostic Interview for Children and Adolescents	Structured syndrome-orientated interview, also parent version (DICA-P) available	Self-report, parent report	6–17	Herjanic & Reich (1982); Welner et al (1987)
CAEF	Children's Anxiety Evaluation Form	Combination of semistructured interview+chart review+direct observation	–	–	Hoehn-Saric et al (1987)
CAPA	Child and Adolescent Psychiatric Assessment	Assesses 30 different categorical disorders, family, peer, academic functioning, life events, service use	Self-report, parent report	8+	Angold & Costello (2000); Angold et al (1995)
CIDI	Composite International Diagnostic Interview	Standardized assessment of symptoms, syndromes and diagnoses of 48 mental disorders according to DSM-IV and ICD-10 criteria along with information about onset, duration, and severity; respond lists to increase validity and to diminish recall bias	Self-report	14–65	Wittchen & Pfister (1997)
CSA	Children's Assessment Schedule	Semistructured psychiatric interview to determine specific diagnoses for clinical practice, or to derive a total score of problems or symptoms, separate scores for specific content areas or symptom complexes	Self-report	6–17	Hodges et al (1982)

Note: References from this table are available from the corresponding author.

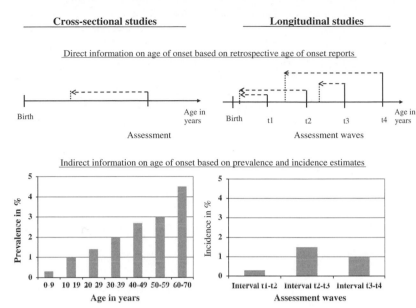

Fig. 1. Assessing onset of anxiety disorders. The age of onset of anxiety disorders can be directly assessed by asking "When was the first time you experienced...." The retrospectively reported ages often reflect the syndrome, rather than disorder onset, and can be subject to recall bias. This fact is indirectly reflected by observations from longitudinal studies whereby different ages of onset are reported for the same condition at various assessment waves. Other sources of information on age of onset are prevalence estimates for disorders in aggregated age groups (mostly reported in cross-sectional studies). More reliably but also more rare, incidence reports from longitudinal studies (ie, the proportion of new cases in a defined time interval) provide insights into the disorder onset.

social phobia, panic disorder, and agoraphobia, which is not seen with the same magnitude in specific phobia or separation anxiety disorder. Confirming retrospective age of onset information, these data allow one to define "core periods of risk" for the first anxiety disorder onset in childhood for the latter conditions and in adolescence for the former conditions. Similar conclusions emerge from incidence estimates (proportions of new-onset cases between 2 assessment waves among those who were previously not affected) from prospective-longitudinal studies.[17,27]

Frequency of Anxiety Disorders
Community prevalence estimates (see **Table 4**) vary slightly due to differences in the studied age groups, assessment instruments (eg, Composite International Diagnostic Interview [CIDI], Kiddie-Schedule for Affective Disorders and Schizophrenia for school-aged children [K-SADS]), information source (eg, self-report, parent/teacher report), method of data aggregation (from multiple information sources or multiple assessment waves), and the diagnostic systems used (ie, DSM-III-R, DSM-IV, ICD-10). In addition, data aggregation from various assessment waves in prospective-longitudinal studies, the number and type of diagnoses included in summary categories (eg, "any" anxiety disorder), and the strictness of application of criteria in generating diagnoses (eg, impairment required or not) are other sources for variance. Differences in prevalence estimates from different countries are unlikely reflective of true regional differences, although it should be noted that most epidemiological

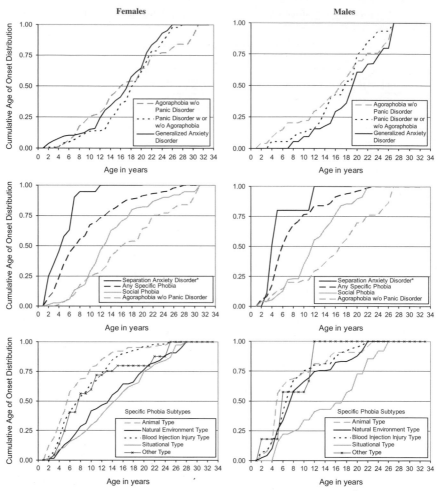

Fig. 2. Patterns of age of onset of anxiety disorders (EDSP; N = 3021). (Note: In phobias impairment was required among subjects aged 18 years or older; *Separation Anxiety Disorder was only assessed in a subsample at T1.)

studies examine prevalence in Western, industrialized countries that may differ from developing countries or other cultures.

Despite notable variation in prevalence estimates that is likely due to method variance, the lifetime prevalence of "any anxiety disorder" in studies with children or adolescents is about 15% to 20%. In particular, it is noteworthy that the period prevalence estimates, for example 1-year or 6-month rates, are not considerably lower than lifetime estimates. This fact indirectly indicates that anxiety disorders exhibit a persisting course or that high rates of forgetting occur for remitted disorders. The most frequent disorders among children and adolescents are separation anxiety disorder (not included in **Table 4**), with estimates of 2.8% and 8%,[28,29,30] and specific and social phobias, with rates up to around 10% and 7%, respectively. Agoraphobia and panic disorder are low-prevalence conditions in childhood (1% or lower); higher prevalences are found in adolescence (2%–3% for panic and 3%–4% for agoraphobia). Of note, considerable controversy surrounds the diagnosis of agoraphobia. Whereas some epidemiological studies find high rates of agoraphobia without evidence of panic attacks, some suggest that this finding reflects diagnostic inaccuracy in epidemiological studies.[31] This issue generally has not been addressed with the same level of rigor in studies of children and adolescents, compared with studies in adults. However, recent findings from the EDSP study among adolescents and young adults suggest that agoraphobia exists as a clinically significant phobic condition independent of panic.[21]

As mentioned before, it is more difficult to provide precise prevalence estimates of GAD in children and adolescents, because this diagnosis only has been applied to youth in DSM-IV, published in 1994.[2] Before 1994, children presenting with worries about multiple events, who typically would receive the DSM-IV diagnosis of GAD, were given the diagnosis of OAD but not GAD. When OAD was subsumed under the diagnosis of GAD in DSM-IV, different criteria were applied to children with multiple worries in DSM-IV, relative to earlier nosologies. This situation complicates attempts to compare earlier to later studies but may explain the lower prevalence rates for GAD than for OAD. Thus, a proportion of children and adolescents who were diagnosed with OAD in the past seem to remain undiagnosed based on current GAD criteria. Similarly, GAD criteria may also identify some children and adolescents who would not meet DSM-III-R criteria for OAD. Data from the EDSP study revealed a cumulative incidence for GAD of 4.3% at age 34 years with relatively few onsets observed in childhood, and the core incidence period being in adolescence and young adulthood.[14]

In terms of sex differences, all anxiety disorders more frequently occur among females than among males. Although sex differences may occur as early as childhood they increase with age,[32] reaching ratios of 2:1 to 3:1 in adolescence (eg, Refs.[28,33]). Fig. 3 depicts the cumulative incidence for anxiety disorders among females and males as assessed in the EDSP study. Unlike for panic attacks (compare Ref.[21]), the sex difference in panic disorder is apparent in cases before the age of 14 but increases further between the ages of 14 and 25 years. The incidence curve for panic disorder reveals a very clear-cut period of increased incidence in females between the ages of 13 and 26 years, whereas males display lower estimates and the period of increased incidence is less pronounced. Agoraphobia revealed a strong and steady incidence increase for females after the age of 6, whereas agoraphobia in males was observed less frequently, with some indication of increased incidence between the ages of 15 and 20 and a leveling off after the age of 25 years. In contrast, a clear sex difference in prevalence was already seen in childhood in the specific phobia animal type (ratio 3:1 by age 10 years).

The choice of appropriate categorical diagnostic thresholds remains a critical issue, giving rise to the consideration of dimensional measures replacing the up to now problematic diagnostic "cutoffs."[34] There is little doubt that the nature of psychopathology is more appropriately conceptualized by dimensional measures and that there is no evidence for a natural point of rarity for most disorders, including anxiety disorders and core anxiety features. In this respect the DSM-IV clinical significance criterion—requiring distress or impairment in social or role functioning—which was introduced to decrease the false-positive problem in psychiatric diagnosis, is particularly problematic.[35] Prevalence rates would markedly increase when the clinical significance criterion threshold simply is lowered or omitted (eg, Ref.[36]). In DSM, such subjects with "subclinical anxiety" would then be classified under "Other Conditions That May Be a Focus of Clinical Attention." As for adults, there is considerable evidence that children and adolescents not meeting the DSM defined clinical significance

Table 4
Prevalence (%) of anxiety disorders in children, adolescents and young adults

Study (Country)	Reference	Instrument	N	Age	Source	Any Anxiety Disorder Lifetime	Period	Specific Phobia Lifetime	Period	Social Phobia Lifetime	Period	Agoraphobia Lifetime	Period	Panic Disorder Lifetime	Period	GAD/OAD Lifetime	Period
DSM-III-R																	
DMHDS (New Zealand)	McGee et al (1990)	DISC	943	15	P/C	–	–	–	3.6[c]	–	1.1[c]	–	–	–	–	–	[5.9][c]
	Feehan et al (1994)	DIS-m-R	930	17–19	C	–	–	–	6.1[c]	–	11.1[c]	–	4.0[c]	–	0.8[c]	–	1.8[c]
	Newman et al (1996)	DIS	961	21	C	–	–	–	8.4[c]	–	9.7[c]	–	3.8[c]	–	0.6[c]	–	1.9[c]
	Kim-Cohen et al (2003)	DIS	967	26	C	–	–	–	7.1[c]	–	10.7[c]	–	–	–	3.9[c]	–	5.5[c]
CHDS (New Zealand)	Fergusson et al (1993)	DISC-P	986	15	P	–	3.9[c]	–	1.3[c]	–	0.7[c]	–	–	–	–	–	1.7 [0.6][c]
		DISC-C	965		C	–	10.8[c]	–	5.1[c]	–	1.7[c]	–	–	–	–	–	4.2 [2.1][a]
	Woodward & Fergusson (2001)	DIS	964	15–16	P/C	29.9	–	20.6	–	2.9	–	1.5[d]	–	–	–	11.0 [4.7]	–
OADP (USA)	Lewinsohn et al (1993)	K-SADS	1710	13–19 (T1)	C	8.8	–	2.0	–	1.4	–	0.7	–	0.8	–	[1.3]	–
				1 year FU (T2)	C	9.2	–	1.5	–	1.5	–	0.6	–	1.2	–	[1.2]	–
Dutch-A (Netherlands)	Verhulst et al (1997)	DISC	780	13–18	P	–	16.5[b]	–	9.2[b]	–	6.3[b]	–	1.9[b]	–	0.3[b]	–	0.7 [1.5][b]
		DISC			C	–	10.0[b]	–	4.5[b]	–	3.7[b]	–	0.7[b]	–	0.2[b]	–	0.6 [1.8][b]
ZESCAP (Switzerland)	Steinhausen et al (1998)	DISC	379	6–17	P	–	11.4[b]	–	5.8[b]	–	4.7[b]	–	1.9[b]	–	–	–	0.5 [2.1][b]
QCMHS (Canada)	Breton et al (1999)	DISC	2400	6–8	C	–	9.2[b]	–	3.2[b]	–	–	–	–	–	–	–	3.9[b]
					P	–	17.5[b]	–	14.6[b]	–	–	–	–	–	–	–	2.7[b]
				9–11	C	–	5.8[b]	–	1.3[b]	–	–	–	–	–	–	–	3.8[b]
					P	–	14.6[b]	–	12.6[b]	–	–	–	–	–	–	–	2.9[b]
				12–14	C	–	12.2[b]	–	10.2[b]	–	–	–	–	–	–	–	1.7[b]
					P	–	12.1[b]	–	7.5[b]	–	–	–	–	–	–	–	5.5[b]
Quebec (Canada)	Romano et al (2001)	DISC	1201	14–17	C	–	8.9[b]	–	1.5[b]	–	4.6[b]	–	1.9[b]	–	–	–	1.1 [2.6][b]
		DISC			P	–	6.5[b]	–	1.0[b]	–	2.9[b]	–	0.9[b]	–	–	–	0.8 [2.3][b]
					P/C	–	14.0[b]	–	2.5[b]	–	6.9[b]	–	2.8[b]	–	–	–	1.7 [4.5][b]
WIC (USA)	Keenan et al (1997)	K-SADS	104	5	C	–	–	11.5	–	4.6	–	–	–	–	–	[1.1]	–

DSM-IV		Interview	N	Age	P/C												
GSMS (USA)	Bittner et al (2007)	CAPA	906	9/11/13	P/C	–	16.1[a]	–	0.6[a]	–	1.5[a]	–	2.5[a]	–	3.1[a]	–	5.8 [6.6][a]
			906	<13	P/C	–	6.6[a]	–	0.4[a]	–	0.5[a]	–	0.1[a]	–	(0.2)[a]	–	1.8 [1.7][a]
			506	>13	P/C	–	10.6[a]	–	0.2[a]	–	1.0[a]	–	2.4[a]	–	(3.0)[a]	–	4.0 [5.5][a]
EDSP (Germany)	Wittchen et al (1998); Wittchen, Stein & Kessler (1999)	CIDI	3021	14–24	C	14.4	3.3[c]	2.3	1.8[c]	3.5	2.6[c]	2.6	1.6[c]	1.6	1.2[c]	0.8	0.5[c]
	Wittchen et al (1999)	CIDI	1395	14–17	C	21.3	14.5[c]	17.1	10.9[c]	3.7	2.5[c]	2.8	2.1[c]	0.7	0.3[c]	0.3	0.2[c]
BJS (Germany)	Essau et al (1998); Essau et al (2000)	CAPI	1035	12–17	C	18.6	11.3[c]	3.5	2.7[c]	1.6	1.4[c]	4.1	2.7[c]	0.5	0.5[c]	0.4	0.2[c]
			380	12–13	C	14.7	8.9[c]	2.6	2.1[c]	0.5	0.5[c]	2.4	1.3[c]	0.0	0.0[c]	0.0	0.0[c]
			350	14–15	C	19.7	12.0[c]	3.1	2.6[c]	2.0	1.1[c]	4.9	3.4[c]	0.9	0.9[c]	0.9	0.3[c]
			305	16–17	C	22.0	13.4[c]	4.9	3.6[c]	2.6	2.6[c]	5.2	3.6[c]	0.7	0.7[c]	0.3	0.3[c]
CCCS (USA)	Angold et al (2002)	CAPA	920	9–17					0.4[a]		1.4[a]		0.5[a]		1.2[a]		–
New Zealand Mental Health Survey (New Zealand)	Wells et al (2006)	CIDI	12,992	16+	C	–	14.8[c]	–	7.3[c]	–	5.1[c]	–	0.6[c]	–	1.7[c]	–	2.0[c]
				16–24	C	–	17.7[c]	–	9.3[c]	–	7.0[c]	–	0.7[c]	–	2.4[c]	–	1.6[c]
IPRP-Study (Puerto Rico)	Canino et al (2004)	DISC	1886	4–17	P/C	6.9[c]		–		–	2.5[c]		–		0.5[c]		–	2.2[c]
Taiwan Epidemiological Study of Mental Disorders in Adolescents (Taiwan)	Gau et al (2005)	K-SADS-E	1070	Seventh grade	C		3.2[a]		5.0[a]		3.4[a]		0.2[a]		0.2[a]		0.7[a]
			1051	Eighth grade	C		7.4[a]		5.6[a]		1.8[a]		0.0[a]		0.1[a]		0.3[a]
			1035	Ninth grade	C		3.1[b]		0.7[a]		2.0[a]		0.0[a]		0.0[a]		0.4[a]

Note: References from this table are available from the corresponding author. GAD, generalized anxiety disorder; OAD, overanxious disorder; [] indicates overanxious disorder; () indicates panic attacks; P, parent report; C, child report.

Study abbreviations in alphabetical order: BJS, Bremer Jugendstudie (Bremen Adolescent Study); CCCS, Caring for Children in the Community Study; CHDS, Christchurch Health and Development Study; DMHDS, Dunedin Multidisciplinary Health and Development Study; Dutch-A, Dutch Adolescents; EDSP, Early Developmental Stages of Psychopathology; GSMS, Great Smoky Mountains Study; IPRP-Study, Island of Puerto Rico Prevalence Study; OADP, Oregon Adolescent Depression Project; QCMHS, Quebec Child Mental Health Survey; ZESCAP, Zurich Epidemiological Study of Child and Adolescent Psychopathology.

Abbreviations of diagnostic interviews: CAPA, Child and Adolescent Diagnostic Assessment; CAPI, Computer Assisted Psychiatric Interview (based on CIDI); CIDI, Composite International Diagnostic Interview; DICA, Diagnostic Interview for Children and Adolescents; CIS, Diagnostic Interview Schedule; DISC, Diagnostic Interview Schedule for Children; K-SADS, Schedule for Affective Disorders and Schizophrenia for School-age Children; SPIKE, Structured Psychopathological Interview and Rating of the Social Consequences for Epidemiology.

[a] 3-month.
[b] 6-month.
[c] 12-month.
[d] Indicates agoraphobia-panic disorder.

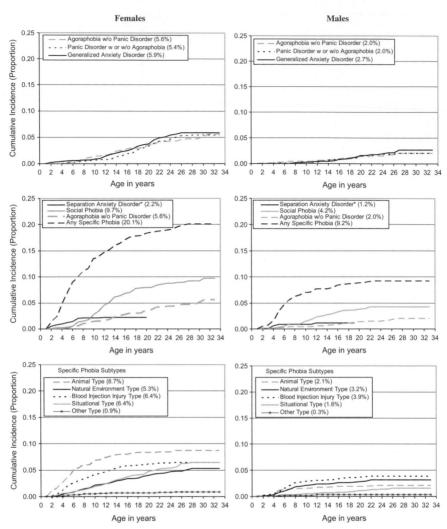

Fig. 3. Cumulative Incidence of anxiety disorders (EDSP; N=3021). (Note: Percentages in the legends refer to the estimated cumulative incidence rate at age 33, *age 19 for Separation Anxiety Disorder which was only assessed in a subsample at T1; in phobias impairment was required among subjects aged 18 years or older.)

threshold might still reveal a similar range of adverse correlates as those meeting the threshold (eg, Ref.[33]). Critical questions therefore are "how can clinical significance or dysfunction be ideally defined" and "what constitutes clinical significance in children versus adolescents versus adults?" Another related concern is that any solution for the distress or impairment criterion that would be applied to anxiety disorders should ideally also be applied to other mental disorders for the reason of consistency.

Similarly, other critical issues relate to symptomatic thresholds required for diagnosis, ie, symptom number, intensity, severity, and temporal thresholds such as duration, persistence, and the clustering of symptoms and criteria in a given time frame.[37] Despite given clinical significance (ie, distress or impairment), such conditions would be classified under the nonspecific residual category "Anxiety Disorder Not Otherwise

Specified." With few exceptions, criteria for children resemble those for adults. Particularly for diagnosis with high symptomatic threshold criteria, it may be clinically relevant to lower the threshold for children (eg, shorter duration requirement, fewer symptoms), to detect affected children early and to provide adequate and focused interventions. Such critical issues have raised significant concerns toward the DSM-V as to whether dimensional and developmental aspects should be specified to provide more clinically relevant information to facilitate diagnosis and treatment.[34,35,37,38,39]

A graphical presentation of the criteria threshold problem is shown in **Fig. 4**. For each of the anxiety diagnoses, DSM-IV provides a specified diagnostic criteria set including symptom count, time/persistence, and clinical significance requirements reflecting the threshold for diagnosis. Falling short of just one criterion leads to nondiagnosis (or nonspecific classification such as "Anxiety Disorder Not Otherwise Specified" or "Other Conditions That May Be a Focus of Clinical Attention") despite the presence of significant specific anxiety pathology (**Fig. 4**A). Thus, the inclusion of dimensional facets in diagnostic systems may facilitate diagnosis and treatment, but it my also complicate the assessment (ie, by use of rating scales or questionnaires, or by the need to develop such scales). Clinicians should also keep in mind that the

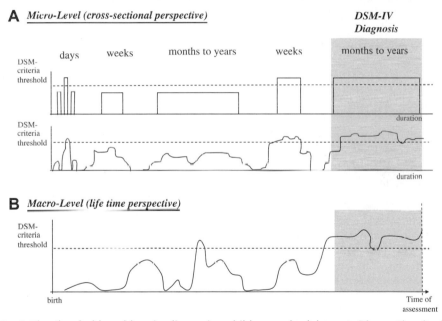

Fig. 4. The threshold problem in diagnosing children and adolescent. Diagnostic criteria define thresholds for diagnoses by specifying type and number of symptoms, the duration and persistence that the symptoms need to be present, and the clinical significance (*A*). Due to the current categorical classification system, being short of just one criterion (eg, only 2 instead of 3 symptoms, only 5 months' instead of 6 months' duration, only 3 instead of 4 days a week, all symptom criteria met but no distress or impairment reported) leads to nondiagnosis (or nonspecific classification as "Anxiety Disorder Not Otherwise Specified" or "Other Conditions That May Be a Focus of Clinical Attention"). The variation of symptoms over time and difficulties in retrospective assessment may negatively affect correct diagnosis. Therefore it is also crucial to take a lifetime approach to diagnosis (*B*). Mere cross-sectional assessment may lead to erroneous nondiagnosis based on transient alleviation of symptoms.

time point and time frame of assessment may be crucial for diagnosis and diagnostic decisions; aspects also essential for interpreting the epidemiological data adequately. Thus, a lifetime diagnostic approach that describes all psychopathological phenomena in a person up to the age of assessment might yield very different diagnostic data than a cross-sectional approach that covers, for example, a 4-week or a 12-month time frame (compare **Fig. 4**B); for some diagnoses (like panic/agoraphobia within the anxiety spectrum or bipolar disorders in the mood disorders) a lifetime approach is essential. Variation in assessment might also affect the rates of "subclinical" or "subsyndromal/subthreshold" conditions, simply because a cross-sectional subthreshold condition may have been threshold at a previous point in time, thus more appropriately labeled as partially remitted.

Natural Course and Longitudinal Outcome

Knowledge on the natural course of anxiety disorders after their first onset is increasing, although several methodological challenges exist. Biases of various sorts are inherent in studies based on clinical samples or in studies using retrospective information on course. Such methods may lead to overestimations of the degree to which anxiety disorders typically seem chronic. Hence, longitudinal studies have clear advantages, particularly when they are based on representative community samples assessed throughout the core high-risk period of first onset and subsequent potential periods of chronic illness. As such, these types of studies represent the method of first choice to study the natural course of anxiety disorders (**Fig. 5**). Although such studies are costly and time consuming, several studies among youth have become available (**Table 5**).

Anxiety disorders seem to take a chronic course based on findings from clinical adult populations (eg, Refs.[40,41]) or retrospective studies (eg, Refs.[42,43]). Prospective epidemiologic follow-up studies among youth from the community only partially support these observations. Thus, on one hand, this work does show that individuals diagnosed with an anxiety disorder, compared with those without, are at statistically increased risk to have the same disorder (eg, Refs.[26,28]; compare **Table 5**) or signs and symptoms of the same disorder[25,44,45] at later points in time ("*homotypic continuity*"). Moreover, follow-back analyses also reveal that those with anxiety disorders in adulthood frequently had the same problems earlier in life (eg, Ref.[46]).

Nevertheless, despite significant longitudinal associations, stability rates (in the form of proportions) of anxiety disorders among youth from the community are overall only low to moderate. For example, in the 15-year prospective multiwave Zurich Cohort study[47] a low stability (4%) was found for *pure* anxiety disorder, defined as GAD or panic disorder. For social phobia no individual met diagnostic criteria continuously at each follow-up assessment, after the disorder had manifested.[48] In the prospective-longitudinal EDSP study, in adolescents aged 14 to 17 at baseline the probability of a positive outcome at 2-year follow-up decreased as a function of severity of baseline anxiety diagnostic status.[45] However, only 19.7% of threshold baseline anxiety cases met threshold anxiety criteria again at follow-up. For the specific diagnoses, considerable variability in outcome was revealed. Taking stable threshold and subthreshold diagnoses at baseline and at follow-up, panic disorder (44%) and specific phobia (30.1%) were found to be most stable, but even here more than 50% of cases were not completely stable. Other disorders showed higher rates of instability, with agoraphobia (13.4%) and social phobia (15.8%) being particularly unstable. Similar trends emerge from clinical studies with youth as well as in an additional series of epidemiological studies (see for review Ref.[49]). For example, Last and colleagues[13,50] found among children and adolescents (aged 5–19 years) with

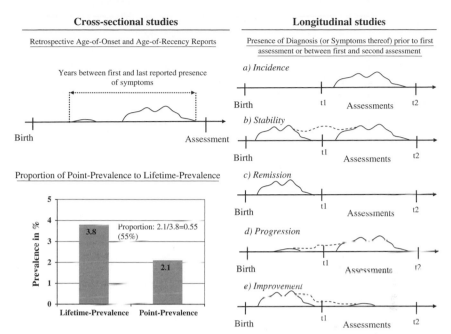

Fig. 5. Assessing the course of anxiety disorders. Several approaches exist to study the course of anxiety disorders. Cross-sectional studies most frequently use retrospective age of onset and age of recency reports to calculate the duration of a condition in years. This approach assumes a continuous disorder course, and may thus overestimate the duration and chronicity because symptom-free intervals are not taken into account. Another indirect measure of disorder chronicity is the proportion of point to lifetime prevalence. The higher the proportion, the higher the chronicity. Because only categorical diagnoses are considered here (no symptomatic improvements below the diagnostic threshold), this may lead to underestimation of chronicity. Overall, cross-sectional studies allow for only crude estimations of course and chronicity of anxiety disorders. Longitudinal studies, in contrast, allow for a more realistic description of the course of a disorder. Taking a prospective approach, the proportion of individuals meeting or not meeting the criteria again at follow-up is frequently used to describe stability and remission. Considering only the full DSM-IV diagnostic level, higher remission rates are possible because improvements below the diagnostic threshold are not taken into account. Thus, the most valid way to describe the course of anxiety disorders is to consider also subthreshold or subsyndromal conditions.

anxiety disorders that over the 3- to 4-year follow-up, 80% had remitted from the anxiety shown initially. Thus overall, among children and adolescents with an anxiety disorder, there is a considerable degree of fluctuation in diagnostic status of the specific anxiety disorder examined; anxiety disorders have a strong tendency to naturally wax and wane over time, particularly in young age groups.[45] It is particularly remarkable that even in disorders that are defined as being chronic, such as GAD, prospective stability rates are only moderate.[51]

Given the limited *homotypic continuity* observed in prospective-longitudinal community studies among youth, the question arises as to whether children and adolescents whose specific anxiety disorder seems to improve or remit are completely healthy in their further course of life. The answer is that this is clearly not the case. For example, in the EDSP only 10% of children and adolescents with specific phobias at baseline had no mental disorder at 10-year follow-up (*full diagnostic remission*); 41% reported the same disorder (*strict homotypic continuity*) and overall, 73% were

Table 5
Course of anxiety disorders from childhood and early adolescence to late adolescence and adulthood (follow-up and follow-back studies)

| Disorder of Interest | Study Characteristics | | | | | | | Outcome | |
Reference	Study (Country)	N	Age at Baseline	FU Duration in Years	Same Disorder	Other Anxiety Disorder	Depressive Disorder	Other Disorders
Social phobia								
Stein et al (2001)	EDSP (Germany)	2548	14–24	5	x	x	x	–
Merikangas et al (2002)	Zurich study (Switzerland)	591	18–19	15	x	x	x	–
Essau, Conradt & Peterman (2002)	BJS (Germany)	1035	12–17	1.3	–	x	–	–
Pine et al (1998)	NYCLS (USA)	776	9–18	9	x	x	–	–
Last et al (1996)	(USA)	247	5–18	34	x	x	n.e.	–
Hale et al (2008)	CONAMORE (Netherlands)	1318	12–16	5	x	n.e.	n.e.	–
Gregory et al (2007)	DMHDS (New Zealand)	1037	11	21	x	x	n.e.	–
Bittner et al (2007)	GSMS (USA)	906	9/11/13	6–10	–	m	–	ADHD (m)
GAD/OAD								
Gregory et al (2007)	DMHDS (New Zealand)	1037	11	21	x	x	n.e.	–
Pine et al (1998)	NYCLS (USA)	776	9–18	9	x	x	x	–
Bittner et al (2004)	EDSP (Germany)	2548	14–24	5	n.e	n.e	x	–

Study	Sample	N	Age	6–10 OAD: 6–10 GAD:				CD (m) Substance use disorders (f)
Bittner et al (2007)	GSMS (USA)	905	9/11/13	6–10 OAD: 6–10 GAD:	f	–	f	–
Hale et al (2008)	CONAMORE (Netherlands)	1318	12–16	5	f	n.a.	n.e.	
Separation anxiety disorder								
Foley et al (2004)	(USA)	161 twins	8–17	1.5	–	x	x	CD, ADHD, ODD
Hale et al (2008)	CONAMORE (Netherlands)	1318	12–16	5	–	n.e.	n.e.	
Bittner et al (2007)	GSMS (USA)	906	9/11/13	6–10	f	f	–	
Bruckl et al (2007)	EDSP (Germany)	1090	14–24	4	n.e.	x	x	Bipolar disorders, pain disorders, alcohol dependence
Pine et al (1998)	NYCLS (USA)	776	9–18	9	n.e.	–	–	–
Agoraphobia								
Gregory et al (2007)	DMHDS (New Zealand)	1037	11	21	x	x	n.e.	–
Specific phobias								
Gregory et al (2007)	DMHDS (New Zealand)	1037	11	21	x	x	n.e.	–
Pine et al (1998)	NYCLS (USA)	776	9–18	9	x	–	–	–
Panic disorder								
Gregory et al (2007)	DMHDS (New Zealand)	1037	11	21	x	x	n.e.	–
Hale et al (2008)	CONAMORE (Netherlands)	1318	12–16	5	–	n.e.	n.e.	–

(continued on next page)

Table 5
(continued)

Disorder of Interest	Study Characteristics					Outcome			
Reference	Study (Country)	N	Age at Baseline	FU Duration in Years	Same Disorder	Other Anxiety Disorder	Depressive Disorder	Other Disorders
Any anxiety disorder								
Last et al (1996)	(USA)	102	5–18	4	x	x	x	Behavioral disorders
Clark et al (2007)	1958 British birth cohort	9727	birth	45	n.e.	n.e.	n.e.	Internalizing and externalizing disorders
Woodward & Fergusson (2001)	CHDS (New Zealand)	964	14–16	21	–	x	x	Substance use disorders
Kim-Cohen et al (2003)	DMHDS (New Zealand)	1037	birth	26	x	x	x	–
Feng et al (2008)	WIC (USA)	290 (boys only)	7–17 months	8	x	x	x	–
Lewinsohn et al (1997)	OADP (USA)	1507	13–19	1	n.e.	x	x	Externalizing disorders (substance use, disruptive behaviors)

Note: References from this table are available from the corresponding author. No associations found. x, positive associations irrespective of gender; f, positive associations only in females; m: positive associations only in males; n.e., not estimated; CD, conduct disorder, ADHD, attention-deficit/hyperactivity disorder; ODD, oppositional defiant disorder.

Study abbreviations: CHDS, Christchurch Health and Development Study; CONAMORE, Conflict and Management of Relationships; DMHDS, Dunedin Multidisciplinary Health and Development Study; EDSP, Early Developmental Stages of Psychopathology; GSMS, Great Smokey Mountain Study; NYCLS, New York Child Longitudinal Study; OADP, Oregon Adolescent Depression Project; WIC, Women Infants Children Program (Pittsburgh).

diagnosed with any anxiety or depressive disorder at subsequent assessments (*heterotypic continuity*).[52] Similarly, only 13% of baseline social phobia cases were free of any diagnosis during the 10-year follow-up; 35% and 64% reported the same disorder and any anxiety/depression respectively. For GAD and PTSD, even all baseline cases revealed either homotypic or heterotypic continuity. Similar findings emerge from other multiwave, prospective-longitudinal studies.[13,28,47,53] Thus, even if for many anxiety cases *strict homotypic continuity* is moderate, there is a substantial degree of continuity of psychopathology as indicated by the later presence of other anxiety disorders (*broad homotypic continuity*) or other disorders (*heterotypic continuity*).

In children and adolescents, there is considerable interanxiety (homotypic) comorbidity with significant association between virtually all specific anxiety disorders, including specific phobia subtypes.[54] The number of "pure" anxiety cases decreases with age in favor of patterns with multiple anxiety disorders by late adolescence or early adulthood. The "load" of anxiety seems to contribute to the development of secondary psychopathological complications. For example, Woodward and Fergusson[55] examined life course outcomes of adolescents with anxiety disorders in a 21-year longitudinal study of a birth cohort of 1265 New Zealand children (CHDS). There were significant associations between the number of anxiety disorders reported in adolescence and later risks of anxiety disorder, major depression, substance dependence, and suicidal behavior. In this study, a higher number of anxiety disorders was also associated with other adverse developmental outcomes such as educational underachievement and early parenthood.

The development of secondary depression seems to be a particularly frequent and concerning heterotypic outcome of anxiety disorders. Is this a characteristic of anxiety in general rather than an issue of specific anxiety disorders or anxiety features (such as panic, avoidance, accumulation of risk factors)? Or is this related to an overarching anxiety or anxiety-depression liability, possibly through shared etiopathogenetic mechanisms (eg, neurobiology)? Cross-sectional and longitudinal studies examined the association between anxiety disorders and depressive disorders[14,55,56,57,58] and concluded that anxiety disorders in general, and also specific types of anxiety disorders (such as phobias, GAD, panic disorder, and so forth) consequently increase the risk for developing a secondary depressive disorder. For example, prospective epidemiological studies found that children and adolescents with specific fears and phobias (especially fear of darkness),[59] social phobia,[18,60,61] or other types of anxiety disorders (agoraphobia, panic disorder, GAD)[14,61] have an increased risk of developing a subsequent depressive disorder. This increased risk for secondary depression seems to be independent of age of onset of anxiety.[18] It could further be shown that certain clinical characteristics of anxiety disorders are associated with secondary depression risk. Onset of depression is more likely in individuals with a higher number of anxiety disorders, a more severe impairment of anxiety disorders, and when panic attacks co-occur.[18,61] Panic attacks among youth have also been shown to be a significant predictor for a wide range of mental disorders and severe psychopathology, particularly as indicated by the incidence of multiple anxiety disorders and substance use disorders.[62]

Besides depression, substance abuse or dependence (alcohol or drugs and medication) is a frequently occurring heterotypic problem among subjects with anxiety disorders.[57,63,64] It has been suggested that substance use is motivated as a possibility to deal with anxiety symptoms, leading to substance-related problems and disorders over the long term.[65] The onset of anxiety disorders precedes that of alcohol and drug disorders at nearly all levels of severity of substance use disorders (use, problems, dependence). Anxiety disorders have been shown to be significant predictors of the subsequent first onset of substance use disorders in cross-sectional and longitudinal analyses.[65,66,67] Although substance use disorders are typically associated with so-called externalizing disorders, such as conduct disorder, attention deficit hyperactivity disorder, or antisocial personality disorder (eg, Ref.[68]), there is also a strong and significant association with "internalizing" disorders, including anxiety disorders.[69] This potentially important pathway has recently been overlooked. Previous research suggests the existence of a second, though less frequent, pathway to substance use disorders originating in early anxiety disorders.[70]

Higher-Order Psychopathological Factors and Metastructure

The frequent observation of comorbidity even in community-based samples has prompted factor analytical studies of higher-order structures of psychopathology. A 2- to 3-factor solution has been repeatedly found when using a limited group of anxiety, depressive, substance use, and antisocial behavior diagnoses.[71,72,73,74,75,76] Anxiety and depressive disorders were consistently loading on an "internalizing" factor that moderately correlates with an "externalizing" factor reflecting substance use and antisocial disorders. The available adult studies frequently revealed 2 additional subfactors for internalizing, namely "fear" (which includes most anxiety disorders) and "anxious-misery" (which includes depressive disorders, but also GAD and PTSD).[71,72,73,74,75] Among youth, this 3-factor structure has so far been replicated using only the EDSP sample.[77]

The finding that all types of anxiety disorders accompany depression is clinically somehow counterintuitive, and therefore several critical concerns have been expressed (see article by Wittchen and colleagues[78] in this issue). Given the differences in incidence patterns of specific anxiety and other mental disorders, and the heterogeneity in the phenomenology within and across disorders, it is questionable whether the structure of psychopathology is stable across development and invariant against the inclusion of more diagnoses. From a developmental perspective it seems plausible that higher-order structure changes over time, particularly among youth. Krueger and colleagues[76] found a good model fit for the 2-factor internalizing-externalizing solution in a young community sample at 2 time points which, however, were only 3 years apart (at ages 18 and 21 years). A similar type of exploration covering longer time frames and age groups is currently under way.[79]

Epidemiology clearly shows that anxiety disorders as early-onset conditions are risk factors for the development of depressive and other disorders occurring later in life. Thus, if one aims to derive a clinically more meaningful taxonomy of mental and anxiety disorders, the need to explore other concepts might arise. For example, one approach, taken from somatic illnesses, might be longitudinal "staging models." Such models would allow one to describe the progression of mental disorders over time from less severe, pure conditions to more complex, severe comorbid stages and thus may have greater potential value for specifying the complexity of developmental patterns of mental disorders.[39] From a clinical perspective, such a view might also facilitate the derivation of secondary prevention and staged intervention.

CORRELATES AND RISK FACTORS FOR ANXIETY DISORDERS

Many variables are considered to be risk factors for anxiety disorders. Attempts to definitively demonstrate that the many correlates of anxiety are, in reality, risk factors face considerable methodological hurdles, because it must be demonstrated that the risk factor is actually present before the onset of the anxiety disorder,[80] and ideally that the probability of onset of a disorder is related to the severity, frequency, or duration of the risk factor. Thus, cross-sectional studies merely allow generation of initial hypotheses about potential risk factors, based on demonstrations of associations between anxiety disorders and a range of potential variables, such as demographic, neurobiologic, family-genetic, personality, or environmental factors; prospective-longitudinal studies are necessary to show that a factor increases the risk for the onset of an anxiety disorder. This problem, of course, does not apply to factors that are present at birth, such as sex or genotype information. Therefore, in the following sections the authors differentiate between evidence for correlates and risk factors for anxiety disorders. Aspects of specificity of these factors for specific anxiety disorders and for anxiety versus depressive disorders are also considered. The focus is primarily on epidemiological studies among youth, as clinical samples may be subject to various biases related to ascertainment;[81] however, such studies are included if no other evidence is available. Findings from epidemiological studies among adults are also included if these allow for the assumption that the variables had an impact in childhood or adolescence.

Demographic Variables

Sex
Female sex consistently emerges as a risk factor for the development of anxiety disorders. Females are about twice as likely as males to develop each of the anxiety disorders (eg, Refs.[28,33,82]). Sex differences in prevalence, if any, are small in childhood but they increase with age.[32]

Education
Most epidemiological studies find higher rates of anxiety disorders among subjects with lower education in comparison with subjects with a higher education (eg, Ref.[33]). It remains unclear to which degree the lower educational performance is a predictor, correlate, or consequence of anxiety. Two adult studies found associations for anxiety but not for depressive disorders.[83,84]

Financial situation
With few exceptions,[85,86] studies consistently find associations between low household income or unsatisfactory financial situations and anxiety disorders (eg, Ref.[33]). However, results from a quasi-experimental study suggest that these associations may not emerge through a risk factor-disorder association; other more complex relationships may explain the associations seen in cross-sectional research.[87]

Urbanization
Degree of urbanization (rural/urban) does not typically emerge as a correlate of anxiety disorders.[33,85,86]

Pathophysiology

Family genetics
Two main approaches have been used to study the familial transmission of anxiety disorders: family studies and twin studies. In family studies, including community studies with linked assessments of familial psychopathology, the familial aggregation of anxiety disorders has been shown to be substantial.[88,89,90,91] Overall, children of parents with at least one anxiety disorder have a substantially increased risk of also having an anxiety disorder.[92] A particular risk emerges for offspring when both parents are affected[88,91] or when the parents suffer from severely impairing, multiple, or early-onset anxiety disorders.[93] Because it is known that anxiety disorders are associated with an increased risk of depression, it is not surprising that parental depression

was also found to be associated with offspring anxiety,[94,95] and that higher rates of depression are also found among offspring of parents with anxiety disorders.[91,96] Such cross-disorder associations have prompted investigations into the specificity of the familial transmission of anxiety and other mental disorders. Although findings are mixed, there is some evidence for specificity. For example, in the longitudinal Oregon study of youth, relatives of subjects with anxiety disorder alone more frequently also had an anxiety disorder alone. The same applied to pure depressive disorders. Relatives of adolescents with comorbid anxiety/depression were more likely to show pure anxiety, pure depression, or comorbid anxiety/depression.[97] Moffitt and colleagues[98] showed in the Dunedin birth cohort that familial depression liability was associated with pure depression but not pure GAD among offspring. In the EDSP study, Beesdo and colleagues[14] showed that parental GAD was associated with anxiety disorders alone and comorbid anxiety/depressive disorders among offspring, but not with depressive disorders alone. Thus, a familial transmission of anxiety at least partly independent from depression is suggested by these findings. Furthermore, some specificity seems to exist in the familial transmission of specific anxiety disorders,[14,99] consistent with findings from the classic family studies. For example, Fyer and colleagues[100] found moderate but specific familial aggregation of simple phobia, social phobia, and panic disorder with agoraphobia in families of subjects who had any of these disorders but no other lifetime anxiety disorder comorbidity.

A meta-analyses of data by Hettema and colleagues[90] from family and twin studies of panic disorder, GAD, and phobias in adults showed that all anxiety disorders have a significant familial aggregation. Twin studies can disentangle the genetic from the shared and nonshared environmental contributions in the familial transmission of anxiety disorders. Findings indicate that the estimated genetic heritabilities across the disorders are generally no more than modest, falling in the range of 30% to 40%. The considerable remaining variance in liability can be attributed primarily to individual (nonshared) environmental factors.[101] Regarding specificity, twin studies indicate that the genetic liability for specific anxiety disorders overlaps partly.[101,102] Furthermore, GAD in particular shares genetic liability with major depression; both disorders, however, can be differentiated based on environmental risk.[103,104]

Psychobiology

Anxiety disorders can be viewed as reflecting individual differences in neural function. Various physiological systems have been examined in animals and humans to document psychobiological substrates of anxiety. However, it is not clear as to what degree many neurobiological factors relate to anxiety and anxiety processing in general, or whether they are specific correlates of anxiety disorders.

Fear-conditioning experiments in animals have demonstrated that the amygdala is involved in the neural circuit of learning to fear a previously neutral/harmless stimulus.[105] Extinction processes have been shown to require communication between the amygdala and the frontal cortex. Other forms of fear develop without prior learning and are regulated by distinct but related neural circuits. Animal research has impressively shown that function of the mature fear circuit, including hypothalamic-pituitary-adrenal (HPA) regulation, also reflects influences during childhood (eg, rearing or stress), but the nature of these influences is likely to be highly complex.[49]

In humans, brain imaging procedures have been used to study brain function related to anxiety. Besides some other brain structures such as the ventrolateral prefrontal cortex,[106,107] amygdala activity has been frequently examined in emotional face-viewing paradigms. Findings are inconsistent, but some studies implicate amygdala hypersensitivity in some forms of anxiety among youth. For example, Thomas and colleagues[108] found enhanced amygdala activation during the viewing of evocative face-emotion displays among children with anxiety disorders. More specifically, McClure and colleagues[107] found among adolescents with GAD increased amygdala responses to fearful facial expressions, particularly when they rated subjective degrees of internal fear. Thus, attention modulates emotion processing and plays an important role in shaping the function of the adolescent human fear circuit. A recent study examined commonalities and differences in amygdala activity in anxious versus depressed adolescents.[109] During fearful-face processing, patients with anxiety and those with major depression both differed in amygdala responses from healthy participants and from each other, but only during a passive viewing condition that did not require a specific attention task. Focusing attention to rate subjectively experienced degrees of fear while viewing fearful faces was associated with similar amygdala hyperactivation in both anxious and depressed adolescents. These data support the view of neural distinctions between depression and anxiety as complex and nuanced, but clearly demonstrable. More work is needed to understand commonalities and differences in neural circuits of the specific anxiety disorders.

Few data are available regarding the question as to whether functional abnormalities occur as correlate of or vulnerability to anxiety disorders. One study compared amygdala activity in adults classified as inhibited or not inhibited in childhood,[110] and found enhanced amygdala activity in the formerly inhibited individuals, implicating amygdala function in risk for anxiety. Another study found that perturbations in amygdala function are evident in adolescents temperamentally at risk for anxiety, and that attention state alters the underlying pattern of neural processing, potentially mediating the observed behavioral patterns across development.[111] More such work is needed to understand to what degree findings of functional neural abnormalities relate to altered processing of anxiety-related cues or reflect the consequences of anxiety disorders, or whether those abnormalities pose a risk for a subsequent anxiety disorder onset. Of particular clinical interest, however, is the finding that brain function abnormalities decrease with successful pharmacological or cognitive-behavioral treatment (eg, Ref.[112]).

Temperament and Personality

Temperamental and personality trait vulnerabilities such as Eysenck's neuroticism, Gray's trait-anxiety, or Kagan's behavioral inhibition, which are likely to be overlapping constructs, are consistently viewed to play an important role in anxiety disorders. In fact one might see these constructs as a precursor condition to the occurrence of prototypical anxiety disorders. The tripartite model conceptualizes general distress or negative affectivity as general higher-order vulnerability factor for anxiety and depression, whereas low positive affectivity is specific to depression, and physiological hyperarousal is specific to anxiety.[113,114] Similarly, in a hierarchical model[115] negative affectivity is the higher-order factor relevant for anxiety and depression, but on a lower level each anxiety disorder contains an additional specific component.

Several studies support the tripartite and the hierarchical models for anxiety and depression symptoms (eg, Refs.[116,117,118]). Twin studies consistently show high correlations between neuroticism and anxiety and depression, as well as their co-occurrence.[119,120] It is estimated that about 50% of the genetic correlations between these disorders derives from the genetic factor for neuroticism. Epidemiological studies are generally in support of these findings, with few indications of specificity between anxiety and depression outcomes.[121,122]

The temperamental concept of behavioral inhibition reflects the consistent tendency to display fear and withdrawal in unfamiliar situations.[123] Behavioral inhibition is at least moderately stable, detectable early in life, and under some genetic control.[124,125] Children with behavioral inhibition are shy with strangers and fearful in unfamiliar situations.[126] With few exceptions,[127,128] behavioral inhibition was shown to be a risk factor for the development of anxiety disorders (eg, Refs.[126,129,130]). There are also indications for specificity in this association within the anxiety disorders (strong associations particularly to social phobia)[126,131,132] and in differentiation to depression.[14,126]

Environmental Factors

Parenting style

Despite the existence of several clinical studies, there are only a few epidemiological studies examining the question as to whether parenting style is an important risk factor for anxiety disorders (for an overview, see Ref.[133]). In the EDSP study among adolescents, parental overprotection and parental rejection were significantly associated with increased rates of social phobia in offspring.[89,99] Other analyses from this study indicate that overprotection increases the risk for anxiety disorders but not "pure" depressive disorders, whereas depressive disorders show associations to rejection.[14] Kendler and colleagues[134] examined 1033 female adult twin pairs, and measured 3 dimensions of parenting (coldness, protectiveness, authoritarianism). High levels of coldness and authoritarianism in parents were modestly associated with increased risk for nearly all disorders. Nevertheless, the impact of protectiveness was more variable. Whereas phobia, GAD, major depression, and panic disorder were significantly associated with protectiveness, bulimia, drug abuse, and alcohol dependence showed no significant associations with this particular parenting dimension. In a clinical sample, Merikangas and colleagues[88] did not find an association between family climate or rearing style and anxiety disorders in offspring of parents with anxiety or substance use disorder. In a prospective-longitudinal design, parent-adolescent disagreements were found to indirectly increase the risk for the onset of anxiety and depressive disorders through their direct association with high symptom levels.[135] Considerable other work finds similar relationships, though using somewhat different procedures.[136,137]

Social learning mechanisms,[138] such as parental modeling of anxious or avoidance behavior, or parental attitudes and actions[139,140,141,142] are discussed as mediating mechanisms of these relationships, reflecting the aspects of the environment in these family-environmental factors. However, recent work suggests that such factors also reflect the influence of genetics, through gene-environment interactions and correlations.[143]

Childhood adversities

Most epidemiological studies find associations between adverse experiences in childhood (eg, loss of parents, parental divorce, physical and sexual abuse) and almost all mental disorders, including anxiety disorders. Kessler and colleagues[144] found associations between retrospectively reported childhood adversities, including loss events (eg, parental divorce), parental psychopathologies (eg, maternal depression), interpersonal traumas (eg, rape), and subsequent onset of DSM-III-R disorders in a large United States community study of adults. These adversities were consistently associated with the onset of anxiety disorders, mood disorders, addictive disorders, and acting out disorders. Also, a history of neglect or abuse was a strong predictor of psychiatric morbidity (ie, anxiety disorders, depression, substance use disorders) in the Netherlands Mental Health Survey and Incidence Study (NEMESIS).[145] In the New Zealand CHDS study, individuals who reported childhood sexual abuse had higher rates of major depression, anxiety disorder, conduct disorder, substance use disorder, and suicidal behavior than those not reporting sexual abuse.[146] Furthermore, there were consistent relationships between the extent of childhood sexual abuse and the risk of mental disorders.

It remains an open question whether the nonspecificity of the findings mainly emerges because of the frequent comorbidity among disorders. Moffitt and colleagues[98] found in the Dunedin birth cohort study that childhood maltreatment was associated with "pure" GAD and "pure" major depression, indicating nonspecificity. In the EDSP, however, childhood separation events were associated only with "pure" anxiety and comorbid anxiety/depression, but not with "pure" depression.[14]

Further questions refer to gender differences. For example, several studies suggest that the relationship between some psychiatric disorders and history of physical or sexual abuse tends to be stronger for women than for men.[147,148]

Life events

Although more consistent findings emerge for depressive disorders,[149,150] several studies showed associations between life events and anxiety disorders. For example, in the EDSP study, preceding DSM-IV defined traumatic events predicted subsequent anxiety and depressive disorders.[151] It has been suggested that experience of threat events tend to precede anxiety disorder, whereas loss events tend to precede depression.[152] In a study that examined the relationship between parental loss before age 17 years and adult pathology in female same-sex twins from a population-based registry, Kendler and colleagues[153] reported that increased risk for GAD was associated with parental separation. Increased risk for phobia was associated with parental death but not parental separation. Moreover, death of persons within the social network were more strongly associated with major depression than with GAD.[154] Moderate specificity in the association between type of life event and type of psychopathology also emerged in a direct comparison of groups with pure major depression, pure GAD, and comorbid major depression and GAD.[155] Loss and humiliation events predicted the onset of pure depression, and the onset of comorbid depression and GAD. Onset of pure GAD was associated with loss and danger events.

Summary of Correlates and Risk Factors

Table 6 summarizes the findings for correlates and risk factors for anxiety disorders, as well as the indications for specificity between the anxiety disorders and between anxiety and depression. Two aspects should be noted. First, this list is not exhaustive; a range of further variables were also found to be of relevance in the etiology/pathogenesis of anxiety disorders (eg, other mental disorders such as attention-deficit/hyperactivity disorder, conduct disorder, depression, somatic conditions, attributional and cognitive styles, neurotransmitter systems, HPA function). Second, beyond the mere identification of risk factors that may increase the probability for the development of anxiety disorders, it is of particular importance to also disentangle interactions between risk factors in the promotion of anxiety disorder onset. For example, Knappe and colleagues[99] showed a combined effect of parental psychopathology and parental rearing on the risk for offspring social phobia, based on prospective-longitudinal community data. More work is needed to identify the core risk variables and to understand their interplay in critical time periods.[156,157,158] Furthermore, intervention studies are needed to elucidate the causality status of risk factors.[80]

Table 6
Selected correlates and risk factors for anxiety disorders

Variables	Association with Anxiety Disorders[a]	Specificity for Particular Anxiety Disorder[b]	Risk Factor Status (Temporal Priority)[b]	Specificity for Anxiety versus Depressive Disorders[b]
Demographics				
Female gender	+++	−	++	−
Lower education	+	−	−	−
Bad financial situation/low household income	+++	−	−	−
Urbanization	+/−	−	+/−	+/−
Pathophysiology				
Family genetics/ familial aggregation	+++	+	+	+
Psychobiology	+++	+	+/−	+
Temperament and personality				
Neuroticism/ negative affectivity	+++	+/−	+	+/−
Behavioral inhibition	+++	+	+	+
Environmental factors				
Parenting style/ family climate	++	−	−	−
Childhood adversities (abuse, neglect, separation from parents, death of parent)	+++	−	+	−
Life events	++	+/−	+	+

[a] Association with anxiety disorders: +++, strong associations in many studies; ++, associations in several studies; +, associations in some studies, but some contrary findings; +/−, contrary findings; −, no associations in many studies.
[b] Specificity for particular anxiety disorder/Risk factor status (temporal priority)/Specificity for anxiety versus depressive disorders: ++, strong evidence; +, some evidence; +/−, contrary findings; −, no evidence.

SUMMARY AND CONCLUSIONS

Anxiety disorders are common and early emerging conditions associated with considerable developmental, psychosocial, and psychopathological complications. Although early anxiety syndromes may remit spontaneously, the vast majority of children and adolescents that have developed a threshold anxiety disorder will be affected by the same condition or other mental disorders (including other anxiety disorders, depressive disorders, or substance use disorders) over the further course of life. The secondary development of depressive disorders is a particularly frequent complication across the range of anxiety disorders, calling for further studies delineating the processes behind this increased depression risk among individuals with anxiety disorders. The identification of early vulnerability and risk factors for anxiety disorders is of crucial importance to facilitate research into the development of targeted prevention or early interventions programs. Although several variables have been identified as potential risk factors for anxiety disorders, such as parental psychopathology, behaviorally inhibited temperament, or early life adversity, more work is needed to identify the most powerful predictors, and to understand their complex biological and psychological mechanisms and interactions in promoting the onset of anxiety disorders, and further, the adverse long-term course, to identify those variables that might provide the best guidance for early intervention. This task is challenging because substantial differences seem to exist between specific anxiety disorders. Moreover, differences exist for different developmental phases. Overall, developmental issues have been largely ignored by the current diagnostic classification systems. The research reviewed in this article suggests incorporation of a developmental perspective into the next revision of the DSM. Such a perspective includes the necessity of explicit information on:

- Differences in symptom presentation across age (children versus adolescents versus adults): what constitutes a disorder given age and context?
- Differences in symptom report as a function of information source (self-report, parent report, teacher report) and guidance on optimal assessment as a function of age and disorder type
- Differences in course, persistence, and outcome as a function of age, age of onset, and disorder type
- Possibilities of dimensional assessments to differentiate degrees of symptom expression in terms of duration, severity, and illness stages

Besides this clinical descriptive perspective, other issues are important, for example the influence of genetic, neurobiologic, or temperamental factors.[159] Developmentally more differentiated information in the DSM would clearly facilitate recognition and diagnosis at all ages, particularly in children in whom the border between normal and pathological phenomena may be particularly narrow. Improved diagnosis also improves allocation of treatment. Many children live with an unrecognized anxiety disorder and are in need of treatment. Psychological and psychopharmacological treatment options are suitable and available for youth; however, more research is needed to further test and improve these interventions.[49] Although considerable evidence has been accumulated on the effectiveness of cognitive-behavior therapy for anxiety disorders among children and adolescents, the data regarding pharmacological treatments such as selective serotonin reuptake inhibitors among youth are still scarce. One major concern with psychopharmacological interventions in children regards the unknown long-term effects of such treatment on neurological development. Across all interventions, open questions also refer to the need to separate specific anxiety disorders. What would be the consequence for clinical research and treatment if all anxiety disorders or even internalizing disorders, including anxiety and depressive disorders, would be lumped into one group in future diagnostic systems? The research reviewed in this article suggests retaining the current degree of specificity in diagnoses as specified in DSM-IV-TR, particularly as related to anxiety disorders in children and adolescents.

REFERENCES

1. Pine DS, Helfinstein SM, Bar-Haim Y, et al. Challenges in developing novel treatments for childhood disorders: lessons from research on anxiety. Neuropsychopharmacology 2009;34(1):213–28.
2. APA. Diagnostic and statistical manual of mental disorders. text revision. 4th edition. Washington, DC: American Psychiatric Press; 2000.
3. Morris RJ, Kratochwill TR. Childhood fears and phobias. In: Kratochwill TR, Morris RJ, editors. The practice of child therapy. 2nd edition. New York: Pergamon; 1991. p. 76–114.
4. Muris P, Merckelbach H, Mayer B, et al. Common fears and their relationship to anxiety disorders symptomatology in normal children. Pers Individ Dif 1998; 24(4):575–8.
5. McCathie H, Spence SH. What is the revised fear survey schedule for children measuring? Behav Res Ther 1991;29(5):495–502.
6. Campbell MA, Rapee RM, Spence SH. Developmental changes in the interpretation of rating format on a questionnaire measure of worry. Clin Psychol 2000; 5(2):49–59.
7. WHO. The ICD-10 classification of mental and behavioural disorders: diagnostic criteria for research. Geneva, Switzerland: World Health Organization; 1993.
8. Schniering CA, Hudson JL, Rapee RM. Issues in the diagnosis and assessment of anxiety disorders in children and adolescents. Clin Psychol Rev 2000;20(4): 453–78.
9. Kendall PC, Hedtke KA, Aschenbrand SG. Behavioral and emotional disorders in adolescents. Nature, assessment and treatment. In: Wolfe DA, Mash EJ, editors. Anxiety disorders. New York: Guilford Press; 2006. p. 259–99.
10. Phillips K, Price LH, Greenberg BD, et al. Should the DSM diagnostic groupings be changed?. In: Phillips K, First MB, Pincus HA, editors. Advancing DSM. Dilemmas in psychiatric diagnosis. Arlington (VA): American Psychiatric Association; 2003. p. 57–87.
11. Henry B, Moffitt TE, Caspi A, et al. On the "remembrance of things past": a longitudinal evaluation of the retrospective method. Psychol Assess 1994;6:92–101.
12. Kessler RC, Berglund P, Demler O, et al. Lifetime prevalence and age-of-onset distributions of DSM-IV disorders in the National Comorbidity Survey Replication. Arch Gen Psychiatry 2005;62:593–602.
13. Last CG, Perrin S, Hersen M, et al. A prospective study of childhood anxiety disorders. J Am Acad Child Adolesc Psychiatry 1996;35:1502–10.
14. Beesdo K, Pine DS, Lieb R, et al. Similarities and differences in incidence and risk patterns of anxiety and depressive disorders: the position of generalized anxiety disorder. Arch Gen Psychiatry, in press.
15. Robins E, Guze SB. Establishment of diagnostic validity in psychiatric illness: its application to schizophrenia. Am J Psychiatry 1970;126(7):983–7.
16. Becker ES, Rinck M, Türke V, et al. Epidemiology of specific phobia subtypes: findings from the Dresden mental health study. Eur Psychiatry 2007;22(2):69–74.
17. Wittchen HU, Lieb R, Schuster P, et al. When is onset? Investigations into early developmental stages of anxiety and depressive disorders. In: Rapoport JL, editor. Childhood onset of "adult" psychopathology. Clinical and research advances. Washington, DC: American Psychiatric Press, Inc.; 1999. p. 259–302.
18. Beesdo K, Bittner A, Pine DS, et al. Incidence of social anxiety disorder and the consistent risk for secondary depression in the first three decades of life. Arch Gen Psychiatry 2007;64(8):903–12.

19. Wittchen H-U, Fehm L. Epidemiology and natural course of social fears and social phobia. Acta Psychiatr Scand 2003;108(Suppl 417):4–18.
20. de Graaf R, Bijl R, Spijker J, et al. Temporal sequencing of lifetime mood disorders in relation to comorbid anxiety and substance use disorders. Soc Psychiatry Psychiatr Epidemiol 2003;38:1–11.
21. Wittchen HU, Nocon A, Beesdo K, et al. Agoraphobia and panic: prospective-longitudinal relations suggest a rethinking of diagnostic concepts. Psychother Psychosom 2008;77:147–57.
22. Ruscio AM, Lane M, Roy-Byrne P, et al. Should excessive worry be required for a diagnosis of generalized anxiety disorder? Results from the US National Comorbidity Survey Replication. Psychol Med 2005;35(12):1761–72.
23. Ruscio AM, Chiu WT, Roy-Byrne P, et al. Broadening the definition of generalized anxiety disorder: effects on prevalence and associations with other disorders in the National Comorbidity Survey Replication. J Anxiety Disord 2007;21: 662–76.
24. Kessler RC, Brandenburg N, Lane M, et al. Rethinking the duration requirement for generalized anxiety disorder: evidence from the National Comorbidity Survey Replication. Psychol Med 2005;35(7):1073–82.
25. Beesdo K. Wie entstehen Generalisierte Ängste? Eine prospektiv-longitudinale, klinisch-epidemiologische Studie bei Jugendlichen und jungen Erwachsenen. [The development of Generalized Anxiety. A prospective-longitudinal, clinicale-pidemiologic study among adolescents and young adults]. Dresden: TUD Press; 2006.
26. Bittner A, Egger HL, Erkanli A, et al. What do childhood anxiety disorders predict? J Child Psychol Psychiatry 2007;48(12):1174–83.
27. Newman DL, Moffitt TE, Caspi A, et al. Psychiatric disorder in a birth cohort of young adults: prevalence, comorbidity, clinical significance, and new case incidence from age 11 to 21. J Consult Clin Psychol 1996;64(3):552–62.
28. Pine DS, Cohen P, Gurley D, et al. The risk for early-adulthood anxiety and depressive disorders in adolescents with anxiety and depressive disorders. Arch Gen Psychiatry 1998;55:56–64.
29. Bowen RC, Offord DR, Boyle MH. The prevalence of overanxious disorder and separation anxiety disorder: results from the Ontario child health study. J Am Acad Child Adolesc Psychiatry 1990;29:753–8.
30. Bolton D, Eley TC, O'Connor TG, et al. Prevalence and genetic and environmental influences on anxiety disorders in 6-year-old twins. Psychol Med 2006; 36(3):335–44.
31. Horwath E, Lish JD, Johnson J, et al. Agoraphobia without panic: clinical reappraisal of an epidemiologic finding. Am J Psychiatry 1993;150(10):1496–501.
32. Craske MG. Origins of phobias and anxiety disorders: why more women than men? Amsterdam: Elsevier; 2003.
33. Wittchen H-U, Nelson CB, Lachner G. Prevalence of mental disorders and psychosocial impairments in adolescents and young adults. Psychol Med 1998;28:109–26.
34. Helzer JE, Kraemer HC, Krueger RF, et al, editors. Dimensional approaches in diagnostic classification. Refining the research agenda for DSM-V. Arlington (VA): APA; 2008.
35. Wakefield JC, First MB. Clarifying the distinction between disorder an nondisorder. Confronting the overdiagnosis (false-positives) problem in DSM-V. In: Phillips K, First MB, Pincus HA, editors. Advancing DSM. Dilemmas in psychiatric diagnosis. Arlington (VA): American Psychiatric Association; 2003. p. 23–55.

36. Shaffer D, Fisher P, Dulcan MK, et al. The NIMH diagnostic interview schedule for children version 2.3 (DISC-2.3): description, acceptability, prevalence rates, and performance in the MECA study. J Am Acad Child Adolesc Psychiatry 1996; 35(7):865–77.

37. Pincus HA, McQueens LE, Elinson L. Subthreshold mental disorders. Nosological and research recommendations. In: Phillips K, First MB, Pincus HA, editors. Advancing DSM. Dilemmas in psychiatric diagnosis. Arlington (VA): American Psychiatric Association; 2003. p. 129–44.

38. Regier DA. Dimensional approaches to psychiatric classification: refining the research agenda for DSM-V: an introduction. Int J Methods Psychiatr Res 2007;16(Suppl 1):S1–5.

39. Shear MK, Bjelland I, Beesdo K, et al. Supplementary dimensional assessment in anxiety disorders. Int J Methods Psychiatr Res 2007;16(Suppl 1):S52–64.

40. Yonkers KA, Bruce SE, Dyck IR, et al. Chronicity, relapse, and illness—course of panic disorder, social phobia, and generalized anxiety disorder: findings in men and women from 8 years of follow-up. Depress Anxiety 2003;17(3):173–9.

41. Bruce SE, Yonkers KA, Otto MW, et al. Influence of psychiatric comorbidity on recovery and recurrence in generalized anxiety disorder, social phobia, and panic disorder: a 12-year prospective study. Am J Psychiatry 2005;162:1179–87.

42. Blazer DG, Hughes D, George LK, et al. Generalized anxiety disorder. In: Robins LN, Regier DA, editors. Psychiatric disorders in America: the Epidemiologic Catchment Area Study. New York: The Free Press; 1991. p. 180–203.

43. Woodman CL, Noyes R, Black DW, et al. A 5-year follow-up study of generalized anxiety disorder and panic disorder. J Nerv Ment Dis 1999;187:3–9.

44. Beesdo K, Knappe S, Höfler M, et al. Stability and persistence of anxiety disorders among youth. A prospective-longitudinal community study. Eur Neuropsychopharmacol, in press.

45. Wittchen H-U, Lieb R, Pfister H, et al. The waxing and waning of mental disorders: evaluating the stability of syndromes of mental disorders in the population. Compr Psychiatry 2000;41(2 Suppl 1):122–32.

46. Gregory AM, Caspi A, Moffitt TE, et al. Juvenile mental health histories of adults with anxiety disorders. Am J Psychiatry 2007;164(2):301–8.

47. Angst J, Vollrath M. The natural history of anxiety disorders. Acta Psychiatr Scand 1991;84:446–52.

48. Merikangas KR, Avenevoli S, Acharyya S, et al. The spectrum of social phobia in the Zurich Cohort Study of young adults. Biol Psychiatry 2002;51:81–91.

49. Pine DS, Klein RG. Anxiety disorders. In: Rutter M, editor. Rutter's child and adolescent psychiatry. John Wiley & Sons; 2008. p. 628–46.

50. Last CG, Hansen C, Franco N. Anxious children in adulthood: a prospective study of adjustment. J Am Acad Child Adolesc Psychiatry 1997;36(5): 645–52.

51. Beesdo K, Wittchen HU, Hoefler M, et al. Risk factors for generalized anxiety: a prospective-longitudinal epidemiological study of adolescents and young adults. Eur Neuropsychopharmacol 2006;16(Suppl 4):s453.

52. Emmelkamp PMG, Wittchen HU. Specific phobias. In: Andrews G, Charney DS, Sirovatka PJ, et al, editors. Stress-induced and fear circuitry disorders. Refining the research agenda for DSM-V. Arlington (VA): APA; 2009. p. 77–101.

53. Wittchen H-U. Der Langzeitverlauf unbehandelter Angststörungen: Wie häufig sind Spontanremissionen? [The long-term course and outcome of untreated anxiety disorders: How frequent are spontaneous remissions?]. Verhaltenstherapie 1991;1(4):273–82.

54. Wittchen H-U, Lecrubier Y, Beesdo K, et al. Relationships among anxiety disorders: patterns and implications. In: Nutt DJ, Ballenger JC, editors. Anxiety disorders. Oxford: Blackwell Science; 2003. p. 25–37.

55. Woodward LJ, Fergusson DM. Life course outcomes of young people with anxiety disorders in adolescence. J Am Acad Child Adolesc Psychiatry 2001; 40(9):1086–93.

56. Fergusson DM, Woodward LJ. Mental health, educational, and social role outcomes of adolescents with depression. Arch Gen Psychiatry 2002;59: 225–31.

57. Kessler RC, Nelson CB, McGonagle KA, et al. Comorbidity of DSM-III-R major depressive disorder in the general population: results from the US National Comorbidity Survey. Br J Psychiatry 1996;168.17–30.

58. Kessler RC, Stang P, Wittchen H-U, et al. Lifetime comorbidities between social phobia and mood disorders in the U.S. National Comorbidity Survey. Psychol Med 1999;29(3):555–67.

59. Pine DS, Cohen P, Brook J. Adolescent fears as predictors of depression. Biol Psychiatry 2001;50(9).721–4.

60. Stein MB, Fuetsoh M, Müller N, et al. Social anxiety disorder and the risk of depression. A prospective community study of adolescents and young adults. Arch Gen Psychiatry 2001;58:251–6.

61. Bittner A, Goodwin RD, Wittchen H-U, et al. What characteristics of primary anxiety disorders predict subsequent major depressive disorder? J Clin Psychiatry 2004;65(5):618–26.

62. Goodwin RD, Lieb R, Höfler M, et al. Panic attack as a risk factor for severe psychopathology. Am J Psychiatry 2004;161;2207–14.

63. Kessler RC, Crum RM, Warner LA, et al. Lifetime co-occurrence of DSM-III-R alcohol abuse and dependence with other psychiatric disorders in the National Comorbidity Survey. Arch Gen Psychiatry 1997;54:313–21.

64. Merikangas KR, Mehta RL, Molnar BE, et al. Comorbidity of substance use disorders with mood and anxiety disorders: results of the international consortium in psychiatric epidemiology. Addict Behav 1998;23:893–907.

65. Zimmermann P, Wittchen HU, Höfler M, et al. Primary anxiety disorders and the development of subsequent alcohol use disorders: a 4-year community study of adolescents and young adults. Psychol Med 2003;33:1211–22.

66. Brückl T, Wittchen H-C, Höfler M, et al. Childhood separation anxiety and the risk for subsequent psychopathology: results from a community study. Psychother Psychosom 2007;76(1):47–56.

67. Crum RM, Pratt LA. Risk of heavy drinking and alcohol use disorders in social phobia: a prospective analysis. Am J Psychiatry 2001;158(10):1693–700.

68. Kim-Cohen J, Caspi A, Moffitt TE, et al. Prior juvenile diagnoses in adults with mental disorder. Arch Gen Psychiatry 2003;60:709–17.

69. Kessler RC, Chiu WT, Demler O, et al. Prevalence, severity, and comorbidity of 12-month DSM-IV disorders in the National Comorbidity Survey Replication. Arch Gen Psychiatry 2005;62:617–27.

70. Wittchen H-U, Frohlich C, Behrendt S, et al. Cannabis use and cannabis use disorders and their relationship to mental disorders: a 10-year prospective-longitudinal community study in adolescents. Drug Alcohol Depend 2007;88(Suppl 1):S60–70.

71. Krueger RF. The structure of common mental disorders. Arch Gen Psychiatry 1999;56:921–6.

72. Cox BJ, Clara IP, Enns MW. Posttraumatic stress disorder and the structure of common mental disorders. Depress Anxiety 2002;15:168–71.

73. Vollebergh WAM, Iedema J, Bijl RV, et al. The structure and stability of common mental disorders. The NEMESIS Study. Arch Gen Psychiatry 2001;58:597–603.

74. Slade T, Watson D. The structure of common DSM-IV and ICD-10 mental disorders in the Australian general population. Psychol Med 2006;36:1593–600.

75. Watson D. Rethinking the mood and anxiety disorders: a quantitative hierarchical model for DSM-V. J Abnorm Psychol 2005;114(4):522–36.

76. Krueger RF, Caspi A, Moffitt TE, et al. The structure and stability of common mental disorders (DSM-III-R): a longitudinal-epidemiological study. J Abnorm Psychol 1998;107:216–27.

77. Beesdo K, Höfler M, Gloster AT, et al. The structure of common mental disorders: a replication study in a community sample of adolescents and young adults submitted.

78. Wittchen H-U, Beesdo K, Gloster A. Anxiety disorders: all the same or sufficiently different? Psychiatr Clin North Am, in press.

79. Wittchen H-U, Beesdo K, Gloster AT, et al. The structure of mental disorders reexamined: Is it developmentally stable and robust against additions? Int J Methods Psychiatr Res, in press.

80. Kraemer HC, Kazdin AE, Offord DR, et al. Coming to terms with the terms of risk. Arch Gen Psychiatry 1997;54(4):337–43.

81. Cohen P, Cohen J. The clinician's illusion. Arch Gen Psychiatry 1984;41(12):1178–82.

82. Costello EJ, Mustillo S, Erkanli A, et al. Prevalence and development of psychiatric disorders in childhood and adolescence. Arch Gen Psychiatry 2003;60:837–44.

83. Kringlen E, Torgersen S, Cramer V. A Norwegian psychiatric epidemiological study. Am J Psychiatry 2001;158(7):1091–8.

84. Meyer C, Rumpf H-J, Hapke U, et al. Lebenszeitprävalenz psychischer Störungen in der erwachsenen Allgemeinbevölkerung. Ergebnisse der TACOS-Studie. [Lifetime prevalence of mental disorders in the adult population: findings from the TACOS study]. Nervenarzt 2000;71:535–42.

85. Canino G, Shrout PE, Rubio-Stipec M, et al. The DSM-IV rates of child and adolescent disorders in Puerto Rico. Arch Gen Psychiatry 2004;61:85–93.

86. Vega WA, Kolody B, Aguilar-Gaxiola S, et al. Lifetime prevalence of DSM-III-R psychiatric disorders among urban and rural Mexican Americans in California. Arch Gen Psychiatry 1998;55:771–8.

87. Costello EJ, Compton SN, Keeler G, et al. Relationships between poverty and psychopathology: a natural experiment. JAMA 2003;290(15):2023–9.

88. Merikangas KR, Avenevoli S, Dierker L, et al. Vulnerability factors among children at risk for anxiety disorders. Biol Psychiatry 1999;46(11):1523–35.

89. Lieb R, Wittchen H-U, Höfler M, et al. Parental psychopathology, parenting styles, and the risk for social phobia in offspring: a prospective-longitudinal community study. Arch Gen Psychiatry 2000;57:859–66.

90. Hettema JM, Neale MC, Kendler KS. A review and meta-analysis of the genetic epidemiology of anxiety disorders. Am J Psychiatry 2001;158(10):1568–78.

91. Johnson JG, Cohen P, Kasen S, et al. Parental concordance and offspring risk for anxiety, conduct, depressive, and substance use disorders. Psychopathology 2008;41:124–8.

92. Wittchen H-U, Kessler RC, Pfister H, et al. Why do people with anxiety disorders become depressed? A prospective-longitudinal community study. Acta Psychiatr Scand 2000;102(Suppl 406):14–23.

93. Schreier A, Wittchen HU, Höfler M, et al. Anxiety disorders in mothers and their children: prospective longitudinal community study. Br J Psychiatry 2008;129: 308–9.
94. Lieb R, Isensee B, Höfler M, et al. Parental major depression and the risk of depressive and other mental disorders in offspring: a prospective-longitudinal community study. Arch Gen Psychiatry 2002;59:365–74.
95. Weissman MM, Wickramaratne P, Nomura Y, et al. Offspring of depressed parents: 20 years later. Am J Psychiatry 2006;163:1001–8.
96. Kendler KS, Davis CG, Kessler RC. The familial aggregation of common psychiatric and substance use disorders in the National Comorbidity Survey: a family history study. Br J Psychiatry 1997;170:541–8.
97. Klein DN, Lewinsohn PM, Rohde P, et al. Family study of co-morbidity between major depressive disorder and anxiety disorders. Psychol Med 2003;33:703–14.
98. Moffitt TE, Caspi A, Harrington H, et al. Generalized anxiety disorder and depression: childhood risk factors in a birth cohort followed to age 32. Psychol Med 2007;37:441–52.
99. Knappe S, Lieb R, Beesdo K, et al. The role of parental psychopathology and family environment for social phobia in the first three decades of life. Depress Anxiety 2009;26(4):363–70.
100. Fyer AJ, Mannuzza S, Chapman TF, et al. Specificity in familial aggregation of phobic disorders. Arch Gen Psychiatry 1995;52:564–73.
101. Hettema JM, Prescott CA, Myers JM, et al. The structure of genetic and environmental risk factors for anxiety disorders in men and women. Arch Gen Psychiatry 2005;62:182–9.
102. Scherrer JF, True WR, Xian H, et al. Evidence for genetic influences common and specific to symptoms of generalized anxiety and panic. J Affect Disord 2000;57(1–3):25–35.
103. Kendler KS. Major depression and generalised anxiety disorder. Same genes, (partly) different environments—revisited. Br J Psychiatry 1996;168(suppl 30):68–75.
104. Kendler KS, Neale MC, Kessler RC, et al. Major depression and generalized anxiety disorder: same genes, (partly) different environments? Arch Gen Psychiatry 1992;49:716–22.
105. LeDoux JE. Emotion circuits in the brain. Annu Rev Neurosci 2000;23:155–84.
106. Guyer AE, Lau JYF, McClure-Tone EB, et al. Amygdala and ventrolateral prefrontal cortex function during anticipated peer evaluation in pediatric social anxiety. Arch Gen Psychiatry 2008;65(11):1303–12.
107. McClure EB, Monk CS, Nelson EE, et al. Abnormal attention modulation of fear circuit function in pediatric generalized anxiety disorder. Arch Gen Psychiatry 2007;64(1):97–106.
108. Thomas KM, Drevets WC, Dahl RE, et al. Amygdala response to fearful faces in anxious and depressed children. Arch Gen Psychiatry 2001;58:1057–63.
109. Beesdo K, Lau JYF, Guyer AE, et al. Common and distinct amygdala-function perturbations in depressed vs anxious adolescents. Arch Gen Psychiatry 2009;66(3):275–85.
110. Schwartz C, Wright C, Shin L, et al. Inhibited and uninhibited infants "grown up": adult amygdalar response to novelty. Science 2003;300(5627):1952–3.
111. Pérez-Edgar K, Roberson-Nay R, Hardin M, et al. Attention alters neural responses to evocative faces in behaviorally inhibited adolescents. Neuroimage 2007;35(4):1538–46.
112. McClure E, Adler A, Monk C, et al. fMRI predictors of treatment outcome in pediatric anxiety disorders. Psychopharmacology 2007;191:97–105.

113. Clark LA, Watson D. Tripartite model of anxiety and depression: psychometric evidence and taxonomic implications. J Abnorm Psychol 1991;100(3):316–36.
114. Clark DA, Steer RA, Beck AT. Common and specific dimensions of self-reported anxiety and depression: implications for the cognitive and tripartite models. J Abnorm Psychol 1994;103:645–54.
115. Zinbarg RE, Barlow DH. Structure of anxiety and the anxiety disorders: a hierarchical model. J Abnorm Psychol 1996;105(2):181–93.
116. Brown TA, Chorpita BF, Barlow DH. Structural relationships among dimensions of the DSM-IV anxiety and mood disorders and dimensions of negative affect, positive affect, and autonomic arousal. J Abnorm Psychol 1998;107(2):179–92.
117. Chorpita BF. The tripartite model and dimensions of anxiety and depression: an examination of structure in a large school sample. J Abnorm Child Psychol 2002;30(2):177–90.
118. Mineka S, Watson D, Clark LA. Comorbidity of anxiety and unipolar mood disorders. Annu Rev Psychol 1998;49:377–412.
119. Hettema JM, Neale MC, Myers JM, et al. A population-based twin study of the relationship between neuroticism and internalizing disorders. Am J Psychiatry 2006;163:857–64.
120. Khan AA, Jacobson KC, Gardner CO, et al. Personality and comorbidity of common psychiatric disorders. Br J Psychiatry 2005;186:190–6.
121. Hayward C, Killen JD, Kraemer HC, et al. Predictors of panic attacks in adolescents. J Am Acad Child Adolesc Psychiatry 2000;39(2):207–14.
122. de Graaf R, Bijl RV, Ravelli A, et al. Predictors of first incidence of DSM-III-R psychiatric disorders in the general population: findings from the Netherlands Mental Health Survey and incidence study. Acta Psychiatr Scand 2002;106:303–13.
123. Kagan J. Temperamental contributions to social behavior. Am Psychol 1989; 44(4):668–74.
124. Robinson JL, Kagan J, Reznick JS, et al. The heritability of inhibited and uninhibited behavior: a twin study. Dev Psychol 1992;28:1030–7.
125. Smoller JW, Rosenbaum JF, Biederman J, et al. Association of a genetic marker at the corticotropin-releasing hormone locus with behavioral inhibition. Biol Psychiatry 2003;54(12):1376–81.
126. Biederman J, Hirshfeld-Becker DR, Rosenbaum JF, et al. Further evidence of association between behavioral inhibition and social anxiety in children. Am J Psychiatry 2001;158(10):1673–9.
127. Johnson SL, Turner RJ, Iwata N. BIS/BAS levels and psychiatric disorder: an epidemiological study. J Psychopathol Behav Assess 2003;25(1):25–36.
128. Caspi A, Moffitt TE, Newman DL, et al. Behavioral observations at age 3 years predict adult psychiatric disorders. Arch Gen Psychiatry 1996;53:1033–9.
129. Rohrbacher H, Hoyer J, Beesdo K, et al. Psychometric properties of the Retrospective Self Report of Inhibition (RSRI) in a representative German sample. Submitted to IJMPR in February 2007. Int J Methods Psychiatr Res 2008;17(2):80–8.
130. Hayward C, Killen JD, Kraemer HC, et al. Linking self-reported childhood behavioral inhibition to adolescent social phobia. J Am Acad Child Adolesc Psychiatry 1998;37:1308–16.
131. Mick MA, Telch MJ. Social anxiety and history of behavioral inhibition in young adults. J Anxiety Disord 1998;12(1):1–20.
132. Schwartz CE, Snidman N, Kagan J. Adolescent social anxiety as an outcome of inhibited temperament in childhood. J Am Acad Child Adolesc Psychiatry 1999; 38(8):1008–15.

133. Rapee RM. Potential role of childrearing practices in the development of anxiety and depression. Clin Psychol Rev 1997;17(1):47–67.
134. Kendler KS, Myers J, Prescott CA. Parenting and adult mood, anxiety and substance use disorders in female twins: an epidemiological, multi-informant, retrospective study. Psychol Med 2000;30:281–94.
135. Rueter MA, Scaramella L, Wallace LE, et al. First onset of depressive or anxiety disorders predicted by the longitudinal course of internalizing symptoms and parent-adolescent disagreements. Arch Gen Psychiatry 1999;56:726–32.
136. Wood JJ, McLeod BD, Sigman M, et al. Parenting and childhood anxiety: theory, empirical findings, and future directions. J Child Psychol Psychiatry 2003;44: 134–51.
137. Pine DS, Klein RG. Anxiety disorders. In: Rutter M, Bishop D, Pine DS, Scott S, Stevenson J, Taylor E, Thapar A, editors. Rutter's child and adolescent psychiatry. 5th edition. Oxford: Blackwell Publishing; 2008. p. 628–69.
138. Ollendick TH, Vasey MW, King NJ, et al. Operant conditioning influences in childhood anxiety. The developmental psychopathology of anxiety. New York: Oxford University Press; 2001. p. 231–52.
139. Muris P, Steerneman P, Merckelbach H, et al. The role of parental fearfulness and modeling in children. Behav Res Ther 1996;34(3):265–8.
140. Gerull F, Rapee RM. Mother knows best: effects of maternal modelling on the acquisition of fear and avoidance behavior in toddlers. Behav Res Ther 2002; 40:279–87.
141. Bögels SM, van Dongen L, Muris PU. Family influences on dysfunctional thinking in anxious children. Infant Child Dev 2003;12(3):243–52.
142. de Rosnay M, Cooper PJ, Tsigaras N, et al. Transmission of social anxiety from mother to infant: an experimental study using a social referencing paradigm. Behav Res Ther 2006;44:1165–75.
143. Rutter M. The interplay of nature, nurture, and development influences. Arch Gen Psychiatry 2002;59:996–1000.
144. Kessler RC, Davis CG, Kendler KS. Childhood adversity and adult psychiatric disorder in the US National Comorbidity Survey. Psychol Med 1997;27: 1101–19.
145. Bijl RV, Ravelli A, Van Zessen G. Prevalence of psychiatric disorder in the general population: results of the Netherlands Mental Health Survey and Incidence Study (NEMESIS). Soc Psychiatry Psychiatr Epidemiol 1998;33:587–95.
146. Fergusson DM, Horwood J, Lynskey MT. Childhood sexual abuse and psychiatric disorder in young adulthood. II. Psychiatric outcomes of childhood sexual abuse. J Am Acad Child Adolesc Psychiatry 1996;35(10):1365–74.
147. Dinwiddie S, Heath AC, Dunne MP, et al. Early sexual abuse and lifetime psychopathology: a co-twin-control study. Psychol Med 2000;30:41–52.
148. MacMillan HL, Fleming JE, Streiner DL, et al. Childhood abuse and lifetime psychopathology in a community sample. Am J Psychiatry 2001;158(11): 1878–83.
149. Pine DS, Cohen P, Johnson J, et al. Adolescent life events as predictors of adult depression. J Affect Disord 2002;68:49–57.
150. Friis RH, Wittchen H-U, Pfister H, et al. Life events and changes in the course of depression in young adults. Eur Psychiatry 2002;17(5):241–53.
151. Perkonigg A, Kessler RC, Storz S, et al. Traumatic events and post-traumatic stress disorder in the community: prevalence, risk factors and comorbidity. Acta Psychiatr Scand 2000;101(1):46–59.

152. Finlay-Jones R, Brown GW. Types of stressful life event and the onset of anxiety and depressive disorders. Psychol Med 1981;11:803–15.
153. Kendler KS, Neale MC, Kessler RC, et al. Childhood parental loss and adult psychopathology in women—a twin study perspective. Arch Gen Psychiatry 1992;49:109–16.
154. Kendler KS, Karkowski LM, Prescott CA. Stressful life events and major depression: risk period, long-term contextual threat, and diagnostic specificity. J Nerv Ment Dis 1998;186(11):661–9.
155. Kendler KS, Hettema JM, Butera F, et al. Life event dimensions of loss, humiliation, entrapment, and danger in the prediction of onsets of major depression and generalized anxiety. Arch Gen Psychiatry 2003;60:789–96.
156. Leonardo ED, Hen R. Anxiety as developmental disorder. Neuropsychopharmacology 2008;33:134–40.
157. Lau JYF, Pine DS. Elucidating risk mechanisms of gene-environment interactions on pediatric anxiety: integrating findings from neuroscience. Eur Arch Psychiatry Clin Neurosci 2008;258:97–106.
158. Rutter M, Moffit TE, Caspi A. Gene-environment interplay and psychopathology: multiple varieties but real effects. J Child Psychol Psychiatry 2006;47(3):226–61.
159. Andrews G, Goldberg DP, Krueger RF, et al. Exploring the feasibility of a meta-structure for DSM-V and ICD-11: could it improve utility and validity? Psychol Med, in press.

First-line Treatment: A Critical Appraisal of Cognitive Behavioral Therapy Developments and Alternatives

Joanna J. Arch, PhD[a],*, Michelle G. Craske, PhD[a,b]

KEYWORDS

- Cognitive behavioral therapy • Anxiety disorders • Exposure
- Mindfulness • Efficacy

Behavioral and cognitive behavioral therapies (CBT) introduced time-limited, relatively effective treatments for anxiety disorders. As a result of ease and efficacy of delivery, CBT developed into the dominant empirically validated therapy for anxiety disorders. This article presents a brief, up-to-date assessment of the successes and challenges of CBT for anxiety disorders. We present a definition of CBT, discuss treatment components, recommendations, and contraindications, review treatment efficacy, and consider multiple remaining challenges, including attrition, long-term follow-up, co-occurring disorders, active treatment comparisons, mediators of change, and broader implementation. We also integrate recent developments in CBT and alternative therapies, including the new science of exposure, unified treatment protocols, and mindfulness and acceptance-based treatments.

COGNITIVE BEHAVIORAL THERAPY DEFINED

Craske[1] defines CBT as follows:

> CBT is an amalgam of behavioral and cognitive interventions... guided by the principles of applied science... The behavioral interventions aim to decrease maladaptive behaviors and increase adaptive ones by modifying their antecedents and consequences and by behavioral practices that result in new learning. The

[a] Department of Psychology, University of California Los Angeles, 1285 Franz Hall, Los Angeles, CA 90095 1563, USA
[b] Department of Psychiatry and Biobehavioral Sciences, University of California Los Angeles, 760 Westwood Plaza, Los Angeles, CA 90095, USA
* Corresponding author.
E-mail address: jarch@ucla.edu (J.J. Arch).

Psychiatr Clin N Am 32 (2009) 525–547
doi:10.1016/j.psc.2009.05.001
0193-953X/09/$ – see front matter © 2009 Elsevier Inc. All rights reserved.

psych.theclinics.com

cognitive interventions aim to modify maladaptive cognitions, self-statements or beliefs… The hallmark features of CBT are problem-focused intervention strategies that are derived from learning theory [as well as] cognitive theory principles…

Therefore, cognitive and behavioral therapies for anxiety disorders aim to help clients reduce distress by changing cognitive and behavioral responses.[2,3] The treatment components of CBT for anxiety disorders vary by the specific intervention but include various combinations of the following: psychoeducation about the nature of fear and anxiety, self-monitoring of symptoms, somatic exercises, cognitive restructuring (eg, logical empiricism and disconfirmation), imaginal and in vivo exposure to feared stimuli while weaning from safety signals, and relapse prevention.

What are the Active and Salient Components of Psychological Interventions for Cognitive Behavioral Therapy?

A functional analysis usually initiates the treatment, establishing the topography of the problem behaviors, emotions, and cognitions, as well as their functional relationships with each other. The aim is to identify the factors that may cause, contribute to, or exacerbate a particular problem. This analysis includes a consideration of the antecedents and consequences of behavior, the stimuli that are eliciting cognitive, emotional, and behavioral conditional responses, and the cognitions that are contributing to the emotions and behaviors. The effect of environmental and cultural contexts on these relationships is evaluated as well. The functional analysis then guides the treatment approach.

Self-monitoring emphasizes the importance of a personal scientist model of learning to observe one's own reactions. Clients are trained to use objective terms and anchors rather than affective-laden terms. For example, clients who have panic disorder are trained to record the intensity of their symptoms on scales of 0 to 10 points instead of using a general description of how "bad" the panic attack felt. The objectivity of recording is assumed to enhance its effectiveness. Then, clients are taught what, when, where, and how to record symptoms. Various types of recording exist, but the most common include event recording (ie, whether an event occurs during a period of recording; that is, did a panic attack occur during a period 2 weeks before treatment) and frequency recording (ie, recording every event during the period of recording, for example every panic attack during the day). There rarely are contraindications to self-monitoring, although the method of monitoring often is modified to suit particular needs and to offset potential pitfalls. For example, the person who has obsessive-compulsive tendencies may benefit from limit setting or tightly abbreviated forms of self-monitoring. Occasionally, anxiety can worsen when it is monitored, although continued monitoring is encouraged to habituate the response.

The goal of psychoeducation is to provide basic information about fear and anxiety, to correct misconceptions about fear and anxiety, and to provide a treatment rationale. Psychoeducation aims to develop an objective and "normalcy-based" understanding to replace anxiety-producing conceptualizations (eg, "I am weird"). Psychoeducation is particularly helpful when clients have specific misappraisals of anxiety symptoms, as often is the case in panic disorder (eg, a racing heart during a panic attack is presumed to lead to a heart attack), posttraumatic stress disorder (PTSD) (eg, flashbacks are viewed as evidence of going crazy), and obsessive-compulsive disorder (OCD) (eg, thoughts about causing harm to others are seen as indicative of risk for actual harm). Psychoeducation is contraindicated when it becomes a safety signal (eg, when a patient carries bibliotherapy at all times to ward off anxiety). As with self-monitoring, psychoeducation sometimes can increase anxiety, although continued exposure to the informational material (albeit perhaps at a slower pace) generally is recommended.

Somatic techniques include progressive muscle relaxation, in its condensed form of 8 to 15 sessions as standardized by Bernstein and Borkovec[4] rather than the lengthy training (30–50 sessions) originally developed by Jacobson.[5] Progressive muscle relaxation training involves tensing and relaxing major muscle groups in progression, followed by deepening relaxation through slow breathing and/or imagery. In systematic desensitization, relaxation is used to counter and inhibit anxiety induced by images of anxiety-provoking scenes.[6] In applied relaxation, relaxation is used as a coping tool when facing anxiety-producing situations. Occasionally, negative reactions can be produced by relaxation, such as relaxation-induced anxiety,[7] which involves intrusive thoughts, fears of losing control, and the experience of unusual and therefore anxiety-producing bodily sensations (such as depersonalization). These negative reactions need not be a contraindication to continued relaxation: discussion of the processes and continued exposure to relaxation and its associated states can be an effective tool for managing relaxation-induced anxiety. Another somatic technique is breathing retraining, which involves slow and diaphragmatic breathing exercises combined with a meditative focus of attention on the sensations of breath and/or words to accompany breathing (eg, counting). Typically, breathing retraining is used as a coping tool as anxiety-producing situations are approached (eg, Barlow and colleagues[8]). Breathing retraining and applied relaxation are discouraged when they may become a means of avoiding feared bodily sensations or a safety signal, as may occur in panic disorder (eg, Barlow & Craske[9]).

Cognitive restructuring begins with a discussion of how cognitive errors contribute to the misconstrual of situations and how they in turn lead to behavioral choices that compound distress and confirm misappraisals, contributing to a self-perpetuating cycle. Next, thoughts are recognized as being hypotheses rather than facts and therefore open to questioning and challenge. This approach is the cognitive technique of "distancing" or the ability to view one's thoughts more objectively and to draw a distinction between "I believe" and "I know." Once relevant anxiety-related cognitions are identified, they are categorized into types of errors, including dichotomous thinking, arbitrary inference, overgeneralization, and magnification, among others. The process of categorization or labeling of thoughts is consistent with a personal scientist model and facilitates an objective perspective by which the validity of the thoughts can be evaluated.

CBT therapists use Socratic questioning to help clients make guided discoveries and question their thoughts. Logical empiricism is employed by which rational consideration is given to the evidence that exists, including ignored evidence, historical data, and alternative explanations for events. As an example, persons who fear dying as a result of panic attacks might be asked to think about the number of times they have panicked and what the result has been in each case. Based on the logical empiricism and data from behavioral experimentation, alternative hypotheses are generated that are more evidence based. For example, the person who misappraises panic attacks as being physically dangerous may generate an alternative appraisal that panic attacks represent a definite change in physiology but one that is not harmful. Or, the person who misappraises a frown as a sign of being ridiculed may generate a variety of alternative appraisals for a frown such as habit, fatigue, misunderstanding, concerns external to the conversation, disagreement, and so on. In addition to surface-level appraisals (eg, "that person is frowning at me because I look foolish"), core level beliefs or schemas (eg, "I am not strong enough to withstand further distress" or "I am unlikable") are challenged and ultimately are replaced with less dysfunctional schemas. Cognitive strategies can extend to meta-cognitions, or beliefs about beliefs, as is characteristic of generalized anxiety disorder (GAD) (eg, the belief that worry represents being out of control) or OCD (eg, the belief that obsessions represent craziness).

Cognitive strategies typically are included with other elements of CBT for panic disorder/agoraphobia, PTSD, social anxiety disorder, and GAD. Cognitive strategies generally are considered less central to the treatment for specific phobia and OCD. As noted later, however, the degree to which the addition of cognitive strategies benefits outcomes from behavioral components of CBT is questionable. In addition, issues of cultural sensitivity arise with cognitive restructuring. Cognitive strategies are closely aligned with the European/North American value of rational thinking. As noted by Hays and Imawasa,[10] emphasis on cognition, logic, verbal skills, and rational thinking can undercut the value many cultures place on spirituality. Related is the emphasis of cognitive strategies on reductionist cause-and-effect relations. In contrast, certain Asian cultural beliefs, for example, emphasize balance (or yin and yang), evaluation of systems holistically, and indirect causes for events. For cognitive strategies to be culturally sensitive, therapists must become knowledgeable about clients' cultural values and beliefs; this understanding could be informed through functional analyses.

Exposure is central to CBT for all anxiety disorders. Exposure therapy involves systematic and repeated approach to feared stimuli, both external, such as agoraphobic situations, and internal, such as feared bodily sensations associated with panic attacks, memories of trauma, or obsessions. Exposure can be conducted in imagination, which is most appropriate for stimuli that are difficult to practice confronting in real life (such as air travel) or are inherently imaginal (such as obsessions in OCD or memories of trauma in PTSD). Another modality gaining popularity is virtual reality; a strength of this modality is the control it provides over the parameters of exposure. For example, in the treatment of the fear of public speaking, virtual reality can provide systematic exposure to audiences of different sizes, to different responses from audiences, and so on. Writing exposure is sometimes used for exposure to traumas in the treatment of PTSD. In vivo (real-life) exposure is used commonly for most anxiety disorders. For example, individuals who have social anxiety are exposed to social situations, whereas individuals who have agoraphobia are exposed to situations such as driving or being away from home. Interoceptive exposure involves repeated and systematic exposure to feared bodily sensations, most applicable to panic disorder (eg, repeated hyperventilation to overcome fears of sensations of shortness of breath and paresthesias). Different modalities of exposure often are combined. For example, writing exposure or imaginal exposure to memories of a trauma can be combined with in vivo exposure to situational reminders of the trauma. Similarly, imaginal exposure to obsessions usually is accompanied by in vivo exposure to obsessional triggers, and virtual reality exposure to phobic situations usually is accompanied by instructions to practice exposure in real-life situations as well.

In models of classical conditioning, the aim of exposure is extinction, whereas in cognitive appraisal models the aim is to gather data to disconfirm distorted thinking. Exposure therapy does not teach skills and therefore is not appropriate when anxiety is related directly to skill deficits, as sometimes occurs in social anxiety or phobias of situations that require skills (eg, phobia of swimming for someone who has not learned how to swim). In the case of skills deficit, exposure therapy may be complemented with behavioral rehearsal strategies. Because exposure typically evokes high levels of anxiety at some point, it generally is not recommended when there are complicating medical conditions that make high levels of autonomic arousal potentially harmful (eg, certain arrhythmias or severe asthma), but systematic desensitization may be considered under these conditions. Because of the potential for high levels of anxiety, attrition is a concern, especially if attrition occurs after initial exposure and before the benefits of exposure have taken place. Thus, careful attention is given to the rationale for exposure and readiness for exposure. Another contraindication is when exposure involves situations that actually are harmful (eg, when exposure places the individual at risk of exposure to an abuser).

Figs. 1 and **2** depict ways in which components of CBT are applied to the treatment of panic disorder and GAD. Panic disorder is believed to be maintained by a fear of bodily sensations that signal the possibility of panic, mediated by interoceptive conditioning and/or catastrophic misappraisals of the bodily sensations, as well as by avoidance behaviors that prevent new learning and sustain panic and anxiety over time (see Craske & Barlow, 2007). CBT involves psychoeducation and cognitive therapy for the misappraisals, exposure to feared bodily sensations and avoided situations, and sometimes breathing retraining as a coping tool for dealing with panic. Generalized anxiety disorder is believed to be maintained by cognitive (attention and judgment) biases toward threat-relevant stimuli and the use of worry (and associated tension) and overly cautious behaviors as a means to avoid catastrophic images (and associated autonomic arousal) (see Craske & Barlow[11]). CBT involves cognitive therapy to address worry and cognitive biases and relaxation to address tension, as well as imaginal exposure to catastrophic images and exposure to stressful situations while response preventing overly cautious behaviors.

Newer therapies for anxiety disorders include mindfulness and acceptance-based therapies such as acceptance and commitment therapy (ACT).[12] These therapies propose different approaches for dealing with anxiety-related cognition, including cognitive defusion (eg, distancing from the content of fear-based thinking) and mindfulness and acceptance,[13] and are more contextually based. To distinguish between traditional CBT approaches that use cognitive restructuring and aim to change the content of anxious thinking versus newer mindfulness and acceptance-based approaches that do not use cognitive restructuring or aim to change the content of anxious thinking, the former are referred to in this article as "CBT" and the latter as "mindfulness and acceptance-based approaches" or "third-wave" behavioral therapies.[14]

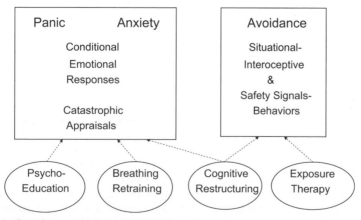

Fig. 1. Panic disorder: maintainers and CBT targets.

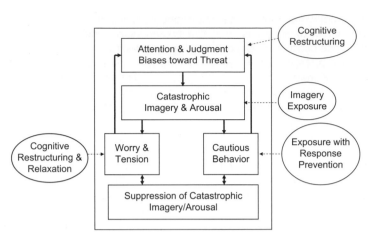

Fig. 2. Generalized anxiety disorder: maintainers and CBT targets.

THE SCIENCE OF EXPOSURE THERAPY

Exposure therapy, a set of procedures involving repeated exposure to feared stimuli, is central to CBT for anxiety disorders. Although originally derived from learning theory, the mechanics of exposure therapy have failed to keep up with advances in the basic science of fear learning and extinction.[15] Instead, contemporary models of exposure therapy have been guided largely by "emotional processing" theory (EPT),[16,17] which emphasizes mechanisms of habituation. EPT purports that the effects of exposure therapy derive from activation of a 'fear structure' and integration of information that is incompatible with it, resulting in the development of a non-fear structure that replaces[16] or competes with[9] the original one. Incompatible information derives first from within-session habituation (WSH), or reduction in fear responding with prolonged exposure to the fear stimulus. WSH is considered a prerequisite for the second piece of incompatible information, which derives from between-session habituation (BSH) over repeated occasions of exposure. BSH is purported to form the basis for long-term learning and to be mediated by changes in "meaning" or lowered probability of harm (ie, risk) and lessened negativity (ie, valence) of the stimulus.

EPT guides clinicians to focus on the initial elevation of fear followed by within- and between-session reductions in fear as signs of treatment success. Although enticing in its face validity, support for the EPT theory has been inconsistent at best.[15] Rather, the evidence suggests that the amount by which fear habituates from the beginning to the end of an exposure practice (WSH) is not a good predictor of overall outcomes, and that evidence for BSH is very mixed.[15]

Thus, the authors have recommended a return to the science of fear learning and extinction to explain the effects of exposure therapy and thereby optimize its implementation.[15] Recent advances indicate that inhibitory learning is central to extinction.[18,19] Within a Pavlovian conditioning approach, inhibitory learning means that the original conditioned stimulus-unconditioned stimulus (CS-US) association learned during fear conditioning is not erased during extinction but rather is left intact as a new, secondary learning about the CS-US develops.[20] By implication, the original association between a conditional stimulus and aversive event is not erased through exposure therapy, but rather a new inhibitory association is developed. Basic research by Bouton[20] indicates that context plays a very important role in determining which set of associations is evoked. If the previously feared stimulus is encountered in a context that is similar to the context in exposure therapy, then the inhibitory association is more likely to be activated, resulting in minimal fear. If the previously feared stimulus is encountered in a context distinctly different from the context of the exposure therapy, however, then the original excitatory association is more likely to be activated, resulting in more fear. Thus, a change in context is assumed to account, at least partially, for the return of fear that sometimes occurs following exposure therapy.[21] Being exposed to a new negative experience that leads to reinstatement or reacquisition of fear[22] also can lead to a return of fear.

Recognition of the role of inhibitory learning in extinction raises interesting questions about how to enhance exposure therapy. Some innovative strategies are being tested that, in contrast to EPT, do not center on the level of expressed fear and its reduction during exposure.[15] For example, inhibitory associations are formed from mismatches between the expectancy of an aversive event and its absence.[23] Such mismatches are assumed to be enhanced by the use of multiple excitatory conditioned stimuli during extinction training.[24,25] This process is called "deepened extinction" and is believed to result in superior learning because of the potency of the mismatch with expectancies provided by the presence of more than one conditional stimulus relative to a single conditional stimulus alone. There have been no direct investigations of this topic in clinical samples to date. The concept of deepened extinction is easily translated into exposure therapy, however, and indeed is the method used in the treatment for panic disorder and agoraphobia when interoceptive exposure to feared physiological sensations (eg, elevated heart rate) and in vivo exposure to feared situations (eg, walking through a shopping mall) subsequently are combined (eg, drinking caffeinated substances while walking through a shopping mall).[26] Given the important clinical implications, direct investigation of deepened extinction in clinical samples is needed.

Another interesting development is the use of biological agents to facilitate the consolidation of inhibitory learning during extinction. Fear extinction is dependent on N-methyl-D-aspartic acid (NMDA)-type glutamate receptors (NMDAr) (reviewed in[23]). NMDAr inhibitors block extinction when given systemically or infused directly into the amygdala during extinction training.[27] Furthermore, systemic or intra-amygdala treatments with D-cycloserine (DCS), an agonist at the glycine binding site of the NMDAr, facilitate extinction in rodents, although not completely.[28,29] The results of investigations combining D-cycloserine with exposure therapy for phobias remain somewhat mixed, with several reports of enhancement of exposure therapy and one report of no effects.[30–32] Nonetheless, further evaluation of this intriguing notion that learning throughout exposure therapy can be enhanced by biological agents is warranted.

The majority of neurobiological research on fear learning and extinction has focused on three general structures: the amygdala, the prefrontal cortex (PFC), and the hippocampus (see[33]). The PFC has long been implicated in executive control and decision making (see[34]). Recent work has revealed that certain parts of the PFC (ie, the ventral medial) also are responsible for emotional regulation and, in particular, for the ability to interpret emotional stimuli and change behavior accordingly (see[33]). Given this role, the ventral medial PFC potentially serves as a prime candidate for a fear extinction structure. In support, extinction in non-primates is associated with neuronal activity primarily within the medial PFC.[35] Research with humans similarly shows that changes in the medial PFC occur during extinction.[36] It has been suggested that the PFC exerts inhibitory control over the amygdala at extinction re-test (see[33]). Hence, behavioral methods for enhancing PFC throughout exposure therapy may prove to be a useful direction for future research. Conceivably, when cognitive restructuring does enhance the benefits of exposure therapy alone, it may do so by activating the PFC. Research on optimal ways of activating the PFC through cognitive-verbal means is warranted.

In addition, the effects of exposure therapy are enhanced by the prevention or removal of "safety signals" or "safety behaviors." Common safety signals and behaviors for clients who have anxiety disorder are the presence of another person, therapists, medications, or food or drink.[37] In the experimental literature, safety signals alleviate distress in the short term, but when they are no longer present, the fear returns,[38] an effect that may derive in part from interference with the development of inhibitory associations. In phobic samples, the availability and use of safety signals and behaviors has been shown to be detrimental to exposure therapy,[39] whereas instructions to refrain from using safety behaviors improved outcomes.[40]

Finally, attention has been given recently to ways of enhancing the retrieval of new inhibitory associations once exposure therapy is completed. One possibility is to conduct exposure therapy in as many contexts as possible (eg,[41]). Another is to provide retrieval cues that remind clients, when they are outside the therapy context, of the new learning that took place in the therapy context[42] or at least to recommend to clients that they actively try to remember what they learned when in the therapy context;[43] both approaches have been shown to offset renewal effects.

EMPIRICAL EFFICACY

Meta-analyses of CBT for anxiety disorders provide a snapshot of efficacy findings across a large number of treatment studies. Meta-analyses use effect-size statistics to capture the magnitude of the differences between disparate types of treatment (or treatment and controls); frequently, treatment differences are measured with Cohen's d effect size (ES) statistics. A Cohen's d effect size of 0.80 or higher is considered a large effect size or difference between groups, 0.50 represents a medium or moderate effect size, and 0.20 represents a small effect size.[44] In translating a moderate effect size to the percentage of clients showing improvement, Heimberg and colleagues[45] demonstrated clinically significant improvement in two thirds of socially anxious patients in a CBT group, versus one third of patients in the active control group.

A review of meta-analyses of randomized, controlled trials by Butler and colleagues[46] demonstrated large effect sizes for CBT in treating a range of anxiety disorders, including panic disorder with or without agoraphobia, GAD, social phobia, and PTSD. Compared with no treatment, wait-list, or placebo controls, the comparison-weighted grand mean effect size of CBT across these anxiety disorders and unipolar depression in adults and children was 0.95 (SD = 0.08) from pre- to posttreatment.[46] These effects are consistent with a second, more recent meta-analysis of CBT for all of the anxiety disorders (with the exception of specific phobia);[47] CBT was more effective than no treatment or "expectancy control" (pill placebo, attentional placebo, nonspecific therapy) conditions across all anxiety disorders. For panic disorder, a meta-analysis by Gould and colleagues[48] found that CBT yielded an effect size of 0.68, particularly when it included interoceptive exposure (effect size = 0.88), that was higher than the effect size for pharmacotherapy (0.47) or combined CBT and pharmacotherapy (0.56). More impressively, CBT showed no slippage of gains at follow-up (usually at 6 months posttreatment, effect size = 0.06), compared with pharmacotherapy (effect size = −0.46) and demonstrated lower attrition rates (6% in CBT versus 20% in pharmacotherapy and 22% in combined treatment). For the treatment of GAD, a carefully conducted meta-analysis by Mitte[49] found that CBT was superior to no treatment (effect size = 0.82) and to medication and therapy placebo (effect size = 0.57), with persistence of effects through the 6-month follow-up.[50] Comparisons of CBT and pharmacotherapy for GAD depended on methodology but found largely equivalent results; however, CBT had significantly lower dropout rates (9%) than pharmacotherapy (~25%), suggesting it was better tolerated.[49] For the treatment of OCD, CBT conferred significant benefits from pre- to posttreatment (effect size = 1.30 to 1.86), and benefits endured at 6-month and 1-year follow-up.[51] CBT for OCD was equivalent in effectiveness to exposure and response prevention, a behavioral therapy often considered the treatment of choice.[52] Replicating the results of a previous meta-analysis,[53] a meta-analysis by Gould and colleagues[54] for social anxiety disorder showed equivalent pre- to posttreatment effects for CBT (effect size = 0.74) and pharmacotherapy (effect size = 0.62). A larger meta-analysis on social anxiety disorder[55] found similar effect sizes for exposure therapy (1.08–3.47) and exposure plus cognitive therapy (0.84–1.80), relative to attention control (1.08–1.24) and pill placebo (0.66–0.81) and showed that the effects of exposure or exposure plus cognitive restructuring were maintained from pretreatment to 6-month follow-up (effect sizes = 1.31 and 0.95, respectively).

For PTSD, a large meta-analysis of CBT and behavioral therapies[56] found that by posttreatment follow-up, 67% of patients who completed treatment no longer met criteria for PTSD, whereas 56% of patients who entered treatment (ie, including drop-outs) no longer met criteria for PTSD. CBT and behavioral therapy were far more effective than wait-list control (effect size of comparison = 1.11–1.53) or supportive therapy (effect size of comparison = 0.83–1.01) (This meta-analysis included eye movement desensitization and reprocessing [EMDR] and did not find significant differences in pre- and posttreatment effect size among traditional CBT, behavioral therapy (expo-sure), and EMDR.)

Excellent CBT outcomes also have been demonstrated for specific phobias.[2] Even in samples of older adults (age > 60 years), for whom CBT yields somewhat less impres-sive results, a recent meta-analysis indicated that CBT was more effective than wait-list (standard mean effect size difference = −0.44, 95% confidence interval [CI] = −0.84 to −0.04) and active control conditions (Active control treatments were defined as treat-ment as usual or as "any other strategies that provided a contact frequency comparable with ... CBT" (p. 405)) (standard mean effect size difference = −0.51, 95 CI = −0.81 to −0.21).[57] Efficacy extends to efforts at prevention of full-fledged anxiety disorders in youths presenting with subclinical and clinical anxiety symptoms.[58,59]

Notwithstanding its demonstrated efficacy across the anxiety disorders, CBT pres-ents challenges on several fronts, most notably in dropout rates and treatment refusal, limited comparisons with other active treatments, and long-term follow-up.

DROPOUT RATES AND TREATMENT REFUSAL

Estimating the number of treatment-seeking patients who refuse to begin CBT is diffi-cult; few studies describe the relevant data. One study, conducted at an anxiety disor-ders outpatient clinic in a university hospital, reported that nearly one third of a large patient sample referred by general medical practitioners or mental health specialists did not begin CBT.[60] In this sample, pretreatment attrition was related to higher levels of depression, referral by a general practitioner rather than by a mental health specialist, and assignment to group therapy rather than to individual therapy. CBT entry rates may be improved by providing preparatory videos or pamphlets that depict CBT methods, a particularly valuable approach for minority groups.[61]

More studies have reported rates of attrition from ongoing CBT, particularly for panic disorder and social anxiety disorder. The average reported CBT attrition rate in panic disorder treatment is 17% of patients (range, 0–54% attrition), and for GAD the CBT attrition rate is 7% (range, 0–17%),[62] although these rates were derived largely from small trials with fewer than 30 patients. A large, randomized, clinical trial (> 150 patients) comparing CBT versus imipramine for panic disorder reported an attrition rate for CBT alone (defined as non-completion of 11 assigned CBT sessions) of 27%.[63] In the treatment of social anxiety disorder, one study also reported a one-third attrition rate and found that higher baseline levels and expressions of anger were associated with attrition.[64] However, most studies fail to find differences between completers and non-completers in terms of sociodemographics or symptom patterns. Limited power to detect differences likely hinders such comparisons. At least for GAD and panic disorder, the addition of pharmacotherapy to CBT results in higher dropout rates than seen with CBT alone.[46,49,65]

LONG-TERM FOLLOW-UP

CBT results often are maintained over follow-up intervals that extend from 6 to 24 months.[46,47,62] For example, in the review of meta-analyses mentioned earlier, Butler and colleagues[46] reported evidence for the maintenance of treatment gains in GAD, panic disorder, social phobia, and OCD. The long-term effects were particularly impressive for panic disorder: the 1-year follow-up rate of relapse was nearly half that of pharmacotherapy. On the other hand, in a university clinic–based study of patients who had panic disorder, 27% of patients who were panic-free by the end of CBT obtained additional treatment for panic disorder over the 2-year follow-up period.[66] Furthermore, long-term CBT effects tend to diminish in non-university, community-based treatment settings.

Few CBT studies examine follow-up beyond a 2-year period. One of the few such studies contacted patients from largely primary care and community-based randomized, controlled trials of brief CBT for panic disorder, GAD, or PTSD. Two to 14 years after treatment, 34% of patients treated for GAD, 26% of patients treated for panic disorder, and 55% of patients treated for PTSD met criteria for the treated disorder.[67] In addition, 52% of the GAD, 48% of the panic disorder, and 74% of the PTSD patients met the *Diagnostic and Statistical Manual of Mental Disorders-IV* criteria for co-occurring psychiatric disorders, and nearly two thirds sought additional treatment for anxiety during the follow-up interval. Interestingly, this study found no relationship between more intensive therapy and long-term outcomes, although more complex/ severe baseline symptoms predicted poorer long-term outcomes. An earlier study[68] focused on long-term (8–14 years) outcomes from two university-based CBT trials for GAD. The patients in the first trial were healthier (eg, had less chronicity, severity, and complexity of illness and greater social resources) than patients in the second trial; at long-term follow-up, 70% of the patients in the first trial did not meet criteria for any psychiatric disorders, 33% to 48% met criteria for full recovery from GAD, and only 3% sought additional treatment during follow-up. In the second trial, only 37% of the patients did not meet criteria for any disorders, 22% to 39% met criteria for full recovery from GAD, and 23% sought additional treatment during follow-up. Treatment with CBT resulted in lower overall psychiatric symptoms and utilization of additional treatment than the combined non-CBT conditions, although there were no differences in diagnostic status (Non-CBT conditions included medication or placebo in Trial 1 and analytic therapy in Trial 2; however, comparisons with individual non-CBT conditions were not made.) The disparate results of the two trials point to possible predictors of long-term CBT outcomes for GAD that are worthy of further study. More targeted research on extended long-term outcomes for anxiety disorders and the factors related to them, especially in real-world settings (eg, therapist characteristics; patient characteristics; socio-economic context; therapeutic alliance;

treatment setting, duration, and adherence; and complexity of treated disorders) is greatly needed.

CO-OCCURRING DISORDERS

Whether CBT for a targeted anxiety disorder diminishes co-occurring disorders remains an important question. Anxiety disorders have high rates of co-occurrence with other Axis I disorders, particularly other anxiety disorders but also major depressive episode, dysthymia, substance abuse, and somatoform disorders (especially hypochondriasis and somatization disorder).[69,70] Several studies have shown that overall rates of co-occurring disorders decrease immediately following CBT for panic disorder[71–74] and GAD.[75] On the other hand, a rigorous analysis of CBT for panic disorder found that, with the exception of GAD, rates of co-occurring disorders decreased immediately following CBT but had increased to approximately pretreatment rates by 2-year follow-up.[66] Although the reasons for this resurgence are not fully known, it may reflect underlying risk factors, such as high levels of neuroticism and poor emotional regulation skills, that cause vulnerability to a variety of mood and anxiety disorders throughout the life span.[76] Methodologies for improving long-term maintenance of treatment gains for primary and/or co-occurring disorders might include following the acute phase of CBT with telephone-delivered or Internet-based booster sessions, which have been found in at least one study to contribute to long-term outcomes.[77] Simultaneous application of CBT for panic disorder and CBT for co-occurring disorders was not found to benefit outcomes over CBT for panic disorder alone, however.[72]

LIMITED TREATMENT COMPARISONS

Although a number of researchers integrate alternative therapeutic approaches, such as interpersonal or acceptance-based approaches, with more traditional CBT or behavioral approaches,[78,79] few directly compare CBT with another treatment approach. In general, the extant randomized control trial literature compares CBT for anxiety disorders with a limited set of alternative treatments such as wait-list control, pill placebo, attention-control placebo, non-directive supportive therapy, or psychoeducation. Except for comparisons with behavior therapy (as discussed later), the meager comparisons of CBT for anxiety disorders with other active, full-treatment conditions such as interpersonal, psychodynamic, or integrative approaches, limits the understanding of the unique or incremental benefits of CBT relative to other active treatments for anxiety disorders.

COMPONENT ANALYSES OF COGNITIVE BEHAVIORAL THERAPY

Longmore and Worrell[80] reviewed the evidence regarding the relative contributions of cognitive and behavioral strategies to treatment outcomes. They concluded that there was no strong evidence that cognitive approaches produced better results than behavioral approaches (ie, behavioral activation and exposure therapy) alone or that cognitive approaches added to the benefit of behavioral approaches. Similarly, a meta-analysis by Norton and Price[47] found no differences across cognitive therapy, exposure therapy, relaxation, or their combination for anxiety disorders. Even self-reported cognitive appraisals and beliefs are changed to the same degree by cognitive and behavioral methods of intervention (eg,[53,81]). Thus, despite occasional demonstrations of superior outcomes from cognitive-based treatments over behavioral treatment alone, as in the case of a recent trial for social phobia,[82] the findings of no differences are broad and compelling and have led several researchers to conclude that the cognitive restructuring component of CBT is superfluous and not necessary (eg,[83]). Another interpretation is that outcomes from mostly cognitive, behavioral, and somatically oriented CBT interventions do not differ because the interventions share much in common. For example, the discussion of intrusive thoughts in cognitive therapy overlaps with exposure therapy, and exposure to feared situations usually involves discussion of appraisals.[1] Nonetheless, if cognitive and cognitive behavioral therapies stipulate that maladaptive thoughts must be challenged, and behavioral therapy obtains roughly equivalent results without doing so, another pathway may be at work. Weighing the evidence for a cognitive pathway to therapeutic change leads directly to a discussion of treatment mediators.

MEDIATORS OF COGNITIVE BEHAVIORAL THERAPY

The cognitive appraisal model of CBT assumes that the active therapeutic mechanism is a change in dysfunctional assumptions and core beliefs toward a more rational and evidence-based orientation. Mediation can be ascribed only when change in cognition is shown to occur before, and becomes a significant predictor of, change in symptom outcomes; very few studies have met these criteria.

Of the available adequate or close-to-adequate studies, the evidence for cognitive mediation of CBT is mixed. Hofmann[84] found that pre- to posttreatment changes in the cognitive variable of estimated social cost, or the projected catastrophic consequences of inept social behavior, mediated reductions in social anxiety at posttreatment and 6 months later in socially anxious individuals treated with CBT. In addition, Kendall and Treadwell[85] found that changes in anxious self-statements mediated treatment gains in children who had anxiety disorders undergoing CBT. On the other hand, Burns and Spangler[86] found no evidence of a mediational link between dysfunctional attitudes and changes in anxiety and depression among a sizable sample of CBT-treated outpatients ($n = 521$). Similarly, a review of the CBT literature by Longmore and Worrell[80] found limited empirical evidence for cognitive mediation of therapeutic change in CBT; in other words, there was limited evidence that change in automatic thoughts, beliefs, or attributions caused symptom improvements. The lack of robust evidence for cognitive mediation of CBT outcomes may stem partly from the inherent limitations of self-report measurement of cognitive change, given the likely demand characteristics and the questionable degree to which self-report data match ongoing, moment-to-moment thinking.[87] Beyond issues of measurement, however, limitations of the cognitive appraisal model are being recognized increasingly. For example, given that the majority of information processing occurs at subconscious levels, without conscious appraisal, the adequacy of attempts to change conscious appraisals has been questioned (eg,[88]). Obviously, attempts to change conscious appraisals form the heart of CBT's cognitive component. Alternative methods for shifting styles of information processing that do not depend on conscious reappraisals now are being tested as complements to or replacements for CBT. These alternatives include mindfulness and acceptance-based approaches, which have been coined the "third wave" of behavioral therapies.[89]

ACCEPTANCE AND MINDFULNESS-BASED APPROACHES TO TREATMENT

Stemming from growing evidence that cognitive strategies are unnecessary in CBT and from a desire to broaden the focus of change and to adopt contextualistic assumptions about the causes of behavior and function of cognition, clinical researchers have developed a new group of treatments, third-wave behavioral therapies. Third-wave therapies integrate mindfulness and acceptance and provide alternatives to the first-order cognitive change strategies (eg, cognitive restructuring) in CBT. ACT, a third-wave behavioral therapy that has been applied to treat anxiety disorders, uses mindfulness and acceptance-based processes such as cognitive defusion, contact with the present moment, and self as context to shift the patient's relationship to cognition, decrease suppression and avoidance of internal experience (known as "experiential avoidance"), increase psychological flexibility, and, ultimately, promote behavior change in the direction of client's chosen values.[83] ACT derives from a basic theory of human cognition and language known as "Relational Frame Theory"[90] and comprises a general set of treatment strategies for application across the full range of psychopathology, including specialized treatment manuals for anxiety disorders.[13] ACT also stems from behavior analysis, which defines behavior as anything one is doing and argues that behavior can understood only be by analyzing the full context in which it occurs. By implication, all psychological symptoms, both internal and external, are relevant targets for treatment in ACT. The context or function of cognition—that patients understand their thoughts to be true and limit valued behaviors accordingly—is emphasized over the content of cognition. Rather than attempt to change the content of thinking directly, as in CBT, the context and function of cognition are modified in ACT, often by helping patients create distance from the literal content of thinking with cognitive defusion (eg, thought content distancing) skills and mindfulness. Mindfulness has been defined as "an open or receptive awareness to what is taking place in the present moment."[91] The related construct of acceptance refers to the quality of "leaning into" and "embracing" rather than judging and suppressing present experience, particularly present internal experience. Acceptance within mindfulness-based treatments is distinguished from acceptance within psychodynamic traditions, which often involves a complex, drawn-out process of acknowledging, analyzing, grieving, and eventually accepting the painful realities and losses in one's past and present to move on to a better future (see[92]). In a mindfulness context, the past is not analyzed, but rather its expressions in the present moment are compassionately acknowledged and accepted.

No randomized trials on ACT for diagnosed anxiety disorders have been published to date, but several published case studies and nonrandomized, baseline control studies outline successful applications of ACT to a variety of anxiety disorders, including social anxiety disorder, OCD, GAD, and PTSD (eg,[93–95]). Although specific anxiety disorders were not diagnosed, another study randomly assigned 101 anxious and depressed patients at a university clinic to ACT or cognitive therapy. Improvements in anxiety, depression, quality of life, and clinician-rated functioning were equivalent across the two treatments.[96] There was some indication that the treatments operated by different pathways, namely, that changes in self-reported avoidance of internal experience, acceptance, and mindful action correlated more with self-reported outcomes in ACT, whereas changes in self-reported observing and describing one's experiences were correlated more with self-reported outcomes in cognitive therapy. Although intriguing, these results should be interpreted cautiously because the temporal precedence for mediation was not established, measures were restricted to self-report scales, and several differences between treatment pathways did not reach full statistical significance.

The degree of difference between ACT and CBT remains a point of debate, however.[97] For example, a recent theoretical analysis[98] concluded that the pathways for ACT and CBT treatment of anxiety disorders may differ, but the overall treatment processes and outcomes seem more similar than distinct. Research using randomized, controlled design is needed to assess ACT for anxiety disorders more carefully, to compare ACT with cognitive therapy and traditional CBT, and to replicate the nascent results described earlier.

Other third-wave mindfulness and acceptance-based interventions have been developed specifically for the treatment of anxiety disorders. For example, Roemer and Orsillo[79] have argued that mindfulness and acceptance may be particularly appropriate for treating future-oriented anxiety, as is characteristic of GAD, that is difficult to dispute by logical argumentation. A pilot study ($n = 16$) of an acceptance-based therapy for GAD demonstrated significant improvements at posttreatment and 3-month follow-up across clinician-rated disorder severity ratings and relevant self-report measures.[99] In addition, others argue that a focus on emotion regulation, emotional avoidance, and/or interpersonal disturbances may prove particularly useful in treating a GAD population.[78,100] For example, Newman and colleagues[101] conducted an open pilot study ($n = 18$) of an integrative CBT therapy that addressed emotional avoidance and interpersonal issues and demonstrated significant improvements at posttreatment and 1-year follow-up.

Finally, interest in Kabat-Zinn's mindfulness-based stress reduction (MBSR),[102] a mindfulness-based intervention without behavioral components, continues to grow. Taught in a group format, MBSR teaches patients multiple mindfulness practices: daily informal mindfulness practices (mindfulness of eating, driving, washing dishes, and other activities), formal sitting meditation (mindfulness of breath), basic Hatha yoga (mindfulness of movement), and a body scan meditation (mindfulness of body). The only randomized, controlled trial to date compared MBSR with CBT group therapy for social anxiety disorder.[103] Results show that both treatments led to significant symptom and mood improvements; however, patients treated with CBT showed significantly higher response and remittance rates and lower scores on clinician- and patient-rated measures of social anxiety. MBSR groups were nearly twice as large as CBT groups, were not led by a mental health professional, and did not include behavioral exposures, factors that may have reduced benefits to this group.

Based on MBSR, Segal and colleagues[104] developed a related treatment known as mindfulness-based cognitive therapy (MBCT), which they successfully applied to reduce relapse/recurrence rates in previously (and frequently) depressed patients.[105,106] One uncontrolled pilot study ($n = 11$) recently applied MBCT to the treatment of GAD,[107] demonstrating significant pre- to posttreatment reductions in anxiety, worry, and depression symptoms. No randomized, controlled trials of MBCT for anxiety disorders have been published to date, however.

In summary, multiple acceptance and mindfulness-based interventions, including ACT, acceptance-based therapy for GAD, MBSR, and MBCT, show initial promise in the treatment of one or more anxiety disorders. Given the popularity of mindfulness and acceptance-based approaches and their growing application to anxiety disorders, additional large, randomized, well-designed studies are essential to expand the understanding of this emerging area.

UNIFIED TREATMENT PROTOCOLS

Another new approach in the treatment of anxiety disorders is the development of unified treatment protocols for use across all the anxiety disorders. Unified treatment protocols are treatment manuals or sets of treatment principles that treat core psychopathological processes common to a broad class of psychiatric disorders, such as anxiety disorders or emotional disorders (eg, anxiety and mood disorders). Barlow and colleagues[108] put forth two rationales to support their unified, CBT-focused treatment protocol for emotional disorders. First, significant co-occurrence among the emotional disorders, mutual response to the same or similar treatments (eg, selective serotonin reuptake inhibitors, CBT) and the response of secondary disorders to treatment of primary disorders suggest common etiologies, risk factors, and treatment pathways among the emotional disorders. Second, the number of treatment manuals for specific emotional disorders has proliferated to such an extent that the dissemination and mastery of extant manuals has grown increasingly burdensome. Integrating decades of scientific evidence against this backdrop, Barlow and colleagues[108] propose three central components for treating emotional disorders: (1) modifying antecedent cognitive appraisals; (2) preventing emotional avoidance; and (3) facilitating opposing action tendencies when the dysregulated emotion arises (ie, encouraging dysregulated patients to behave the opposite way that they feel). The treatment involves standard emotional exposure and mood-induction exercises and tailors these exercises to the particulars of a given presentation. The efficacy of the unified treatment protocol for emotional disorders has not been tested rigorously, although the authors report that several small groups of heterogeneous patients treated with the unified protocol seemed to do as well as or better than disorder-specific treatment groups.[108]

Other researchers have employed unified, also known as "transdiagnostic," treatment protocols in the treatment of mixed anxiety disorder groups. For example, Norton[109] applied a transdiagnostic CBT group treatment within a mixed anxiety disorder sample ($n = 52$), mostly comprising patients who had panic disorder and social anxiety disorder. Patients improved significantly during treatment, demonstrating clinically significant decreases in state anxiety, and improvements did not differ by diagnostic group. Results should be interpreted cautiously, however, because the study was uncontrolled and used only a single outcome measure (eg, state anxiety). A larger study by Erikson and colleagues[110] randomly assigned diagnostically mixed patients who had anxiety disorders ($n = 152$) to a CBT group for (any) anxiety disorders or a wait-list control group. The transdiagnostic group that received CBT evidenced superior outcomes compared to the wait-list control group at posttreatment assessment and 6-month follow-up. In summary, although more research is needed, the preliminary evidence demonstrates initial efficacy for transdiagnostic CBT in mixed anxiety disorder groups, relative to baseline and wait-list control conditions.

As noted earlier, ACT provides a unified set of treatment principles and technologies to apply across diverse psychopathologies. Eifert and Forsyth[13] developed a unified treatment protocol that applies ACT to the treatment of all anxiety disorders. A series of case studies support its effectiveness;[95] randomized, controlled trials have yet to be published.

Potential advantages of unified or transdiagnostic treatment protocols include ease and flexibility of delivery, particularly within treatment groups of diagnostically diverse patients, and adeptness in treating complex, multi-issue patients. Unified protocols have not yet been fully tested against diagnostic-specific protocols, however, and may lack the degree of specificity needed to treat individual anxiety disorders as effectively. Ensuring that unified protocols are at least as effective as, if not more effective than, diagnostic-specific protocols will be an important step in assessing their utility. Nonetheless, the focus on common treatment factors invites researchers to consider shared underlying etiologies and mechanisms of change in the treatment of emotional disorders.

BROADER IMPLEMENTATION

A continuing challenge is the implementation of CBT in real-world settings, such as primary care settings where anxiety disorders are particularly prevalent,[111] costly,[112] and poorly treated,[113] with anxious patients often dissatisfied because of perceived unmet needs.[114] Adapting CBT to these settings requires consideration of several factors, including the limited training in CBT available to therapists and health care providers, limited client motivation, and limited clinic resources.

One option is to provide expert CBT therapists in primary care and other real-world settings (eg,[73]) although this option is costly and unlikely to be sustained over time. Another option is to train local therapists, an approach that becomes especially viable with computerized technology as a way of offsetting training costs.[115] A third option is a computerized system approach the authors developed for supporting delivery of CBT for anxiety disorders by novice clinicians, called "CALM Tools for Living."[116] This CBT approach addresses the four most common anxiety disorders in primary care settings: panic disorder with or without agoraphobia, GAD, social anxiety disorder, and PTSD. In this program, the core elements of CBT are the same across the four anxiety disorders, but other elements are tailored to the features unique to each anxiety disorder through branching mechanisms. Preliminary results indicate that the computerized program is well liked by novice clinicians.[116] The computer program aids them by providing the structure for delivering CBT and helping clinicians remain on target and maintain CBT fidelity. The computer program is designed to help the clinician to guide the patient as opposed to a patient self-directed program.

Another dissemination strategy is self-directed treatment, mostly recently delivered by computer and Internet technology. These programs have been found to be generally acceptable to clients and effective in treating depression and anxiety (eg,[117]) as well as specific anxiety disorders, including panic disorder (eg,[118]) social anxiety disorder,[119] PTSD,[120] and OCD.[121] Solely computerized/Internet treatments are problematic, however, because they are associated with higher rates of dropout or refusal and lower rates of satisfaction with therapy, compared with a live clinician.[122] Computerized programs are more acceptable and more successful when clinician involvement is offered (eg,[123]).

Finally, preparatory techniques and motivational interviewing have the potential to increase attendance and participation in CBT sessions within real-world settings. For example, providing three sessions of motivational interviewing before CBT treatment of anxiety disorders has been shown to enhance treatment compliance and response among patients in a public hospital mental health clinic.[124]

SUMMARY AND FUTURE DIRECTIONS

This article has presented both the challenges and recent developments in CBT and alternative therapies. Numerous research developments are underway, including greater linkage of exposure therapy to basic science and learning theory, more rigorous testing of mindfulness and acceptance-based treatments, distilling CBT approaches into a single set of treatment principles, and bringing CBT fully into primary care and community settings. All represent exciting new directions and/or expansions of classic CBT for anxiety disorders. Several of these developments are founded on a return to basic scientific theory and research and, from this perspective, share common aims. The article has noted the paucity of research on anxiety disorders that directly attempts to prevent posttreatment relapse and/or the re-emergence of co-occurring disorders, an area of burgeoning success in major depression.[104–106] In addition, relatively little is known about the patient, therapist, treatment, or contextual factors associated with CBT refusal and attrition and few interventions aim to prevent these problems. Finally, to conclude on a note of promise, investigating the neural underpinnings of CBT-related improvements may aid in more precisely understanding and targeting the central pathways of therapeutic change in future research on anxiety disorders.

REFERENCES

1. Craske MG. Cognitive-behavioral therapy. APA books, in press.
2. Craske MG. Anxiety disorders: psychological approaches to theory and treatment. Boulder (CO): Westview Press; 1999.
3. Craske MG, Barlow DH. Panic disorder and agoraphobia. In: Barlow DH, editor. Clinical handbook of psychological disorders: a step-by-step treatment manual. 2nd edition. New York: Guilford Press; 1993. p. 1.
4. Bernstein DA, Borkovec TD. Progressive relaxation training: A manual for the helping professions. Champaign (IL): Research Press; 1973.
5. Jacobson F. Progressive muscle relaxation. Chicago, IL: University of Chicago Press; 1938.
6. Wolpe J. Psychotherapy by reciprocal inhibition. Oxford: Stanford University Press; 1958.
7. Heide FJ, Borkovec TD. Relaxation-induced anxiety: Paradoxical anxiety enhancement due to relaxation training. J Consult Clin Psychol 1983;51:171–82.
8. Barlow DH, Craske MG, Cerny JA, Klosko JS. Behavioral treatment of panic disorder. Behav Ther 1989;20:261–82.
9. Barlow DH, Craske MG. Mastery of your anxiety and panic. 4th edition. New York, NY: Oxford Univ Press; 2007.
10. Hays PA, Iwamasa GY. Culturally responsive cognitive-behavioral therapy: Assessment, practice, and supervision. . Washington DC. American Psychological Association; 2006.
11. Craske MG, Barlow DH. Master of your anxiety and worry: Client workbook. 2nd edition. New York, NY: Oxford Univ Press; 2005.
12. Hayes SC, Strosahl KD, Wilson KG. Acceptance and commitment therapy: an experiential approach to behavior change. New York: Guilford Press; 1999.
13. Eifert GH, Forsyth JP. Acceptance and commitment therapy for anxiety disorders. a practitioner's treatment guide to using mindfulness, acceptance, and values-based behavior change strategies. New York: Guilford Press; 2005.
14. Hayes SC, Follette VM, Linehan MM, editors. Mindfulness and acceptance: expanding the cognitive-behavioral tradition. New York: The Guilford Press; 2004.
15. Craske MG, Kircanski K, Zelikowsky M, et al. Optimizing inhibitory learning during exposure therapy. Behav Res Ther 2008;46:5.
16. Foa EB, Kozak MJ. Emotional processing of fear: exposure to corrective information. Psychol Bull 1986;99:20–35.
17. Foa EB, McNally R. Mechanisms of change in exposure therapy. In: Rapee RM, editor. Current controversies in the anxiety disorders. New York: The Guilford Press; 1996. p. 329.
18. Myers KM, Davis M. Mechanisms of fear extinction. Mol Psychiatry 2007;12:120.
19. Rescorla RA, Wagner AR. A theory of Pavlovian conditioning: variations in the effectiveness of reinforcement and nonreinforcement. In: Black AH, Prokasy WF, editors. Classical conditioning II. New York: Appleton-Century-Crofts; 1972. p. 64.
20. Bouton ME. Context, time and memory retrieval in the interference paradigms of Pavlovian learning. Psychol Bull 1993;114:80–99.
21. Craske MG, Mystkowski JL. Exposure therapy and extinction: clinical studies. In: Craske M, Hermans D, Vansteenwegen D, editors. Fear and learning: from basic

processes to clinical implications. Washington, DC: American Psychological Association; 2006.

22. Hermans D, Craske MG, Mineka S, et al. Extinction in human fear conditioning. Biol Psychiatry 2006;60:361–8.

23. Walker DL, Davis M. The role of amygdala glutamate receptors in fear learning, fear- potentiated startle, and extinction. Pharmacol Biochem Behav 2002;71:379 (Special Issue: Functional role of specific systems within the extended amygdala and hypothalamus).

24. Rescorla RA. Experimental extinction. In: Mowrer RR, Klein SB, editors. Handbook of contemporary learning theories. Mahwah (NJ): Lawrence Erlbaum Associates; 2001. p. 199.

25. Rescorla RA. Extinction can be enhanced by a concurrent excitor. J Exp Psychol Anim Behav Process 2000;26:251.

26. Barlow DH, Craske M. Mastery of your anxiety and panic. Albany (NY): Graywind Publications; 1988.

27. Walker DL, Ressler KJ, Lu KT, et al. Facilitation of conditioned fear extinction by systemic administration or intra-amygdala infusions of D-cycloserine as assessed with fear- potentiated startle in rats. J Neurosci 2002;22:2343.

28. Vervliet B. Learning and memory in conditioned extinction: effects of D-cycloserine. Acta Psychol, in press.

29. Woods AM, Bouton ME. D-cycloserine facilitates extinction but does not eliminate renewal of the conditioned emotional response. Behav Neurosci 2006; 120:1159.

30. Guastella AJ, Dadds MR, Lovibond PF, et al. A randomized controlled trial of the effect of D-cycloserine on exposure therapy for spider fear. J Psychiatr Res 2007;41:466.

31. Hofmann SG, Pollack MH, Otto MW. Augmentation treatment of psychotherapy for anxiety disorders with D-cycloserine. CNS Drug Rev 2006;12:208.

32. Ressler KJ, Rothbaum BO, Tannenbaum L, et al. Cognitive enhancers as adjuncts in psychotherapy: use of D-cycloserine in phobic individuals to facilitate extinction of fear. Arch Gen Psychiatry 2004;61:1136.

33. Sotres-Bayon F, Cain CK, LeDoux JE. Brain mechanisms of fear extinction: historical perspectives on the contribution of prefrontal cortex. Biol Psychiatry 2006;60:329.

34. Stuss DT, Knight RT. Principles of frontal lobe function. New York: Oxford University Press; 2002.

35. Rauch SL, Shin LM, Phelps EA. Neurocircuitry models of posttraumatic stress disorder and extinction: human neuroimaging research—past, present and future. Biol Psychiatry 2006;60:376.

36. Phelps EA. The human amygdale and awareness: interactions between emotion and cognition. In: Gazzaniga MS, editor. The cognitive neurosciences. Cambridge (MA): MIT Press; 2004. p. 1005.

37. Barlow DH. Anxiety and its disorders: the nature and treatment of anxiety and panic. New York: Guilford Press; 1988.

38. Lovibond PF, Davis NR, O'Flaherty AS. Protection from extinction in human fear conditioning. Behav Res Ther 2000;38:967.

39. Sloan T, Telch MJ. The effects of safety-seeking behavior and guided threat reappraisal on fear reduction during exposure: an experimental investigation. Behav Res Ther 2002;40:235.

40. Salkovskis PM. The importance of behaviour in the maintenance of anxiety and panic: a cognitive account. Behav Psychother 1991;19:6.

41. Vansteenwegen D, Vervliet B, Iberico C, et al. The repeated confrontation with videotapes of spiders in multiple contexts attenuates renewal of fear in spider anxious students. Behav Res Ther 2007;46:1169.

42. Collins BN, Brandon TH. Effects of extinction context and retrieval cues on alcohol cue reactivity among nonalcoholic drinkers. J Consult Clin Psychol 2002;70:390.

43. Mystkowski JL, Craske MG, Echiverri AM, et al. Mental reinstatement of context and return of fear in spider phobia. Behav Ther 2006;37:49.

44. Cohen J. A power primer. Psychol Bull 1992;112:155.

45. Heimberg RG, Dodge CS, Hope DA, et al. Cognitive behavioral group treatment for social phobia: comparison with a credible placebo control. Cognit Ther Res 1990;14:1.

46. Butler AC, Chapman JE, Forman EM, et al. The empirical status of cognitive-behavioral therapy: a review of meta-analyses. Clin Psychol Rev 2006; 26:17.

47. Norton PJ, Price EC. A meta-analytic review of adult cognitive-behavioral treatment outcome across the anxiety disorders. J Nerv Ment Dis 2007;195:521.

48. Gould RA, Otto MW, Pollack MH. A meta-analysis of treatment outcome for panic disorder. Clin Psychol Rev 1995;15:819.

49. Mitte K. Meta-analysis of cognitive-behavioral treatments for generalized anxiety disorder: a comparison with pharmacotherapy. Psychol Bull 2005; 131:785.

50. Gould RA, Otto MW, Pollack MH, et al. Cognitive behavioral and pharmacological treatment of generalized anxiety disorder: a preliminary meta-analysis. Behav Ther 1997;28:285.

51. van Balkom AJLM, van Oppen P, Vermeulen AWA, et al. A meta-analysis on the treatment of obsessive compulsive disorder. Clin Psychol Rev 1994;14: 359.

52. Abramowitz JS. Effectiveness of psychological and pharmacological treatments for obsessive-compulsive disorder: a quantitative review. J Consult Clin Psychol 1997;65:44.

53. Feske U, Chambless DL. Cognitive behavioral versus exposure only treatment for social phobia: a meta-analysis. Behav Ther 1995;26:695.

54. Gould RA, Buckminster S, Pollack MH, et al. Cognitive-behavioral and pharmacological treatment for social phobia: a meta-analysis. Clin Psychol Sci Pract 1997;4:291.

55. Fedoroff IC, Taylor S. Psychological and pharmacological treatments of social phobia: a meta-analysis. J Clin Psychopharmacol 2001;21:311.

56. Bradley R, Greene J, Russ E, et al. A multidimensional meta-analysis of psychotherapy for PTSD. Am J Psychiatry 2005;162:214.

57. Hendriks GJ, Oude Voshaar RC, Keijsers GP, et al. Cognitive-behavioural therapy for late-life anxiety disorders: a systematic review and meta-analysis. Acta Psychiatr Scand 2008;117:403.

58. Barrett PM, Duffy AL, Dadds MR, et al. Cognitive-behavioral treatment of anxiety disorders in children: long-term (6-year) follow-up. J Consult Clin Psychol 2001; 69:135.

59. Barrett PM, Turner C. Prevention of anxiety symptoms in primary school children: preliminary results from a universal school-based trial. Br J Clin Psychol 2001; 40:399.

60. Issakidis C, Andrews G. Pretreatment attrition and dropout in an outpatient clinic for anxiety disorders. Acta Psychiatr Scand 2004;109:426.

61. Organista KC. Cognitive-behavioral therapy with Latinos and Latinas. In: Hays PA, Iwamasa GY, editors. Culturally responsive cognitive-behavioral therapy: assessment, practice, and supervision. Washington, DC: American Psychological Association; 2006. p. 73.

62. Haby MM, Donnelly M, Corry J, et al. Cognitive behavioural therapy for depression, panic disorder and generalized anxiety disorder: a meta-regression of factors that may predict outcome. Aust N Z J Psychiatry 2006;40:9.

63. Barlow DH, Gorman JM, Shear MK, et al. Cognitive-behavioral therapy, imipramine, or their combination for panic disorder: a randomized controlled trial. JAMA 2000;283:2529.

64. Erwin BA, Heimberg RG, Schneier FR, et al. Anger experience and expression in social anxiety disorder: pretreatment profile and predictors of attrition and response to cognitive-behavioral treatment. Behav Ther 2003;34:331.

65. Furukawa TA, Watanabe N, Churchill R. Combined psychotherapy plus antidepressants for panic disorder with or without agoraphobia. Cochrane Database Syst Rev 2007;(1):CD004364.

66. Brown TA, Barlow DH. Long-term outcome in cognitive-behavioral treatment of panic disorder: clinical predictors and alternative strategies for assessment. J Consult Clin Psychol 1995;63:754.

67. Durham RC, Chambers JA, Power KG, et al. Long-term outcome of cognitive behaviour therapy clinical trials in central Scotland. Health Technol Assess 2005;9:1.

68. Durham RC, Chambers JA, MacDonald RR, et al. Does cognitive-behavioural therapy influence the long-term outcome of generalized anxiety disorder? An 8–14 year follow-up of two clinical trials. Psychol Med 2003;33:499.

69. Brown TA, Campbell LA, Lehman CL, et al. Current and lifetime comorbidity of the DSM-IV anxiety and mood disorders in a large clinical sample. J Abnorm Psychol 2001;110:585.

70. Kessler RC, Chiu WT, Demler O, et al. Prevalence, severity, and comorbidity of 12-month DSM-IV disorders in the National Comorbidity Survey Replication. Arch Gen Psychiatry 2005;62:617.

71. Brown TA, Antony MM, Barlow DH. Diagnostic comorbidity in panic disorder: effect on treatment outcome and course of comorbid diagnoses following treatment. J Consult Clin Psychol 1995;63:408.

72. Craske MG, Farchione TJ, Allen LB, et al. Cognitive behavioral therapy for panic disorder and comorbidity: more of the same or less of more? Behav Res Ther 2007;45:1095.

73. Roy-Byrne PP, Craske MG, Stein MB, et al. A randomized effectiveness trial of cognitive-behavioral therapy and medication for primary care panic disorder. Arch Gen Psychiatry 2005;62:290.

74. Tsao JC, Mystkowski JL, Zucker BG, et al. Effects of cognitive-behavioral therapy for panic disorder on comorbid conditions: replication and extension. Behav Ther 2002;33:493.

75. Borkovec TD, Abel JL, Newman H. Effects of psychotherapy on comorbid conditions in generalized anxiety disorder. J Consult Clin Psychol 1995;63:479.

76. Craske MG. Origins of phobias and anxiety disorders: why more women than men? Oxford (UK): Elsevier Ltd; 2003.

77. Craske MG, Roy-Byrne P, Stein MB, et al. CBT intensity and outcome for panic disorder in a primary care setting. Behav Ther 2006;37:112.

78. Borkovec TD, Newman MG, Castonguay LG. Cognitive-behavioral therapy for generalized anxiety disorder with integrations from interpersonal and experiential therapies. CNS Spectr 2003;8:382.

79. Roemer L, Orsillo SM. Expanding our conceptualization of and treatment for generalized anxiety disorder: integrating mindfulness/acceptance-based approaches with existing cognitive-behavioral models. Clin Psychol Sci Pract 2002;9:54.
80. Longmore RJ, Worrell M. Do we need to challenge thoughts in cognitive behavioral therapy? Clin Psychol Rev 2007;27:173.
81. Arntz A. Cognitive therapy versus interoceptive exposure as treatment of panic disorder without agoraphobia. Behav Res Ther 2002;40:325.
82. Clark DM, Ehlers A, Hackmann A, et al. Cognitive therapy versus exposure and applied relaxation in social phobia: a randomized controlled trial. J Consult Clin Psychol 2006;74:568.
83. Hayes SC, Luoma JB, Bond FW, et al. Acceptance and commitment therapy: model, processes and outcomes. Behav Res Ther 2006;44·1
84. Hofmann SG. Cognitive mediation of treatment change in social phobia. J Consult Clin Psychol 2004;72:392.
85. Kendall PC, Treadwell KR. The role of self-statements as a mediator in treatment for youth with anxiety. J Consult Clin Psychol 2007;75:380.
86. Burns DD, Spangler DL. Do changes in dysfunctional attitudes mediate changes in depression and anxiety in cognitive behavioral therapy? Behav Ther 2001;32:337.
87. Jarrett R, Vittengl J, Doyle K, et al. Changes in cognitive content during and following cognitive therapy for recurrent depression: substantial and enduring, but not predictive of change in depressive symptoms. J Consult Clin Psychol 2007;75:432.
88. Teasdale JD, Barnard PJ. Affect, cognition, and change: re-modelling depressive thought. In: Essays in cognitive psychology. Hillsdale (NJ): Lawrence Erbaum Associates, Inc.; 1993. p. xv.
89. Hayes SC. Acceptance and commitment therapy and the new behavior therapies: mindfulness, acceptance, and relationship. In: Hayes SC, Follette VM, Linehan MM, editors. Mindfulness and acceptance: expanding the cognitive behavioral tradition. New York: The Guilford Press; 2004. p. 1.
90. Hayes SC, Barnes-Holmes D, Roche B, editors. Relational frame theory: a post-Skinnerian account of human language and cognition. New York: Plenum Press; 2001.
91. Brown KW, Ryan RM, Creswell JD. Mindfulness: theoretical foundations and evidence for its salutary effects. Psychol Inq 2007;18:211.
92. McWilliams N. Psychoanalytic case formulation. New York: Guilford Press; 1999.
93. Dalrymple K, Herbert JD. Acceptance and commitment therapy for generalized social anxiety disorder: a pilot study. Behav Modif 2007;31:543.
94. Twohig MP, Hayes SC, Masuda A. Increasing willingness to experience obsessions: Acceptance and commitment therapy as a treatment for obsessive compulsive disorder. Behavior Therapy 2006;37:3–13.
95. Eifert GH, Forsyth JP, Arch JJ, Espejo E, Keller M, Langer D. Acceptance and commitment therapy for anxiety disorders: Three case studies exemplifying a unified treatment protocol. Cognitive and Behavioral Therapy, in press.
96. Forman EV, Herbert JD, Moitra E, et al. A randomized controlled effectiveness trial of acceptance and commitment therapy and cognitive therapy for anxiety and depression. Behav Modif 2007;31:772.
97. Hayes SC. Climbing our hills: a beginning conversation on the comparison of acceptance and commitment therapy and traditional cognitive behavioral therapy. Clinical Psychology: Science and Practice 2008;15:286.

98. Arch JJ, Craske MG. ACT and CBT for anxiety disorders: different treatments, similar mechanisms? Clinical Psychology: Science and Practice, in press.

99. Roemer L, Orsillo SM. An open trial of an acceptance-based behavior therapy for generalized anxiety disorder. Behav Ther 2007;38:72.

100. Mennin DS, Heimberg RG, Turk CL, et al. Preliminary evidence for an emotion dysregulation model of generalized anxiety disorder. Behav Res Ther 2005;43:1281.

101. Newman MG, Castonguay LG, Borkovec TD, et al. An open trial of integrative therapy for generalized anxiety disorder. Psychother Theor Res Pract Train 2008;45:135 Special Issue: New treatments in psychotherapy.

102. Kabat-Zinn J. Full catastrophe living: using the wisdom of your body and mind to face stress, pain, and illness. New York: Delta; 1990.

103. Koszycki D, Benger M, Shlik J, et al. Randomized trial of a mindfulness-based stress reduction program and cognitive behavior therapy in generalized social anxiety disorder. Behav Res Ther 2007;45:2518.

104. Segal ZV, Williams JM, Teasdale JD. Mindfulness-based cognitive therapy for depression. New York: Guilford Press; 2002.

105. Ma SH, Teasdale JD. Mindfulness-based cognitive therapy for depression: replication and exploration of differential relapse prevention effects. J Consult Clin Psychol 2004;72:31.

106. Teasdale JD, Segal ZV, Williams JM, et al. Prevention of relapse/recurrence in major depression by mindfulness-based cognitive therapy. J Consult Clin Psychol 2000;68:615.

107. Evans S, Ferrando S, Findler M, et al. Mindfulness-based cognitive therapy for generalized anxiety disorder. J Anxiety Disord 2008;22:716.

108. Barlow DH, Allen LB, Choate ML. Toward a unified treatment for emotional disorders. Behav Ther 2004;35:205.

109. Norton PJ. An open trial of a transdiagnostic cognitive-behavioral group therapy for anxiety disorder. Behav Ther 2008;39:242.

110. Erickson DH, Janeck AS, Tallman K. A cognitive-behavioral group for patients with various anxiety disorders. Psychiatr Serv 2007;58:1205.

111. Mergl R, Allgaier A, Seidscheck I, et al. Anxiety & somatoform disorders in primary care: prevalence and recognition. Depress Anxiety 2007;24:185–95.

112. Marcus S, Olfson M, Pincus H, et al. Self-reported anxiety, general medical conditions, and disability bed days. Am J Psychiatry 1997;154:1766.

113. Stein MB, Sherbourne CD, Craske MG, et al. Quality of care for primary care patients with anxiety disorders. Am J Psychiatry 2004;161:2230.

114. Craske MG, Edlund MJ, Sullivan G, et al. Perceived unmet need for mental health treatment and barriers to care among patients with panic disorder. Psychiatr Serv 2005;56:988.

115. Gega L, Norman IJ, Marks IM. Computer-aided vs. tutor-delivered teaching of exposure therapy for phobia/panic: randomized controlled trial with pre-registration nursing students. Int J Nurs Stud 2007;44:397.

116. Craske MG, Rose R, Lang AJ, et-al. Computer-assisted delivery of cognitive behavioral therapy for anxiety disorders in primary care settings. Depress Anxiety, in press.

117. Proudfoot J, Goldberg D, Mann A, et al. Computerized, interactive, multimedial cognitive behavioural program for anxiety and depression in general practice. Psychol Med 2003;33.

118. Carlbring P, Bohman S, Brunt S, et al. Remote treatment of panic disorder: a randomized trial of Internet-based cognitive behavior therapy supplemented with telephone calls. Am J Psychiatry 2006;163:2119–25.

119. Botella C, Hofmann SG, Moscovitch DA. A self-applied, internet-based intervention for fear of public speaking. J Clin Psychol 2004;60:821.
120. Lange A, van de Ven J, Schrieken B, et al. Interapy: treatment of posttraumatic stress through the internet: a controlled trial. J Behav Ther Exp Psychiatry 2001; 32:73.
121. Greist JH, Marks IM, Baer L, et al. Behavior therapy for obsessive-compulsive disorder guided by a computer or by a clinician compared with relaxation as a control. J Clin Psychiatry 2002;63:138.
122. Christensen H, Griffiths K, Jorm A. Delivering interventions for depression using the internet randomized controlled trial. Br Med J 2004;328:265.
123. Spek V, Cuijpers P, Nyklicek I, et al. Internet-based cognitive behavioural therapy for symptoms of depression and anxiety: a meta-analysis. Psychol Med 2007;37:319.
124. Westra HA, Dozois DJA. Preparing clients for cognitive behavioral therapy: a randomized pilot study of motivational interviewing for anxiety. Cognit Ther Res 2006;30:481.

The Neurobiology of Anxiety Disorders: Brain Imaging, Genetics, and Psychoneuroendocrinology

Elizabeth I. Martin, PhD[a],*, Kerry J. Ressler, MD, PhD[b,c],
Elisabeth Binder, MD, PhD[d,e,f], Charles B. Nemeroff, MD, PhD[a]

KEYWORDS

- Amygdala • Generalized anxiety disorder
- Posttraumatic stress disorder • Panic disorder
- Social anxiety disorder • Corticotropin-releasing factor

This work was supported by National Institute of Health (NIH) grants MH-541380, MH-77083, MH-69056, MH-58922, MH-42088, MH071537, and DA-019624; the Doris Duke Clinical Scientist Award, and the Burroughs Wellcome Fund. K.J.R. has received awards and/or funding support from Lundbeck, Burroughs Wellcome Foundation, Pfizer, the National Alliance for Research in Schizophrenia and Depression (NARSAD), the National Institute of Mental Health (NIMH), and the National Institute on Drug Abuse and has a consulting agreement with Tikvah Therapeutics for N-methyl-D-aspartic acid–based therapeutics. C.B.N currently serves on the scientific advisory boards of American Foundation for Suicide Prevention (AFSP), AstraZeneca, NARSAD, Quintiles, Janssen/Ortho-McNeil, and PharmaNeuroboost. He holds stock/equity in Corcept, Revaax, NovaDel Pharma, CeNeRx, and PharmaNeuroboost. He is on the board of directors of the AFSP, George West Mental Health Foundation, NovaDel Pharma, and Mt. Cook Pharma, Inc. He holds a patent on the method and devices for transdermal delivery of lithium (US 6,375,990 B1) and the method for estimating serotonin and norepinephrine transporter occupancy after drug treatment using patient or animal serum (provisional filing April, 2001). In the past year, he also served on the Scientific Advisory Board for Forest Laboratories, received grant support from the NIMH, NARSAD, and AFSP, and served on the Board of Directors of the American Psychiatric Institute for Research and Education. E.B. is co-inventor on the following patent applications: FKBP5: a novel target for antidepressant therapy, international publication number: WO 2005/054500; and Polymorphisms in ABCB1 associated with a lack of clinical response to medicaments, international application number: PCT/EP2005/005194. She receives grant support from NARSAD and the Doris Duke Charitable Foundation. In the past 2 years, she has received grant support from Pfizer Pharmaceuticals (Young Investigator award) and GlaxoSmithKline.

[a] Laboratory of Neuropsychopharmacology, Department of Psychiatry and Behavioral Sciences, Emory University, Atlanta, GA, USA
[b] Howard Hughes Medical Institute, Chevy Chase, MD, USA
[c] Department of Psychiatry and Behavioral Sciences, Yerkes Research Center, Emory University, Atlanta, GA, USA
[d] Max-Planck Institute of Psychiatry, Munich, Germany
[e] Department of Psychiatry and Behavioral Sciences, Emory University School of Medicine, Atlanta, GA, USA
[f] Department of Human Genetics, Emory University School of Medicine, Atlanta, GA, USA
* Corresponding author.
E-mail address: eimarti@emory.edu (E.I. Martin).

Psychiatr Clin N Am 32 (2009) 549–575
doi:10.1016/j.psc.2009.05.004
psych.theclinics.com

INTRODUCTION TO EMOTIONAL PROCESSING

Mood and anxiety disorders are characterized by a variety of neuroendocrine, neuro-transmitter, and neuroanatomical disruptions. Identifying the most functionally relevant differences is complicated by the high degree of interconnectivity between neurotransmitter- and neuropeptide-containing circuits in limbic, brain stem, and higher cortical brain areas. Furthermore, a primary alteration in brain structure or function or in neurotransmitter signaling may result from environmental experiences and underlying genetic predisposition; such alterations can increase the risk for psychopathology.

Functional Anatomy

Symptoms of mood and anxiety disorders are thought to result in part from disruption in the balance of activity in the emotional centers of the brain rather than in the higher cognitive centers. The higher cognitive centers of the brain reside in the frontal lobe, the most phylogenetically recent brain region. The prefrontal frontal cortex (PFC) is responsible for executive functions such as planning, decision making, predicting consequences for potential behaviors, and understanding and moderating social behavior. The orbitofrontal cortex (OFC) codes information, controls impulses, and regulates mood. The ventromedial PFC is involved in reward processing[1] and in the visceral response to emotions.[2] In the healthy brain, these frontal cortical regions regulate impulses, emotions, and behavior via inhibitory top-down control of emotional-processing structures (eg,[3]).

The emotional-processing brain structures historically are referred to as the "limbic system" (**Fig. 1**). The limbic cortex is part of the phylogenetically ancient cortex. It includes the insular cortex and cingulate cortex. The limbic cortex integrates the sensory, affective, and cognitive components of pain and processes information regarding the internal bodily state.[4,5] The hippocampus is another limbic system structure; it has tonic inhibitory control over the hypothalamic stress-response system and plays a role in negative feedback for the hypothalamic–pituitary–adrenal (HPA) axis. Hippocampal volume and neurogenesis (growth of new cells) in this structure have been implicated in stress sensitivity and resiliency in relationship to mood and anxiety disorders. An evolutionarily ancient limbic system structure, the amygdala, processes emotionally salient external stimuli and initiates the appropriate behavioral response. The amygdala is responsible for the expression of fear and aggression as well as species-specific defensive behavior, and it plays a role in the formation and retrieval of emotional and fear-related memories. (**Fig. 2** depicts the amygdala's involvement in fear circuitry). The central nucleus of the amygdala (CeA) is heavily interconnected with cortical regions including the limbic cortex. It also receives input from the hippocampus, thalamus, and hypothalamus.

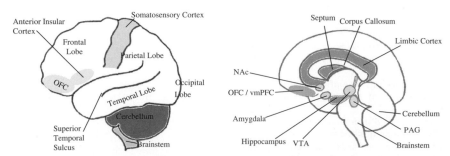

Fig. 1. The limbic system. (*A*) Lateral view of cortex. (*B*) Sagittal view of slice through midline. NAc, nucleus accumbens; OFC, orbital frontal cortex; PAG, periaqueductal gray; VTA, ventral tegmental area.

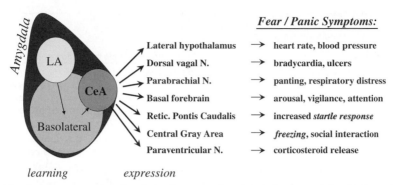

Fig. 2. The fear response is a hardwired process involving the amygdala. (*Adapted from* Davis M. The role of the amygdala in fear and anxiety. Ann Rev Neurosci 1992;15:356; with permission.)

Neuroendocrine and Neurotransmitter Pathways

In addition to the activity of each brain region, it also is important to consider the neurotransmitters providing communication between these regions. Increased activity in emotion-processing brain regions in patients who have an anxiety disorder could result from decreased inhibitory signaling by γ-amino-butyric-acid (GABA) or increased excitatory neurotransmission by glutamate.

Well-documented anxiolytic and antidepressant properties of drugs that act primarily on monoaminergic systems have implicated serotonin (5-hydroxytryptamine, 5-HT), norepinephrine (NE), and dopamine (DA) in the pathogenesis of mood and anxiety disorders. Genes whose products regulate monoaminergic signaling have become a prime area of research in the pathophysiology of mood and anxiety disorders, and they are thought to be critical for the mechanism of action of antidepressant drugs. Monoaminergic regulators include transmitter receptors; vesicular monoamine transporter (vMAT), which packages these neurotransmitters into vesicles; the transmitter-specific reuptake transporters serotonin transporter (SERT), neurotonin transporter, and dopamine transporter; the enzyme monoamine oxidase, which degrades 5-HT, DA, and NE; and the enzyme catecholamine-O-methyltransferase (COMT), which degrades DA and NE.

In the central nervous system, classic neurotransmitters often are packaged and co-released with neuropeptides, many of which are expressed in limbic regions where they can influence stress and emotion circuitry (**Table 1**). The functional implications of these limbic co-localizations have been addressed in numerous reviews (eg,[6–12]). Neuropeptides with particularly strong links to psychopathology include cholecystokinin (CCK), galanin, neuropeptide Y (NPY), vasopressin (AVP), oxytocin, and corticotropin-releasing factor (CRF), among others. CCK is found in the gastrointestinal system and vagus nerve and is located centrally in numerous limbic regions (reviewed in[13]). Galanin is co-localized with monoamines in brainstem nuclei. It influences pain processing and feeding behavior and also regulates neuroendocrine and cardiovascular systems.[14–16] NPY is known for its orexigenic effects and is expressed abundantly in the central nervous system, where it is co-localized with NE in the hypothalamus, hippocampus, and amygdala (reviewed in[13]). Centrally, oxytocin regulates reproductive, maternal, and affiliative behavior.[17,18] Central AVP regulates fluid homeostasis but also can co-localize with oxytocin to influence affiliative behavior[19] or with CRF to regulate the HPA axis.

CRF in parvocellular neurons of the hypothalamic paraventricular nucleus is the primary secretagogue for the HPA axis in response to a threatening stimulus. AVP

Table 1
Neuropeptides in stress and psychopathology

Neuropeptide	Role in Stress-neurobiology	Role in Psychopathology
Cholecystokinin (CCK) (Brawman-Mintzer et al., 1997; Koszycki et al., 2004)	Weak ACTH secretagogue	Anxiogenic Exogenous CCK evokes anxiety; patients who have anxiety disorders are hypersensitive
Galanin (Gal) (Barrera et al., 2005; Karlsson and Holmes, 2006)	Increased by physiological and psychological stress and pain	Depressogenic Galanin antagonists are being developed and possess antidepressant properties
Neuropeptide Y (NPY) (Hashimoto et al., 1996; Heilig, 2004; Martin, 2004; Sajdyk et al., 2004; Hou et al., 2006; Yehuda et al., 2006; Karl and Herzog, 2007)	Increased during stress Endogenous alarm system Stress-induced increase in feeding Modulate behavior to cope with chronic stress.	Antidepressant and anxiolytic in laboratory animals Depressed patients have low plasma concentrations of NPY, especially in first episode Plasma NPY concentration is normalized by antidepressants
Oxytocin (OT) Gimpl and Fahrenholz, 2001)	Weak ACTH secretagogue	Low OT in CSF is associated with depression in women
Vasopressin (AVP) (van Londen et al., 1997; Ma et al., 1999; Wigger et al., 2004; Goekoop et al., 2006)	Increased by stress Moderate ACTH secretagogue synergize to stimulate ACTH production and release	Potentially elevated in depression
Corticotropin-releasing factor	Increased by stress Primary ACTH secretagogue	Elevated in MDD, PD, PTSD; associated with HPA axis hyperactivity in MDD and HPA axis hypoactivity in PTSD

synergizes with CRF in HPA axis activation. In the HPA axis, CRF is released from the paraventricular nucleus and acts on receptors in the anterior pituitary to elicit production and release of adrenocorticotropic hormone (ACTH), which is released systemically and activates production and release of glucocorticoids from the adrenal cortex. In humans, the main stress steroid is cortisol; in rats it is corticosterone. HPA axis activity is regulated by numerous other limbic system structures, including the amygdala, which enhances HPA axis activity, and the hippocampus, which suppresses HPA axis activation (**Fig. 3**).

Standardized endocrine challenge tests to assess HPA axis activity include the dexamethasone suppression test and the CRF stimulation test. In the dexamethasone suppression test, systemic administration of dexamethasone, a synthetic glucocorticoid, decreases (ie, suppresses) plasma ACTH and cortisol concentrations via negative feedback at the level of the pituitary gland. In the CRF stimulation test, intravenously administered CRF (which does not enter the central nervous system) elevates plasma ACTH and cortisol concentrations by stimulating CRF_1 receptors in the anterior pituitary. A combination of the dexamethasone suppression test and the CRF stimulation test, the Dex/CRF test, developed by Holsboer and colleagues, generally is considered to be the most sensitive measure of HPA axis activity.

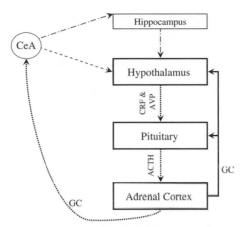

Fig. 3. The HPA axis. Black line- Suppression connection; dotted line- Facilitory connection; dots and dashes line- Suppression connection indirect pathway (via BNST and other limbic regions); and dashed lines- Facilitory connection indirect pathway (via BNST and other limbic regions).

Genetic Contribution to Emotionality

Each anxiety disorder, as well as major depressive disorder (MDD), has both genetic and environmental contributions to vulnerability. In attempts to identify the genetic contribution for psychopathology, the candidate genes have largely been the same across diagnoses. Researchers have tended to concentrate on the genes whose products regulate the HPA axis and monoaminergic signaling. Ongoing research supports the hypothesis that a genetic predisposition may be shared among mood and anxiety disorders, with the individual clinical manifestation being a product of both genetic and environmental influences. In particular, epigenetic factors may permit a remarkably complex range of gene–environment interactions.

Among the limited longitudinal studies available, there is much support for a "developmental dynamic pattern" regarding the influence of genetic factors on individual differences in symptoms of depression and anxiety. In this model, the impact of genes on psychopathology changes so that different developmental stages are associated with a unique pattern of risk factors. This model is in sharp contrast to a "developmental stable model" in which the genetic contribution to psychopathology is mediated by one set of risk factors that do not change with the age of the subject.[20]

Another approach for assessing the impact of genes on risk for psychopathology focuses not on diagnostic class but on more circumscribed phenotypic characteristics. A recent study assessed anxious behavioral characteristics in children between 7 and 9 years of age. They found shared and specific genetic effects on anxiety-related behavior but no single underlying factor, supporting the hypothesis that genes are involved in the general predisposition for anxiety-related behavior and also for specific symptom subtypes.[21]

PANIC DISORDER
Anatomical and Neuroimaging Findings in Panic Disorder

Neuroimaging in patients who have panic disorder (PD) under resting conditions and under anxiety- or panic-provoking conditions has identified neuroanatomical alterations associated with symptom severity or treatment response.

Single-photon emission computed tomography (SPECT) identified lower metabolism in the left inferior parietal lobe and overall decreased bilateral cerebral blood flow (CBF) in patients who had PD as compared with control subjects, and this decrease corresponded with symptom severity.[22] Other studies, however, have demonstrated elevated glucose uptake in the amygdala, hippocampus, thalamus, midbrain, caudal pons, medulla, and cerebellum as measured by positron emission tomography (PET). These elevations normalize after successful pharmacological or behavioral therapy, suggesting that the increased glucose uptake in these regions is state dependent. Patients who had PD had decreased frontal activity bilaterally but increased activity in the right medial and superior frontal lobe in SPECT studies. Interestingly, the CBF asymmetry and shift to the right hemisphere correlated with disorder severity in individual patients (reviewed in[23]).

After administration of the respiratory stimulant doxapram, patients who had PD exhibited a greater decrease in PFC activity but a larger increase in cingulate gyrus and amygdala activity while experiencing panic than control subjects. In patients who had PD who were administered sodium lactate to provoke a panic attack, functional MRI (fMRI) demonstrated elevated CBF in the right OFC and left occipital cortex but decreased CBF in the hippocampus and amygdala (reviewed in[23]). Other studies have shown that patients who do not experience a panic attack after sodium lactate infusion show no differences in CBF compared with control subjects. Interestingly, when a spontaneous panic attack was observed in an fMRI study, the panic was associated with significantly increased activity in the right amygdala.[24]

Imaging analyses of patients who have PD who are in an anxious (but not panicked) state also have provided important data. Upon presentation of threatening words in fMRI studies, the left posterior cingulate and left medial frontal cortex were activated in these patients.[25] Others have shown that presentation of negative emotional words elicits activations in the right amygdala and right hippocampus in patients who have PD.[26] When patients who have PD are presented with anxiety-provoking visual stimuli, they exhibit increased activity in the inferior frontal cortex, hippocampus, anterior cingulate cortex (ACC), posterior cingulate cortex (PCC), and OFC.[27] Compared with healthy control subjects, patients who had PD exhibited less activation in the ACC and amygdala when shown pictures of angry faces. These latter results were interpreted as a blunted response caused by chronic hyperactivity in these circuits in patients who had PD.[28]

Neuroendocrine and Neurotransmitter Signaling in Panic Disorder

Amino acid neurotransmitters

Decreased inhibitory signaling has been hypothesized to play an important pathophysiological role in PD. In drug-free patients who had PD, increased benzodiazepine binding in the temporal cortex and right lateral frontal gyrus[29] but decreased binding in the left hippocampus[30,31] has been observed. In patients who have PD and comorbid MDD treated with antidepressant medications, benzodiazepine binding was decreased in the lateral temporal lobes, left medial inferior temporal lobe, and bilateral OFC. Binding in the insular cortex bilaterally was negatively correlated with panic severity and with comorbid depression.[32]

Magnetic resonance spectroscopy (MRS) has demonstrated decreased GABA concentrations in the occipital cortex,[33] ACC, and basal ganglia[34] in patients who have PD compared with control subjects. Although there is no evidence for differences in plasma or cerebrospinal fluid (CSF) GABA concentrations in patients who have PD,[33] low baseline CSF GABA concentrations did correlate with a poor therapeutic response to the triazolobenzodiazepine alprazolam or the tricyclic antidepressant imipramine. Interestingly, patients who have PD and who have a family history of mood and anxiety disorders exhibit decreased cortical GABA concentrations (reviewed in[35]).

Elevated excitatory glutamatergic signaling is associated with panicogenicity, and drugs that reduce glutamate availability are hypothesized to possess anxiolytic properties. For example, LY354740, an agonist on presynaptic metabotropic glutamate receptors (mGluR II), leads to decreased release of glutamate. This drug decreases anxiety-like behavior in the fear-potentiated startle paradigm in experimental animals.[36] LY354740 and other presynaptic metabotropic glutamate agonists also exert neuroprotective effects. In human studies, LY354740 and related drugs decrease subjective anxiety in a conditioned-fear paradigm in healthy volunteer subjects. In patients who have PD, mGluR II agonists are protective against panicogenic agents such as carbon dioxide inhalation (reviewed in[37]).

Monoamines

Monoaminergic drugs, including tricyclic antidepressants and selective serotonin-reuptake inhibitors (SSRIs), are effective in the treatment of PD. Two SSRIs, fluvoxamine and paroxetine, had a more rapid onset of action and a better therapeutic response on PD symptoms than achieved with cognitive behavioral therapy (CBT) (reviewed in[38]). The dose of paroxetine needed to treat PD optimally is higher than that required for MDD, suggesting that the mechanism by which SSRIs reduce panic symptoms may be distinct from their mechanism of antidepressant action.[39] Patients who have PD exhibit an increased anxiogenic response to administration of the $5\text{-}HT_{2c}/5\text{-}HT_3$ agonist meta-chlorophenylpiperazine (mCPP).[40] In PET studies, $5HT_{1A}$ receptor binding is decreased in the cingulate cortex and raphe nucleus of patients who have PD. SPECT studies have revealed decreased SERT binding in the midbrain, bilateral temporal lobe, and thalamus. The magnitude of the decrease correlates with symptom severity and also normalizes in patients who have PD in remission (reviewed in[35]). Together, these data support a role for serotonergic circuits in the pathogenesis of PD.

Noradrenergic involvement in PD is evidenced by challenge with the $\alpha2$ antagonist yohimbine. Yohimbine-elicited panic-like anxiety in patients who have PD is associated with elevated cardiovascular activity and increased serum NE concentrations. There is some evidence that the $\alpha2$ agonist clonidine has an anxiolytic effect. Patients who have anxiety disorders, including PD, often exhibit a blunted growth hormone response to clonidine administration, suggesting that presynaptic NE autoreceptors are supersensitive (reviewed in[35]). Overall, these data suggest that patients who have PD have alterations in NE circuits, and this system therefore may represent a target for novel treatment development.

Neuropeptides

Although CCK is a well-known panic-inducing agent even in healthy volunteers, few studies have specifically addressed the role of CCK in panic disorder. Chronic imipramine treatment decreases the acute anxiety-inducing effects of CCK, but this finding does not speak to a role for endogenous CCK systems in PD (reviewed in[13]).

A recent study also identified an association between galanin and symptom severity in female patients who had PD but had no effect on risk for PD. The associated single-nucleotide polymorphisms (SNPs) were within CpG dinucleotides of the galanin promoter, suggesting that epigenetic factors could explain the influence of galanin on PD severity.[41]

Corticotropin-releasing factor and the hypothalamic-pituitary-adrenal axis

Patients who have PD have been reported to exhibit increased baseline plasma cortisol concentration, which is positively correlated with the risk for a panic attack after lactate administration. These data suggest that elevated baseline plasma cortisol represents a state of anticipatory anxiety, but not panic itself. The underlying biology of elevated basal cortisol concentrations may be related to increases in CRF concentrations in the CSF of patients who have PD (reviewed in[35]).

The HPA axis in patients who have PD has been assessed at rest over a full circadian cycle, before and after activation by a panicogenic agent that does not independently activate the HPA axis (doxapram) and before and after administration of a panicogenic agent that does activate the HPA axis (the CCK-B agonist pentagastrin). Increased overnight plasma cortisol concentrations corresponding to sleep disruption have been noted in subjects who have PD; this increase is a trait rather than a state-dependent marker of PD. In the doxapram challenge study, an exaggerated increase in plasma ACTH was observed in the patients who had PD. Compared with healthy control subjects, plasma ACTH concentrations were elevated following pentagastrin administration in patients who had PD. Taken together, these data support the hypothesis that patients who have PD are hypersensitive to the HPA axis–activating effects of situations that are novel, threatening, and uncontrollable. After the basal state was established reliably, the ACTH response to CRF administration was not altered in patients who had PD, suggesting that the previous studies were confounded by the effects of the novel environment on the HPA axis (reviewed in[42]).

Genetic Contribution to Panic Disorder

PD is thought to be the most heritable of the anxiety disorders. First-degree relatives of proband patients who have PD have a sevenfold increased likelihood for PD and also have an increased risk for phobic disorders.[43–45] Twin studies suggest that 30% to 40% of the variance in vulnerability for PD is derived from genetic factors and the remainder from individual-specific, but not shared, environment/life experiences.[43]

Linkage studies in families that have PD have been hampered by non-replication and small numbers.[45,46] A large analysis including 120 pedigrees with more than 1500 individuals revealed two loci with genome-wide significance on chromosomes 2q and 15q, but these results await further replication.[47] A large number of genetic association studies for PD have been published, implicating many genes. A recent review compiled the genes that have been associated with PD in more than one study thus far, although in some cases different polymorphisms within these genes have been associated with PD in different studies, complicating any attempt to draw causal conclusions from these data (reviewed in[45]). The genes associated with PD in multiple studies are:

1. COMT
2. *Adenosine 2A receptor*
3. *CCK*
4. CCK Receptor B
5. $5HT_{2A}$ receptor
6. Monoamine oxidase-A

In addition to the aforementioned target genes, polymorphisms in *SLC6A4*, the gene for the serotonin transporter, also have been associated with PD. The association, however, is not with the well-studied promoter-length polymorphism.[48] Rather, SNPs within the serotonin transporter gene show association with PD and comorbid PD/social anxiety disorder (SAD). Subjects who have at least one copy of haplotype A-A-G from rs3794808, rs140701, and rs4583306 have 1.7 times the odds of PD than subjects with no copy of this haplotype.[49] In combination with associations of other genes within the monoamine system mentioned earlier in this article, these data support the hypothesis that monoaminergic systems are involved in anxiety disorders as a group; their exact role may be disorder specific.

Although most genetic-association studies have investigated only single polymorphism contributions, it is very likely that a combination of polymorphisms in sets of candidate genes act in concert to increase the risk for this disorder. In fact, a recent study investigating the contribution of genetic variants in the CRF and AVP system reported that the strongest results were the combined effects of rs878886 in CRF_1 and rs28632197 in the gene encoding the vasopressin 1B receptor (AVP_{1B}).[50] A model with two SNPs showed significant associations with PD in both samples separately, and significance improved to $P = .00057$ in the combined sample of 359 cases and 794 controls. Both SNPs are of potential functional relevance, because rs878886 is located in the 3' untranslated region of the CRF_1 gene, and rs28632197 leads to an arginine-to-histidine amino acid exchange at position 364 of AVP_{1B}, which is located in the intracellular C-terminal domain of the receptor and probably is involved in G-protein coupling. These genetic data support the large body of evidence demonstrating interactions of AVP and CRF systems in anxiety. Another family-based study failed to find an association of four polymorphisms in the CRF_1 locus with PD, but fewer CRF_1 polymorphisms and no AVP_{1B} polymorphisms were tested in this study.[51]

POSTTRAUMATIC STRESS DISORDER
Anatomical and Neuroimaging Findings in Posttraumatic Stress Disorder

Activation of the amygdala is important for the fear learning associated with PTSD symptoms and with extinction learning associated with PTSD treatment. Amygdala hyperresponsiveness has been identified in numerous studies of patients who have PTSD (reviewed in[37]). Greater activation of the amygdala in response to viewing fearful faces corresponded with poor prognosis in CBT;[52] other studies have shown that severity of PTSD symptoms predicts the magnitude of amygdala activation when encoding memories unrelated to the traumatic event.[53]

A recent study examined the neural correlates of responsiveness to CBT in Iraq war veterans who had PTSD. Avoidance symptoms of PTSD are thought to result from conditioned fear-like encoding of the environment surrounding a traumatic event. CBT in PTSD attempts to override the conditioned fear with extinction learning. In patients who had recently diagnosed PTSD, rostral ACC volume predicted a successful CBT response. It is possible that decreased rostral ACC volume results in a decreased ability for extinction learning. Thus, patients who have PTSD and who have a smaller ACC volume may be less able to regulate fear during therapy, rendering the CBT process less effective.[54] Functional imaging studies have shown that greater activation of the ventral ACC in response to viewing fearful faces corresponded with a poorer response to CBT.[52]

It has been hypothesized that symptoms of PTSD, including intrusive thoughts and re-experiencing trauma, result from an inability of higher cognitive structures to repress negative emotional memories. This imbalance is obvious in functional imaging studies with tasks that require interrelated executive and emotional processing systems. In healthy subjects and in recently deployed veterans of war who have PTSD, presentation of emotional stimuli, as compared with neutral stimuli, elicits activation in ventral frontolimbic brain regions, including the ventromedial PFC, inferior frontal gyrus, and ventral anterior cingulate gyrus. In patients who have PTSD, the magnitude of ventral activation is positively correlated with symptom severity. Furthermore, compared with neutral stimuli, combat-related stimuli produced enhanced activation of this ventral emotional system. The amplitude of this increase also correlated with the severity of PTSD symptoms.[55] During executive tasks, healthy controls and patients who have PTSD activate a dorsal executive network that includes the middle frontal gyrus, dorsal anterior cingulate gyrus, and inferior parietal lobule. In patients who have PTSD, reduced activation of the dorsal executive network correlates with symptom severity. The middle frontal gyrus, a component of the dorsal executive network, also is activated when patents who have PTSD view combat-related images. These results suggest that brain areas that are restricted to executive functioning in healthy subjects are used for emotional/affective processing in patients who have PTSD, thereby diminishing the capacity of executive control.[55]

Similarly, sensory gating deficits in patients who have PTSD may result from information processing systems being overpowered by hypervigilance for threat-related stimuli and hyperarousal. A task requiring subjects to inhibit a primed motor response has demonstrated deficits of inhibitory control in patients who have PTSD. In control subjects, inhibitory processing activated the right frontotemporoparietal cortical network. In patients who had PTSD, the left ventrolateral PFC (vlPFC) was activated, and the frontotemporoparietal cortical network was less active. In terms of the behavioral response, increased error correlated with PTSD symptom severity. Increased symptom severity may result in increasingly overwhelmed inhibitory networks. Conversely, decreasing ability to recruit inhibitory control networks may result in more intense symptoms.[56]

Neurotransmitter and Neuroendocrine Signaling in Posttraumatic Stress Disorder

Amino acid neurotransmitters

Glutamate plays a critical role in hippocampal-dependent associative learning and in amygdala-dependent emotional processing in stressful conditions or following stress exposure. Inappropriate glutamate signaling therefore could contribute to the processing distortion experienced by many patients who have PTSD. In support of the glutamate hypothesis of PTSD, the N-methyl-D-aspartic acid receptor antagonist ketamine is well known for its ability to induce dissociative and perceptual distortions, similar to the processing distortion in patients who have PTSD (reviewed in[37]).

Recent research has explored the possible therapeutic potential of glutamatergic targets in PTSD. One such drug is the anticonvulsant topiramate. Topiramate inhibits excitatory transmission at kainate and α-amino-3-hydroxy-5-methyl-4-isoxazole propionate (AMPA) receptors and has demonstrated anxiolytic properties at lower doses than required for anticonvulsant effects, suggesting a unique mechanism of action. Open-label studies using topiramate as either adjunctive or monotherapy have demonstrated some efficacy in diminishing nightmares and flashbacks and in improving overall PTSD symptoms.[37]

Monoamines

There are numerous reports of hyperactive noradrenergic signaling in PTSD. For example, NE is robustly secreted after exposure to acute physiological stress, and CSF concentrations of NE are tonically elevated in PTSD veterans. There is no evidence of a correlation between NE concentration and symptom severity, however (reviewed in[57]). As with patients who have PD, yohimbine elicits panic-like anxiety associated with cardiovascular symptoms and increased serum NE in patients who have PTSD relative to healthy control subjects (reviewed in[35]). Furthermore, patients who have PTSD have been shown to exhibit elevated 24-hour urinary catecholamine excretion.[58] Some of the effects of NE on PTSD symptoms may be mediated by interactions between NE and glucocorticoids (eg,[59]). Drugs targeting the NE system have been assessed in PTSD with varying degrees of success for individual PTSD symptoms (see[57] for a thorough review).

SSRIs have been demonstrated to be of moderate efficacy in PTSD, and sertraline is approved by the Food and Drug Administration to treat this disorder. In patients who had non–combat-related PTSD, paroxetine treatment improved hyperarousal and avoidance symptoms by 8 weeks and improved re-experiencing symptoms by the end of the 12-week study.[60] The Institute of Medicine report on treatment of PTSD did not consider the efficacy data on SSRIs to be sufficient when compared with the psychotherapy data.[61]

Neuropeptides

In healthy soldiers during intense military training, interrogation stress led to an increase in plasma NPY concentrations; plasma NPY concentrations were correlated with cortisol concentrations and with behavioral performance. Combat-exposed men who did not develop PTSD tended to have higher concentrations of plasma NPY than combat-exposed men who had PTSD. These data suggest that NPY could be a neural correlate of resiliency.[62]

A recent review article identified a potential role for neurokinins in PTSD.[35] Neuro-kinin 2 antagonists did not exhibit anxiolytic properties in preclinical tests in which benzodiazepines were active. The latter are of limited use in PTSD, however. Expression of galanin has been demonstrated to be stress responsive, in that it is decreased by acute stress but returns to normal within several days. If the stress continues and becomes chronic, galanin expression increases. It has been suggested that elevated galanin expression induced by chronic stress leads to increased autoinhibition of NE cell bodies in the locus coeruleus (LC); decreased tonic LC activity could contribute to depressive symptoms in patients who have PTSD (reviewed in[35]).

Corticotropin-releasing factor and the hypothalamic-pituitary-adrenal axis

Numerous studies have identified HPA axis disruption in patients who have PTSD.[63–68] Compared with healthy control subjects, and in contrast to patients who have MDD, cortisol concentration is decreased in plasma, in saliva upon awakening, and in 24-hour urinary measures in combat-exposed patients who have PTSD.[69] In a more recent study, a mixed population of civilian patients who had PTSD also exhibited decreased cortisol concentrations; lower plasma cortisol corresponded with greater symptom severity.[70] Importantly, there also have been studies showing no difference in circadian salivary or 24-hour urinary cortisol concentrations (eg,[71,72]).

As in patients who have MDD, CSF concentrations of CRF were found to be higher in patients who had PTSD than in comparison subjects in two studies.[73,74] Patients who have MDD typically exhibit a blunted HPA axis response in the CRF-stimulation test, and in veterans of the Vietnam or Korean wars hospitalized for PTSD, the ACTH response to ovine CRF injection also was blunted relative to control subjects and was independent of comorbid MDD diagnosis.[75] In contrast, although dexamethasone non-suppression often is observed in patients who have MDD, patients who have PTSD exhibit greater suppression of plasma ACTH and cortisol concentrations.[76] Negative findings also have been reported.[77] Dexamethasone hypersuppression in patients who have PTSD may result from sensitized central glucocorticoid receptors (GRs) secondary to chronic elevations in CRF. This finding is in sharp contrast to patients who have MDD, in whom chronic CRF overexpression is thought to result eventually in GR desensitization and reduced negative feedback (reviewed in[35]). Alterations in CRFergic signaling and the HPA axis could result from insufficient glucocorticoid signaling caused by decreased hormone bioavailability or from decreased hormone receptor sensitivity.[78]

Genetic Contribution to Posttraumatic Stress Disorder

The heritability for PTSD has an estimated range of 30% to 40%, probably resulting from a variety of genes, each with relatively small contributions to the genetic predisposition for this disorder.[79–83] Because of the importance of the environmental impact for this disorder, linkage studies in pedigrees cannot be conducted easily. Candidate gene association studies also are confounded by the problem of matching for environmental exposure and largely have been limited by small sample size ($n < 100$); therefore these studies would able to detect only large genetic effects.

Because PTSD is the only anxiety diagnosis requiring a prior traumatic event, much research has been devoted to examining gene-by-environment interactions in patients who have PTSD. A complex-repeat polymorphism in the 5' upstream region of SLC6A4, the gene encoding the serotonin transporter (serotonin transporter-linked polymorphic region, 5-HTTLPR), has been studied in depth by numerous groups. This polymorphism consists of a repetitive region containing 16 imperfect repeat units of 22 bp, located approximately 1000 bp upstream of the transcriptional start site.[48,84] The 5-HTTLPR is polymorphic because of the insertion/deletion of units 6 through 8, which produces a short (S) allele that is 44 bp shorter than the long (L) allele. The 5-HTTLPR has been associated with different basal expression and functional activity of the transporter, most likely related to differential transcriptional activity.[48,84] The L-allele of this polymorphism has been shown to lead to a higher serotonin reuptake by the transporter and thus less serotonin in the synaptic cleft. The short SERT allele has been shown to interact with stressful life events (including abuse in childhood) to increase the risk for depression later in life.[85–91] This polymorphism recently has been shown to play a role in the genetic underpinnings of PTSD. In hurricane victims, the SERT polymorphism interacts with severity of trauma and level of social support toward the development of PTSD.[92]

Other genes interacting with early-life stress (ELS) also are strong candidates for influencing susceptibility for PTSD. Preclinical studies indicate that the persistent hyperactivity of the HPA axis associated with ELS is mediated by a hyperactive CRF_1 system, with chronic overactivity of CRF_1 in limbic brain regions.[93,94] In fact, the authors have shown that a haplotype within the gene encoding CRF_1 interacts with child abuse to predict depression severity in adults.[95] These polymorphisms, however, did not interact with ELS to predict PTSD symptoms.[96]

Polymorphisms in genes regulating GR activity may alter sensitization of the stress-response pathway during development so that victims of ELS have increased risk for PTSD following traumatic events in adulthood. FKBP5, a co-chaperone of heat shock protein 90, plays a role in regulating the expression of glucocorticoid-responsive genes.[97] Increased expression of FKBP5 has been shown to reduce glucocorticoid binding affinity[98] and to reduce nuclear translocation of the GR,[99] resulting in resistance to glucocorticoid activation. In humans, the rare alleles of the FKBP5, SNPs rs4613916, rs1360780, and rs3800373, were associated with higher FKBP5 expression in blood monocytes as well as with a stronger induction of FKBP5 mRNA by cortisol.[100] As an important candidate gene in trauma-related HPA axis disturbances, the putative functional SNPs in FKBP5 are hypothesized to moderate the development of PTSD and/or to alter the impact of early trauma or PTSD on GR.[100–102]

In support of this hypothesis, there seems to be a positive correlation between the upregulation of FKBP5 mRNA in peripheral blood mononuclear cells induced by acute trauma and the development of the PTSD 4 months later.[103] Furthermore, when exposed to medical trauma, pediatric patients who had the rs3800373 and rs1360780 alleles were more likely to exhibit peritraumatic dissociation,[104] a strong predictor of PTSD in adulthood.[105] In the largest genetics study in PTSD conducted thus far, the authors' group showed that the same alleles increased the risk for adult PTSD symptom severity in adults who had been exposed to child abuse but not to trauma as adults.[96] Additional research will be necessary to clarify the gene–environment relationship between early-life trauma versus adult trauma.

SOCIAL ANXIETY DISORDER
Anatomical and Neuroimaging Findings in Social Anxiety Disorder

As with PD and PTSD, amygdala activation has been implicated in symptoms of SAD. Social-cue tasks, such as the viewing of harsh faces, were associated with hyperreactivity in the amygdala and other limbic areas in patients who had SAD. Similarly, in response to viewing negative (but not neutral or positive) affective faces, patients who have SAD exhibited bilateral amygdala activation, which positively correlated with symptom severity and which reversed upon successful treatment. In anticipation of public speaking, subcortical, limbic, and lateral paralimbic activity is increased in patients who have SAD, suggesting elevations in automatic emotional processing. Decreased activity in the ACC and PFC in these subjects suggests a decreased ability for cognitive processing (reviewed in[23]).

In contrast to the social-cue studies, activity in the left hippocampus and right amygdala was decreased during script-guided mental imagery tasks that provoke social anxiety. This decrease may reflect active blunting of the emotional and autonomic response to improve overall functioning during social situations that provoke anxiety.[106] Furthermore, anxiety-provoking imagery (compared with neutral imagery) was associated with increased activation in the left postcentral gyrus and putamen and in the right inferior frontal and middle temporal gyri. Relative decreased activity was observed in the right middle temporal gyrus, left precuneus, and posterior cingulate gyrus. After 8 weeks of treatment with nefazodone, both remitted and partially improved social anxiety was associated with decreased regional CBF (rCBF) in the lingual gyrus, left superior temporal gyrus, and right vlFC and with increased rCBF in the left middle occipital gyrus and inferior parietal cortex. In subjects who achieved remission following nefazodone treatment, posttreatment testing revealed decreased rCBF in the ventral and dorsal ACC, left vlPFC, dorsolateral PFC, and brainstem and increased rCBF in the middle cingulate cortex, left hippocampus, parahippocampal gyrus, subcallosal orbital, and superior frontal gyri.[106]

The combined results of imaging analysis in subjects who have SAD suggest dysfunction of a cortico-striato-thalamic network: hyperactivity in the right PFC, striatal dysfunction, and increased hippocampal and amygdala activity with left lateralization. It has been suggested that hyperactivity in the frontolimbic system, including the ACC, which processes negative emotional information and anticipation of aversive stimuli, could result in misinterpretation of social cues (reviewed in[23,107]).

Neurotransmitter and Neuroendocrine Signaling in Social Anxiety Disorder

Amino acid neurotransmitters
Increased excitatory glutamatergic activity has been reported in patients who have SAD. Compared with matched control subjects, patients who had SAD had a 13.2% higher glutamate/creatine ratio in the ACC as measured by MRS. The glutamate/creatine ratio correlated with symptom severity, suggesting a causal role between excitatory signaling in the ACC and psychopathology (reviewed in[37]).

Monoamines
In addition to benzodiazepines, SSRIs, SNRIs, and monoamine oxidase inhibitors are effective in the treatment of SAD. That SSRI treatment is successful in treating SAD

symptoms and reversing some brain abnormalities (eg, elevated amygdala activity) has been cited as evidence for a serotonergic role in the etiology of SAD.[107] Data supporting the hypothesis of disrupted monoaminergic signaling in patients who have SAD include decreased $5HT_{1A}$ receptor binding in the amygdala, ACC, insula, and dorsal raphe nucleus (DRN). Moreover, trait and state anxiety is elevated in patients who have SAD who have one or two copies of the short SERT allele, and this patient population exhibits amygdala hyperactivity in anxiety-provocation paradigms. Neuroimaging analyses also have revealed decreased density of the dopamine transporter and decreased binding capacity for the D_2 receptor (reviewed in[23]). A role for DA in SAD is supported by the finding that patients who have Parkinson's disease have high rates of comorbid SAD (reviewed in[107]). This co-morbidity, however, could result from insecurity regarding display of the physical symptoms of this movement disorder rather than a common etiology of DA malfunction.

A recent study assessed whether a DA agonist (pramipexole, 0.5 mg) or antagonist (sulpiride, 400 mg) influenced response to anxiogenic challenge such as verbal tasks and autobiographical scripts in patients who had SAD. The anxiogenic effect of the behavioral challenges was significantly increased in patients who had untreated SAD following administration of either drug. After successful treatment with SSRIs, however, administration of pramipexole seemed to dampen the behavioral provocation-induced anxiety, whereas sulpiride administration continued to enhance the anxiogenic effects of these tasks. These authors suggested that instability in the dopaminergic response to social stress contributes to anxiety severity and is normalized only partly by successful treatment, perhaps via SSRI-induced desensitization of postsynaptic D_3 receptors.[108]

Neuropeptides

As key effectors of social behavior, the neuropeptides oxytocin and vasopressin are of particular interest in SAD and autistic spectrum disorders. Recently direct oxytocin administration to the amygdala in laboratory animals was shown to decrease activation in this region and to dampen amygdala–brainstem communications, which are known to play a role in the autonomic and behavioral components of fear. Furthermore, preliminary data have shown that genetic variants in the central vasopressin and oxytocin receptors (AVP_{1A} and $OXTR$, respectively) influence amygdalar activity. These data support the hypothesis of amygdala hyperactivity in SAD. Future research in this area may elucidate neural underpinning of human social behavior and the genetic risk for disorders including SAD and autism.[18]

Corticotropin-releasing factor and the hypothalamic-pituitary-adrenal axis

Some evidence indicates sensitization of the HPA axis in patients who have SAD. Psychosocial stress produces a greater increase in plasma cortisol, but not ACTH, in patients who have SAD than in control patients despite similar baseline cortisol concentrations.[109] Compared with healthy control subjects or patients who have PTSD, subjects who have SAD tend toward an elevated cortisol response in the Trier Social Stress Test (TSST). The degree of cortisol elevation was correlated with increased avoidance behavior in the approach–avoidance task and the predicted stress-induced increased social avoidance above and beyond effects of blood pressure and subjective anxiety.[110] Negative findings also have been reported, however (eg,[111,112]). For example, an earlier study found that adolescent girls who had social phobia and control subjects exhibited an equal elevation in salivary cortisol following the TSST. To the authors' knowledge, there are no endocrine-challenge studies (Dex-Suppression, CRF-Stimulation, or Dex/CRF) in patients who have SAD.

Genetic Contribution to Social Anxiety Disorder

Unfortunately, there are very few studies specifically examining the genetic underpinnings of SAD. Available data suggest that SAD has a high degree of familial aggregation. In a recent meta-analysis in which SAD was grouped with specific phobia and agoraphobia, an association between phobia in probands and their first-degree relatives was identified.[43]

Twin studies in social phobics suggest that additive genetics is responsible for increased incidence of SAD in monozygotic compared with dizigotic twins and suggest no role for common environmental experiences. Adult twin studies of combined phobia diagnoses (including social phobics) suggest that the additive genetics accounts for 20% to 40% of the variance in diagnosis. This result corresponds with a population based twin study of adolescents diagnosed with social phobia, MDD, and alcoholism, in which genetics accounted for 28% of the risk variance for SAD. Again, the remaining risk was derived from non-shared environmental experiences. Unlike MDD and PTSD, there is little evidence that early-life trauma influences the risk for developing SAD in adulthood.[43]

The one genome-wide linkage analysis of SAD implicated a region on chromosome 16 near the gene encoding the norepinephrine transporter. Other genes associated with SAD include (1) a functional variant in *ADRB1*, the gene encoding the β1-adrenergic receptor, and (2) two SNPs and a 3-SNP haplotype in the gene for COMT in female patients who have SAD (reviewed in[107]). Because SAD is such a complex phenotype, it has been suggested that it may be more fruitful to search for susceptibility genes by examining intermediate phenotypes, quantitative traits, and comorbidity with other illnesses. In fact, SAD heritability includes disorder-specific but also nonspecific genetic factors. SAD is associated with behavioral inhibition in childhood, low extroversion, and high neuroticism. These personality traits are not SAD specific but are hypothesized to contribute to a spectrum of psychopathology inclusive of mood and anxiety disorders. Furthermore, behavioral inhibition, low extroversion, and high neuroticism are each known to be highly heritable and may largely account for the genetic contribution to SAD.

Genes associated with high behavioral inhibition include *CRF* and *SERT*. Internalizing neuroticism is associated with the gene encoding glutamic acid decarboxylase, the rate-limiting enzyme in the synthesis of GABA from glutamate (reviewed in[107]).

GENERALIZED ANXIETY DISORDER
Anatomical and Neuroimaging Findings in Patients who Have Generalized Anxiety Disorder

Structural imaging studies have shown high ratios of gray matter to white matter in the upper temporal lobe of pediatric patients who have generalized anxiety disorder (GAD).[113] Pediatric patients who have GAD also exhibit increased amygdala volume, which may correspond to the stress-induced amygdalar hypertrophy observed in laboratory animal studies (reviewed in[37]).

In functional imaging studies of adolescent patients who have GAD, resting vlPFC activity is elevated relative to healthy control subjects. Because the vlPFC activity correlates negatively with symptom severity, the elevation in vlPFC metabolism is interpreted as a compensatory response rather than an underlying cause of GAD.[114] Because of observed hypermetabolism in the PFC of patients who have GAD, neuronal viability has been assessed in this region as measured by the ratio of *N*-acetylasparate to creatine using proton MRS. For patients who had GAD, neuronal viability was increased in the right dorsolateral PFC in those without early-life stress but was decreased in those who self-reported early-life trauma.[115]

Functional brain imaging results obtained under resting conditions in patients who have GAD have tended to be inconsistent; provocative anxiety-inducing tasks have produced more robust and interpretable fMRI results. The pattern of brain activity in anxious patients who have GAD correlates well with results from laboratory animal studies in which limbic circuits, particularly the amygdala, play an important role in the fear response (eg,[116,117]; see[118] for a review). In fact, many imaging studies of patients who have GAD show elevated amygdala and insula activation during negative emotional processing (reviewed in[23,119,120]). In response to viewing angry faces, adolescent patients who had GAD exhibited an elevated right amygdala response; this activation correlated positively with symptom severity. The overactivity in the right amygdala also was correlated negatively with activity in the right vlPFC, suggesting top-down disinhibition as a potential mechanism for elevated amygdala activity.[121] Interestingly, strong pretreatment activation of the left amygdala in pediatric patients who had GAD predicted a positive therapeutic response to fluoxetine or CBT.[122] These results have been interpreted to suggest that a greater amygdaloid response to negative emotions represents a healthier signal-to-noise ratio. When adult patients who have GAD view fearful faces, lower pretreatment amygdala activity and higher ACC activity predict a positive treatment response to venlafaxine.[123] Additional studies will be crucial in determining whether amygdala activation has clinical utility in predicting treatment outcome.

Interconnectivity with brain regions responsible for interpreting social behavior may be one mechanism by which the amygdala plays a substantial role in anxiety disorders. The brain regions responsible for interpreting social behavior include the superior temporal gyrus, thalamus, and PFC. Amygdala hyperactivity may mediate the inaccurate interpretations of social behavior in patients who have GAD.[120]

Neurotransmitter and Neuroendocrine Signaling in Generalized Anxiety Disorder

Amino acid neurotransmitters

The observed limbic overactivity in patients who have GAD could result from decreased inhibitory neurotransmission, increased excitatory neurotransmission, or a combination of these two processes. Dysregulation of GABA inhibitory neurotransmission has been documented in several anxiety disorders (reviewed in[124]). $GABA_A$ receptor downregulation is observed in patients who have GAD and has been hypothesized to play a role in the etiology of this illness (reviewed in[68]). In support of this hypothesis is the finding that symptoms of GAD, including excessive worry, hypervigilance, and psychomotor agitation, are treated effectively with $GABA_A$ facilitators such as benzodiazepines and barbiturates (reviewed in[124]). Furthermore, treatment with riluzole, an anti-glutamatergic agent, seems to improve GAD symptoms.[125,126]

Monoamines

Although all the SSRIs have shown efficacy in GAD, the drug most frequently studied in anxiety is paroxetine, which decreases symptoms of harm avoidance. It is important to note that GAD often is comorbid with other disorders, including MDD, PD, and SAD, each of which also has shown responsiveness to SSRI treatment.[39]

More concrete evidence supporting a role for 5-HT circuitry in GAD includes challenge with the $5-HT_{2c}/5-HT_3$ agonist mCPP, which elicits anxiety and anger in patients who have GAD (reviewed in[68]).

Further evidence for a serotonergic component of GAD is provided by functional brain imaging studies that have found that midbrain SERT density correlates negatively with symptom severity.[127,128] Recent studies have replicated the negative correlation between SERT density and anxiety symptoms in GAD, but there is no difference in SERT density in subjects who have GAD as compared with controls.[127]

Neuropeptides

Patients who have GAD are hypersensitive to exogenously administered CCK agonists,[129,130] leading to the study of CCK receptor–selective antagonists as a putative novel class of anxiolytics. One such drug was developed but was not demonstrated to possess anxiolytic efficacy.[131] Additional research and development of unique CCK antagonists will be an important step in clarifying the role of CCK in anxiety and its potential as a therapeutic target.

To the authors' knowledge, no studies have specifically examined the role of NPY in GAD. NPY does possess anxiolytic effects in laboratory animals (reviewed in[132]). These anxiolytic effects may be caused by NPY–CRF interactions; these two neuropeptides are co-localized in numerous limbic regions and exert opposing effects on the amygdala, LC, and periaqueductal gray matter, the last region is responsible for the motor output for the behavioral stress response.[133]

Corticotropin-releasing factor and the hypothalamic-pituitary-adrenal axis

Although very few studies have specifically examined HPA axis reactivity in patients who have GAD, there is no evidence of hypercortisolism, dexamethasone non-suppression, or increased CSF CRF concentrations.[67,68] That CRF and the HPA axis seem to play a less prominent role in GAD than in other anxiety disorders and MDD is perhaps surprising given that CRF antagonists have been demonstrated to possess anxiolytic effects ([134–136]; reviewed in[137]). It is possible that the lack of evidence for a pathophysiological role for CRF circuits in GAD is an artifact of the paucity of endocrine studies in these patients. It is equally likely, however, that the difference in CRF/HPA axis observations in patients who have MDD and patients who have GAD represents a critical biological distinction between these two syndromes.

Genetic Contribution to Generalized Anxiety Disorder

Overall the genetic contribution is thought to be less substantial in GAD than in other anxiety disorders. Studies have shown that first-degree relatives of GAD probands have elevated rates of mood and anxiety disorders in general[138] and perhaps have a specifically increased risk for GAD.[43] A recent study of more than 3000 twin pairs found modest familial aggregation of GAD with equal heritability in males and females in same-sex or opposite-sex twin pairs; there was no evidence for gender-specific genetic underpinnings of GAD.[139] Results from twin studies estimate that approximately 32% of the variance for liability to GAD is caused by additive genetics in male and female twins and that the remaining variance is explained by environment specific to the individual, rather than the shared environment of the twin pair (reviewed in[43]). Only a handful of genetic-association studies specific for GAD have been reported, and all are thus far unreplicated (eg,[140–142]).

SUMMARY AND GUIDANCE FOR THE DIAGNOSTIC AND STATISTICAL MANUAL OF MENTAL DISORDERS, EDITION FIVE
Functional Neuroanatomy

Commonalities in anxiety disorders include functional hyperactivity in limbic regions, particularly the amygdala, and the inability of higher cortical executive areas to normalize the limbic response to stimuli (**Table 2**). In contrast to MDD, in which amygdala

Table 2
Functional anatomy of normal and pathological sadness and anxiety

Anatomic Area	Normal and Pathological Sadness	Normal and Pathological Anxiety
Insular cortex	Acute sadness activates dorsal insula	Acute anxiety activates ventral insula
Cingulate cortex	Pregenual ACC deactivated in euthymic MDD Pregenual ACC activated in acute MDD Subgenual ACC normal in acute MDD but hypoactive in patients who have remitted MDD ACC and PCC activated by acute sadness	Acute anxiety has no effect on ACC but deactivates the PCC
Amygdala	Overactive at rest in primary mood disorders Magnitude of activity correlates to severity Overactivity without conscious perception Normal activity after treatment Smaller volume of left amygdala versus controls	Not overactive at rest Overactive during symptom provocation Right amygdala most relevant to anxiety

hyperactivity is observed under resting conditions, provocation paradigms are required to identify amygdalar hyperactivity in patients who have an anxiety disorder.

Additional neuroimaging studies must focus not on individual brain regions but on corticolimbic circuits. Between-laboratory consistency must become a priority throughout the research community to allow interpretation of results across studies. Perhaps most importantly, neuroimaging research must place more emphasis on hypothesis-driven studies. It is hoped that such increased consistency and clear goals will lead to more reliable and robust observations that finally can piece together the diagnosis-specific clinical implications of functional and structural alterations in patients who have mood and anxiety disorders.

Neurotransmitter and Neuroendocrine Signaling

Disruption in neurotransmitter, neuropeptide, and neuroendocrine signaling is not unique to mood and anxiety disorders; a great deal of overlap between diagnostic syndromes should be expected. For example, dysregulation of the generalized stress response is common to numerous medical and psychiatric diagnoses. Repeated, prolonged, or particularly severe stress could increase the magnitude and duration of CRF, glucocorticoid, and catecholaminergic signaling, and these three signaling classes can explain the psychiatric, circulatory, metabolic, and immune manifestations of stress-related illness. In contrast, hypoactivation of the HPA axis as a compensatory mechanism for chronic/severe stress exposure may occur also. HPA axis hyperactivity is seen in MDD, OCD, PD, anorexia, and alcoholism (to name a few), whereas HPA axis hypoactivity is observed in chronic fatigue, fibromyalgia, nicotine withdrawal, PTSD, and the postpartum period. Importantly, the direction of the HPA axis disruption depends on the nature, duration, predictability, and severity of the stressor and also on the age of the subject, individual genetic background, and previous experiences (reviewed in[58]).

The clinical implications of altered monoaminergic signaling probably are influenced by an equally long list of factors. A closer relationship between preclinical and clinical research is essential before it will be possible to begin to piece together the relationship between each of these factors.

Genetic Contribution

When attempting to identify the genetic contribution toward susceptibility for psychopathology, the candidate genes are largely the same across diagnoses and tend to be genes whose products regulate the HPA axis and monoaminergic signaling. These similarities, however, do not preclude important clinical distinctions between diagnostic classes within anxiety disorders or between anxiety disorders and MDD. Some genetic factors are nonspecific but influence the risk for psychopathology in general. Others are diagnosis specific. Moreover, the impact of individual diagnosis-specific genetic risk factors may vary over time, depending on the developmental stage and previous experience of each subject.

Overall, the decision to classify MDD, PD, PTSD, SAD, and GAD as distinct disorders must be based not only on clinical phenomenology but also on pathophysiology, genetics, course of illness, and treatment response data. Neuroendocrine, neurotransmitter, and neuroanatomical differences between patients who have mood or anxiety disorders and healthy control subjects must be interpreted with care (**Table 3**). Brain regions and neurotransmitter systems implicated in mood and anxiety disorders have wide-ranging functions, many of which may be unrelated to

Table 3
Summary of select neurotransmitter abnormalities in MDD, GAD, and normal sadness and anxiety

Neurotransmitter	Normal and Pathological Sadness	Normal and Pathological Anxiety
GABA	Inconsistent GABA-A agonists not approved for MDD by the Food and Drug Administration	Decreased GABA-A receptor density in GAD; GABA-A agonists are anxiolytic Affinity for GABA-A predicts efficacy of benzodiazepines
Serotonin	Decreased 5HIAA CSF concentrations in suicide victims Normal in non-suicidal MDD patients Blunted prolactin response to 5-HT agonists	Decreased 5HIAA CSF concentrations in some studies
SERT	Decreased density in midbrain Density correlates negatively with anxiety symptoms in MDD	Density correlates negatively with anxiety symptoms in GAD
5HT1A	—	Anxiolytic as DRN autoreceptors Anxiogenic as hippocampus postsynaptic receptors
5HT2	Desensitized by antidepressants	Anxiogenic Antagonists are anxiolytic
Norepinephrine	Elevated in CSF and plasma of patients who have severe melancholic MDD Unchanged in patients who have non-melancholic MDD Blunted growth hormone response to clonidine Blunted rapid-eye-movement response to clonidine	Unchanged in GAD

the etiology of psychiatric disorders. Finally each of these disorders clearly represents the result of complex gene–environment interactions. The clinical phenotype may well be determined largely by individual differences in multiple genes that exhibit functional polymorphisms. It is hoped that continued research will begin to uncover more consistent findings across laboratories, methodologies, and subjects. At that point, a new discussion of diagnostic criteria may be relevant.

REFERENCES

1. Keedwell PA, Andrew C, Williams SC, et al. The neural correlates of anhedonia in major depressive disorder. Biol Psychiatry 2005;58:843–53.
2. Drevets WC. Neuroimaging and neuropathological studies of depression: implications for the cognitive-emotional features of mood disorders. Curr Opin Neurobiol 2001;11:240–9.
3. Miller EK, Cohen JD. An integrative theory of prefrontal cortex function. Annu Rev Neurosci 2001;24:167–202.
4. Treede RD, Kenshalo DR, Gracely RH, et al. The cortical representation of pain. Pain 1999;79:105–11.
5. Vogt BA, Finch DM, Olson CR. Functional heterogeneity in cingulate cortex: the anterior executive and posterior evaluative regions. Cereb Cortex 1992;2:435–43.
6. Gysling K, Forray MI, Haeger P, et al. Corticotropin-releasing hormone and urocortin: redundant or distinctive functions? Brain Res Brain Res Rev 2004;47:116–25.
7. Barrera G, Echevarria DJ, Poulin JF, et al. One for all or one for one: does cotransmission unify the concept of a brain galanin "system" or clarify any consistent role in anxiety? Neuropeptides 2005;39:289–92.
8. Honkaniemi J, Pelto-Huikko M, Rechardt L, et al. Colocalization of peptide and glucocorticoid receptor immunoreactivities in rat central amygdaloid nucleus. Neuroendocrinology 1992;55:451–9.
9. Palkovits M. Stress-induced expression of co-localized neuropeptides in hypothalamic and amygdaloid neurons. Eur J Pharmacol 2000;405:161–6.
10. Watts AG. The impact of physiological stimuli on the expression of corticotropin-releasing hormone (CRH) and other neuropeptide genes. Front Neuroendocrinol 1996;17:281–326.
11. Cole RL, Sawchenko PE. Neurotransmitter regulation of cellular activation and neuropeptide gene expression in the paraventricular nucleus of the hypothalamus. J Neurosci 2002;22:959–69.
12. Holmes A, Heilig M, Rupniak NM, et al. Neuropeptide systems as novel therapeutic targets for depression and anxiety disorders. Trends Pharmacol Sci 2003;24:580–8.
13. Schatzberg AF, Nemeroff CB, editors. Textbook of psychopharmacology. ed. 3. Washington (DC): The American Psychiatric Publishing; 2004. p. 717–65, 847–68, 913–35.
14. Lang R, Gundlach AL, Kofler B. The galanin peptide family: receptor pharmacology, pleiotropic biological actions, and implications in health and disease. Pharmacol Ther 2007;115:177–207.
15. Liu HX, Hokfelt T. The participation of galanin in pain processing at the spinal level. Trends Pharmacol Sci 2002;23:468–74.
16. Bedecs K, Berthold M, Bartfai T. Galanin 10 years with a neuroendocrine peptide. Int J Biochem Cell Biol 1995;27:337–49.
17. Gimpl G, Fahrenholz F. The oxytocin receptor system: structure, function, and regulation. Physiol Rev 2001;81:629–83.

18. Meyer-Lindenberg A. Impact of prosocial neuropeptides on human brain function. Prog Brain Res 2008;170:463–70.
19. Egashira N, Tanoue A, Matsuda T, et al. Impaired social interaction and reduced anxiety-related behavior in vasopressin V1a receptor knockout mice. Behav Brain Res 2007;178:123–7.
20. Kendler KS, Gardner CO, Lichtenstein P. A developmental twin study of symptoms of anxiety and depression: evidence for genetic innovation and attenuation. Psychol Med 2008;38:1567–75.
21. Hallett V, Ronald A, Rijsdijk F, et al. Phenotypic and genetic differentiation of anxiety-related behaviors in middle childhood. Depress Anxiety 2009;26: 316–24.
22. Lee YS, Hwang J, Kim SJ, et al. Decreased blood flow of temporal regions of the brain in subjects with panic disorder. J Psychiatr Res 2006;40:528–34.
23. Engel K, Bandelow B, Gruber O, et al. Neuroimaging in anxiety disorders. J Neural Transm 2009;116:703–16.
24. Pfleiderer B, Zinkirciran S, Arolt V, et al. fMRI amygdala activation during a spontaneous panic attack in a patient with panic disorder. World J Biol Psychiatry 2007;8:269–72.
25. Maddock RJ, Buonocore MH, Kile SJ, et al. Brain regions showing increased activation by threat-related words in panic disorder. Neuroreport 2003;14: 325–8.
26. van den Heuvel OA, Veltman DJ, Groenewegen HJ, et al. Disorder-specific neuroanatomical correlates of attentional bias in obsessive-compulsive disorder, panic disorder, and hypochondriasis. Arch Gen Psychiatry 2005;62. 922–33.
27. Bystritsky A, Pontillo D, Powers M, et al. Functional MRI changes during panic anticipation and imagery exposure. Neuroreport 2001;12:3953–7.
28. Pillay SS, Gruber SA, Rogowska J, et al. fMRI of tearful facial affect recognition in panic disorder: the cingulate gyrus-amygdala connection. J Affect Disord 2006; 94:173–81.
29. Malizia AL, Cunningham VJ, Bell CJ, et al. Decreased brain GABA(A)-benzodiazepine receptor binding in panic disorder: preliminary results from a quantitative PET study. Arch Gen Psychiatry 1998;55:715–20.
30. Bremner JD, Innis RB, Southwick SM, et al. Decreased benzodiazepine receptor binding in prefrontal cortex in combat-related posttraumatic stress disorder. Am J Psychiatry 2000;157:1120–6.
31. Bremner JD, Innis RB, White T, et al. SPECT [I-123]iomazenil measurement of the benzodiazepine receptor in panic disorder. Biol Psychiatry 2000;47: 96–106.
32. Kaschka W, Feistel H, Ebert D. Reduced benzodiazepine receptor binding in panic disorders measured by iomazenil SPECT. J Psychiatr Res 1995;29: 427–34.
33. Goddard AW, Mason GF, Appel M, et al. Impaired GABA neuronal response to acute benzodiazepine administration in panic disorder. Am J Psychiatry 2004; 161:2186–93.
34. Ham BJ, Sung Y, Kim N, et al. Decreased GABA levels in anterior cingulate and basal ganglia in medicated subjects with panic disorder: a proton magnetic resonance spectroscopy (1H-MRS) study. Prog Neuropsychopharmacol Biol Psychiatry 2007;31:403–11.
35. Kent JM, Mathew SJ, Gorman JM. Molecular targets in the treatment of anxiety. Biol Psychiatry 2002;52:1008–30.

36. Helton DR, Tizzano JP, Monn JA, et al. Anxiolytic and side-effect profile of LY354740: a potent, highly selective, orally active agonist for group II metabotropic glutamate receptors. J Pharmacol Exp Ther 1998;284:651–60.

37. Cortese BM, Phan KL. The role of glutamate in anxiety and related disorders. CNS Spectr 2005;10:820–30.

38. Pull CB, Damsa C. Pharmacotherapy of panic disorder. Neuropsychiatr Dis Treat 2008;4:779–95.

39. Vaswani M, Linda FK, Ramesh S. Role of selective serotonin reuptake inhibitors in psychiatric disorders: a comprehensive review. Prog Neuropsychopharmacol Biol Psychiatry 2003;27:85–102.

40. Neumeister A, Young T, Stastny J. Implications of genetic research on the role of the serotonin in depression: emphasis on the serotonin type 1A receptor and the serotonin transporter. Psychopharmacology (Berl) 2004;174:512–24.

41. Unschuld PG, Ising M, Erhardt A, et al. Polymorphisms in the galanin gene are associated with symptom-severity in female patients suffering from panic disorder. J Affect Disord 2008;105:177–84.

42. Abelson JL, Khan S, Liberzon I, et al. HPA axis activity in patients with panic disorder: review and synthesis of four studies. Depress Anxiety 2007;24: 66–76.

43. Hettema JM, Neale MC, Kendler KS. A review and meta-analysis of the genetic epidemiology of anxiety disorders. Am J Psychiatry 2001;158:1568–78.

44. Hettema JM, Prescott CA, Myers JM, et al. The structure of genetic and environmental risk factors for anxiety disorders in men and women. Arch Gen Psychiatry 2005;62:182–9.

45. Smoller JW, Gardner-Schuster E, Covino J. The genetic basis of panic and phobic anxiety disorders. Am J Med Genet C Semin Med Genet 2008;148: 118–26.

46. Finn CT, Smoller JW. The genetics of panic disorder. Curr Psychiatry Rep 2001;3: 131–7.

47. Fyer AJ, Hamilton SP, Durner M, et al. A third-pass genome scan in panic disorder: evidence for multiple susceptibility loci. Biol Psychiatry 2006;60:388–401.

48. Lesch KP, Bengel D, Heils A, et al. Association of anxiety-related traits with a polymorphism in the serotonin transporter gene regulatory region. Science 1996;274:1527–31.

49. Strug LJ, Suresh R, Fyer AJ, et al. Panic disorder is associated with the serotonin transporter gene (SLC6A4) but not the promoter region (5-HTTLPR). Mol Psychiatry 2008.

50. Keck ME, Kern N, Erhardt A, et al. Combined effects of exonic polymorphisms in CRHR1 and AVPR1B genes in a case/control study for panic disorder. Am J Med Genet B Neuropsychiatr Genet 2008;147B:1196–204.

51. Hodges LM, Weissman MM, Haghighi F, et al. Association and linkage analysis of candidate genes GRP, GRPR, CRHR1, and TACR1 in panic disorder. Am J Med Genet B Neuropsychiatr Genet 2009;150B:65–73.

52. Bryant RA, Felmingham K, Kemp A, et al. Amygdala and ventral anterior cingulate activation predicts treatment response to cognitive behaviour therapy for post-traumatic stress disorder. Psychol Med 2008;38:555–61.

53. Dickie EW, Brunet A, Akerib V, et al. An fMRI investigation of memory encoding in PTSD: influence of symptom severity. Neuropsychologia 2008;46:1522–31.

54. Bryant RA, Felmingham K, Whitford TJ, et al. Rostral anterior cingulate volume predicts treatment response to cognitive-behavioural therapy for posttraumatic stress disorder. J Psychiatry Neurosci 2008;33:142–6.

55. Morey RA, Petty CM, Cooper DA, et al. Neural systems for executive and emotional processing are modulated by symptoms of posttraumatic stress disorder in Iraq war veterans. Psychiatry Res 2008;162:59–72.

56. Falconer E, Bryant R, Felmingham KL, et al. The neural networks of inhibitory control in posttraumatic stress disorder. J Psychiatry Neurosci 2008;33:413–22.

57. Strawn JR, Geracioti TD Jr. Noradrenergic dysfunction and the psychopharmacology of posttraumatic stress disorder. Depress Anxiety 2008;25:260–71.

58. Pervanidou P. Biology of post-traumatic stress disorder in childhood and adolescence. J Neuroendocrinol 2008;20:632–8.

59. Hurlemann R. Noradrenergic-glucocorticoid mechanisms in emotion-induced amnesia: from adaptation to disease. Psychopharmacology (Berl) 2008;197: 13–23.

60. Marshall RD, Schneier FR, Fallon BA, et al. An open trial of paroxetine in patients with noncombat-related, chronic posttraumatic stress disorder. J Clin Psychopharmacol 1998;18:10–8.

61. Committee on Treatment of Posttraumatic Stress Disorder, Institute of Medicine. Treatment of posttraumatic stress disorder: an assessment of the evidence. Washington (DC): National Academies Press; 2008.

62. Yehuda R, Brand S, Yang RK. Plasma neuropeptide Y concentrations in combat exposed veterans: relationship to trauma exposure, recovery from PTSD, and coping. Biol Psychiatry 2006;59:660–3.

63. Yehuda R. Biology of posttraumatic stress disorder. J Clin Psychiatry 2001; 62(17):41–6.

64. Yehuda R, Giller EL, Southwick SM, et al. Hypothalamic-pituitary-adrenal dysfunction in posttraumatic stress disorder. Biol Psychiatry 1991;30:1031–48.

65. de Kloet CS, Vermetten E, Geuze E, et al. Assessment of HPA-axis function in posttraumatic stress disorder: pharmacological and non-pharmacological challenge tests, a review. J Psychiatr Res 2006;40:550–67.

66. Risbrough VB, Stein MB. Role of corticotropin releasing factor in anxiety disorders: a translational research perspective. Horm Behav 2006;50:550–61.

67. Fossey MD, Lydiard RB, Ballenger JC, et al. Cerebrospinal fluid corticotropin-releasing factor concentrations in patients with anxiety disorders and normal comparison subjects. Biol Psychiatry 1996;39:703–7.

68. Nutt DJ. Neurobiological mechanisms in generalized anxiety disorder. J Clin Psychiatry 2001;62(11):22–7 [discussion: 28].

69. Yehuda R, Southwick SM, Nussbaum G, et al. Low urinary cortisol excretion in patients with posttraumatic stress disorder. J Nerv Ment Dis 1990;178:366–9.

70. Olff M, Guzelcan Y, de Vries GJ, et al. HPA- and HPT-axis alterations in chronic posttraumatic stress disorder. Psychoneuroendocrinology 2006;31:1220–30.

71. Rasmusson AM, Lipschitz DS, Wang S, et al. Increased pituitary and adrenal reactivity in premenopausal women with posttraumatic stress disorder. Biol Psychiatry 2001;50:965–77.

72. Lipschitz DS, Rasmusson AM, Yehuda R, et al. Salivary cortisol responses to dexamethasone in adolescents with posttraumatic stress disorder. J Am Acad Child Adolesc Psychiatry 2003;42:1310–7.

73. Baker DG, Ekhator NN, Kasckow JW, et al. Plasma and cerebrospinal fluid interleukin-6 concentrations in posttraumatic stress disorder. Neuroimmunomodulation 2001;9:209–17.

74. Bremner JD, Licinio J, Darnell A, et al. Elevated CSF corticotropin-releasing factor concentrations in posttraumatic stress disorder. Am J Psychiatry 1997; 154:624–9.

75. Smith MA, Davidson J, Ritchie JC, et al. The corticotropin-releasing hormone test in patients with posttraumatic stress disorder. Biol Psychiatry 1989;26:349–55.
76. Yehuda R, Halligan SL, Grossman R, et al. The cortisol and glucocorticoid receptor response to low dose dexamethasone administration in aging combat veterans and holocaust survivors with and without posttraumatic stress disorder. Biol Psychiatry 2002;52:393–403.
77. Kudler H, Davidson J, Meador K, et al. The DST and posttraumatic stress disorder. Am J Psychiatry 1987;144:1068–71.
78. Raison CL, Miller AH. When not enough is too much: the role of insufficient glucocorticoid signaling in the pathophysiology of stress-related disorders. Am J Psychiatry 2003;160:1554–65.
79. Segman RH, Shalev AY. Genetics of posttraumatic stress disorder. CNS Spectr 2003;8:693–8.
80. Yehuda R, Halligan SL, Bierer LM. Relationship of parental trauma exposure and PTSD to PTSD, depressive and anxiety disorders in offspring. J Psychiatr Res 2001;35:261–70.
81. Yehuda R, Halligan SL, Grossman R. Childhood trauma and risk for PTSD: relationship to intergenerational effects of trauma, parental PTSD, and cortisol excretion. Dev Psychopathol 2001;13:733–53.
82. Koenen KC, Lyons MJ, Goldberg J, et al. A high risk twin study of combat-related PTSD comorbidity. Twin Res 2003;6:218–26.
83. Stein MB, Jang KL, Taylor S, et al. Genetic and environmental influences on trauma exposure and posttraumatic stress disorder symptoms: a twin study. Am J Psychiatry 2002;159:1675–81.
84. Heils A, Teufel A, Petri S, et al. Allelic variation of human serotonin transporter gene expression. J Neurochem 1996;66:2621–4.
85. Caspi A, Sugden K, Moffitt TE, et al. Influence of life stress on depression: moderation by a polymorphism in the 5-HTT gene. Science 2003;301:386–9.
86. Eley TC, Sugden K, Corsico A, et al. Gene-environment interaction analysis of serotonin system markers with adolescent depression. Mol Psychiatry 2004;9: 908–15.
87. Grabe HJ, Lange M, Wolff B, et al. Mental and physical distress is modulated by a polymorphism in the 5-HT transporter gene interacting with social stressors and chronic disease burden. Mol Psychiatry 2005;10:220–4.
88. Kaufman J, Yang BZ, Douglas-Palumberi H, et al. Social supports and serotonin transporter gene moderate depression in maltreated children. Proc Natl Acad Sci U S A 2004;101:17316–21.
89. Kendler KS, Kuhn JW, Vittum J, et al. The interaction of stressful life events and a serotonin transporter polymorphism in the prediction of episodes of major depression: a replication. Arch Gen Psychiatry 2005;62:529–35.
90. Gillespie NA, Whitfield JB, Williams B, et al. The relationship between stressful life events, the serotonin transporter (5-HTTLPR) genotype and major depression. Psychol Med 2005;35:101–11.
91. Kaufman J, Yang BZ, Douglas-Palumberi H, et al. Brain-derived neurotrophic factor-5-HTTLPR gene interactions and environmental modifiers of depression in children. Biol Psychiatry 2006;59:673–80.
92. Kilpatrick DG, Koenen KC, Ruggiero KJ, et al. The serotonin transporter genotype and social support and moderation of posttraumatic stress disorder and depression in hurricane-exposed adults. Am J Psychiatry 2007;164:1693–9.
93. Ladd CO, Huot RL, Thrivikraman KV, et al. Long-term behavioral and neuroendocrine adaptations to adverse early experience. Prog Brain Res 2000;122:81–103.

94. Plotsky PM, Thrivikraman KV, Nemeroff CB, et al. Long-term consequences of neonatal rearing on central corticotropin-releasing factor systems in adult male rat offspring. Neuropsychopharmacology 2005;30:2192–204.
95. Bradley RG, Binder EB, Epstein MP, et al. Influence of child abuse on adult depression: moderation by the corticotropin-releasing hormone receptor gene. Arch Gen Psychiatry 2008;65:190–200.
96. Binder EB, Bradley RG, Liu W, et al. Association of FKBP5 polymorphisms and childhood abuse with risk of posttraumatic stress disorder symptoms in adults. JAMA 2008;299:1291–305.
97. Davies TH, Ning YM, Sanchez ER. A new first step in activation of steroid receptors: hormone-induced switching of FKBP51 and FKBP52 immunophilins. J Biol Chem 2002;277:4597–600.
98. Denny WB, Valentine DL, Reynolds PD, et al. Squirrel monkey immunophilin FKBP51 is a potent inhibitor of glucocorticoid receptor binding. Endocrinology 2000;141:4107–13.
99. Wochnik GM, Ruegg J, Abel GA, et al. FK506-binding proteins 51 and 52 differentially regulate dynein interaction and nuclear translocation of the glucocorticoid receptor in mammalian cells. J Biol Chem 2005;280:4609–16.
100. Binder EB, Salyakina D, Lichtner P, et al. Polymorphisms in FKBP5 are associated with increased recurrence of depressive episodes and rapid response to antidepressant treatment. Nat Genet 2004;36:1319–25.
101. Newport DJ, Heim C, Bonsall R, et al. Pituitary-adrenal responses to standard and low-dose dexamethasone suppression tests in adult survivors of child abuse. Biol Psychiatry 2004;55:10–20.
102. Yehuda R, Golier JA, Halligan SL, et al. The ACTH response to dexamethasone in PTSD. Am J Psychiatry 2004;161:1397–403.
103. Segman RH, Shefi N, Goltser-Dubner T, et al. Peripheral blood mononuclear cell gene expression profiles identify emergent post-traumatic stress disorder among trauma survivors. Mol Psychiatry 2005;10:500–13, 425.
104. Koenen KC, Saxe G, Purcell S, et al. Polymorphisms in FKBP5 are associated with peritraumatic dissociation in medically injured children. Mol Psychiatry 2005;10:1058–9.
105. Ozer EJ, Best SR, Lipsey TL, et al. Predictors of posttraumatic stress disorder and symptoms in adults: a meta-analysis. Psychol Bull 2003;129:52–73.
106. Kilts CD, Kelsey JE, Knight B, et al. The neural correlates of social anxiety disorder and response to pharmacotherapy. Neuropsychopharmacology 2006;31:2243–53.
107. Stein MB, Stein DJ. Social anxiety disorder. Lancet 2008;371:1115–25.
108. Hood S, Potokar J, Davies S, et al. Dopaminergic challenges in social anxiety disorder: evidence for dopamine D3 desensitisation following successful treatment with serotonergic antidepressants. J Psychopharmacol 2008; Oct 6. [Epub ahead of print].
109. Condren RM, O'Neill A, Ryan MC, et al. HPA axis response to a psychological stressor in generalised social phobia. Psychoneuroendocrinology 2002;27:693–703.
110. Roelofs K, van Peer J, Berretty E, et al. Hypothalamus-pituitary-adrenal axis hyperresponsiveness is associated with increased social avoidance behavior in social phobia. Biol Psychiatry 2009;65:336–43.
111. van Veen JF, van Vliet IM, Derijk RH, et al. Elevated alpha-amylase but not cortisol in generalized social anxiety disorder. Psychoneuroendocrinology 2008;33:1313–21.

112. Martel FL, Hayward C, Lyons DM, et al. Salivary cortisol levels in socially phobic adolescent girls. Depress Anxiety 1999;10:25–7.
113. De Bellis MD, Keshavan MS, Shifflett H, et al. Superior temporal gyrus volumes in pediatric generalized anxiety disorder. Biol Psychiatry 2002;51:553–62.
114. Monk CS, Nelson EE, McClure EB, et al. Ventrolateral prefrontal cortex activation and attentional bias in response to angry faces in adolescents with generalized anxiety disorder. Am J Psychiatry 2006;163:1091–7.
115. Mathew SJ, Mao X, Coplan JD, et al. Dorsolateral prefrontal cortical pathology in generalized anxiety disorder: a proton magnetic resonance spectroscopic imaging study. Am J Psychiatry 2004;161:1119–21.
116. Herry C, Ciocchi S, Senn V, et al. Switching on and off fear by distinct neuronal circuits. Nature 2008;454:600–6.
117. Izumi T, Inoue T, Kato A, et al. Changes in amygdala neural activity that occur with the extinction of context-dependent conditioned fear stress. Pharmacol Biochem Behav 2008;90:297–304.
118. Davis M, Walker DL, Myers KM. Role of the amygdala in fear extinction measured with potentiated startle. Ann N Y Acad Sci 2003;985:218–32.
119. Anand A, Shekhar A. Brain imaging studies in mood and anxiety disorders: special emphasis on the amygdala. Ann N Y Acad Sci 2003;985:370–88.
120. Rauch SL, Shin LM, Wright CI. Neuroimaging studies of amygdala function in anxiety disorders. Ann N Y Acad Sci 2003;985:389–410.
121. Monk CS, Telzer EH, Mogg K, et al. Amygdala and ventrolateral prefrontal cortex activation to masked angry faces in children and adolescents with generalized anxiety disorder. Arch Gen Psychiatry 2008;65:568–76.
122. McClure EB, Adler A, Monk CS, et al. fMRI predictors of treatment outcome in pediatric anxiety disorders. Psychopharmacology (Berl) 2007;191:97–105.
123. Whalen PJ, Johnstone T, Somerville LH, et al. A functional magnetic resonance imaging predictor of treatment response to venlafaxine in generalized anxiety disorder. Biol Psychiatry 2008;63:858–63.
124. Nemeroff CB. The role of GABA in the pathophysiology and treatment of anxiety disorders. Psychopharmacol Bull 2003;37:133–46.
125. Mathew SJ, Amiel JM, Coplan JD, et al. Open-label trial of riluzole in generalized anxiety disorder. Am J Psychiatry 2005;162:2379–81.
126. Pittenger C, Coric V, Banasr M, et al. Riluzole in the treatment of mood and anxiety disorders. CNS Drugs 2008;22:761–86.
127. Maron E, Kuikka JT, Ulst K, et al. SPECT imaging of serotonin transporter binding in patients with generalized anxiety disorder. Eur Arch Psychiatry Clin Neurosci 2004;254:392–6.
128. Malison RT, Price LH, Berman R, et al. Reduced brain serotonin transporter availability in major depression as measured by [123I]-2 beta-carbomethoxy-3 beta-(4-iodophenyl)tropane and single photon emission computed tomography. Biol Psychiatry 1998;44:1090–8.
129. Koszycki D, Copen J, Bradwejn J. Sensitivity to cholecystokinin-tetrapeptide in major depression. J Affect Disord 2004;80:285–90.
130. Brawman-Mintzer O, Lydiard RB, Bradwejn J, et al. Effects of the cholecystokinin agonist pentagastrin in patients with generalized anxiety disorder. Am J Psychiatry 1997;154:700–2.
131. Pande AC, Greiner M, Adams JB, et al. Placebo-controlled trial of the CCK-B antagonist, CI-988, in panic disorder. Biol Psychiatry 1999;46:860–2.
132. Heilig M. The NPY system in stress, anxiety and depression. Neuropeptides 2004;38:213–24.

133. Sajdyk TJ, Shekhar A, Gehlert DR. Interactions between NPY and CRF in the amygdala to regulate emotionality. Neuropeptides 2004;38:225–34.
134. Lelas S, Wong H, Li YW, et al. Anxiolytic-like effects of the corticotropin-releasing factor1 (CRF1) antagonist DMP904 [4-(3-pentylamino)-2,7-dimethyl-8-(2-methyl-4-methoxyphenyl)-pyrazolo-[1,5-a]-pyrimidine] administered acutely or chronically at doses occupying central CRF1 receptors in rats. J Pharmacol Exp Ther 2004;309:293–302.
135. Millan MJ, Brocco M, Gobert A, et al. Anxiolytic properties of the selective, non-peptidergic CRF(1) antagonists, CP154,526 and DMP695: a comparison to other classes of anxiolytic agent. Neuropsychopharmacology 2001;25:585–600.
136. Chaki S, Nakazato A, Kennis L, et al. Anxiolytic- and antidepressant-like profile of a new CRF1 receptor antagonist, R278995/CRA0450. Eur J Pharmacol 2004; 485:145–58.
137. Holsboer F, Ising M. Central CRH system in depression and anxiety—evidence from clinical studies with CRH1 receptor antagonists. Eur J Pharmacol 2008;583:350–7.
138. Ninan PT. Recent perspectives on the diagnosis and treatment of generalized anxiety disorder. Am J Manag Care 2001;7:S367–76.
139. Hettema JM, Prescott CA, Kendler KS. A population-based twin study of generalized anxiety disorder in men and women. J Nerv Ment Dis 2001;189:413–20.
140. Tadic A, Rujescu D, Szegedi A, et al. Association of a MAOA gene variant with generalized anxiety disorder, but not with panic disorder or major depression. Am J Med Genet B Neuropsychiatr Genet 2003;117B:1–6.
141. You JS, Hu SY, Chen B, et al. Serotonin transporter and tryptophan hydroxylase gene polymorphisms in Chinese patients with generalized anxiety disorder. Psychiatr Genet 2005;15:7–11.
142. Koenen KC, Amstadter AB, Ruggiero KJ, et al. RGS2 and generalized anxiety disorder in an epidemiologic sample of hurricane-exposed adults. Depress Anxiety 2009;26:309–15.

Specific Phobias

Alfons O. Hamm, PhD

KEYWORDS

- Phobias • Fear • Exposure therapy • Behavior therapy
- Conditioning • Relaxation

What was called phobic disorders (phobic neurosis) in the past has been split in the Diagnostic and Statistical Manual of Mental Disorders, Revised Third Edition (DSM-III-R) and later in Diagnostic and Statistical Manual of Mental Disorders, Fourth Edition (DSM-IV) into descriptively and phenomenologically three different groups of phobias:

Agoraphobia (not a codable disorder)
Social anxiety disorder
Specific phobias

The latter were further subtyped into animal type, blood injection injury type, situational type, and natural environment type. All phobic disorders essentially share the same set of criteria despite minor differences in the description of criteria It is unclear, however, whether the differences are essential and well grounded or accidentally different.[1] Overall, phobic disorders and particularly specific phobias are characterized by marked and persistent fear cued by a specific object or situation accompanied by the compelling desire to avoid such object or situation. There is general consensus among experts that systematic exposure to the feared object or situation is the method of choice for treating specific phobias. Despite this consensus, there is also consensus that only a very small percentage of those who suffer from specific phobias receive this form of treatment.[2]

EXPOSURE-BASED THERAPIES

Joseph Wolpe, the pioneer of behavior therapy, took this view when he developed the systematic desensitization, the first behaviorally oriented approach for treating specific phobias. During systematic desensitization, patients are confronted with their feared situation in sensu (ie, they are instructed to imagine the fearful objects or situations with increasing intensity or proximity of the threat). Systematic empirical research, however, not only has questioned the mechanisms of change of systematic desensitization postulated by Wolpe[3] but also proven to be less clinically effective than exposure to the feared situation in reality. As a consequence of these developments, systematic desensitization has fallen out of favor, and behavior therapy of

Department of Clinical Psychology, University of Greifswald, Franz-Mehring-Strasse 47, D-17487 Greifswald, Germany
E-mail address: hamm@uni-greifswald.de

Psychiatr Clin N Am 32 (2009) 577–591
doi:10.1016/j.psc.2009.05.008
0193-953X/09/$ – see front matter © 2009 Elsevier Inc. All rights reserved.

specific phobias has shifted to exposure in vivo, in which patients are confronted with their feared situations or objects in reality (eg, patients are encouraged to approach and touch the feared animal until the fear subsides,[4] or patients climb the highest building in the area together with the therapist and practice standing at the top without touching the railings).[5]

Exposure in Vivo

Exposure in vivo therapy of specific phobias normally comprises three different phases.

1. Instruction phase. Here patients first will be given a plausible model of their phobia and an explanation why their phobic fear was maintained for such long period of time. Patients will be instructed that one reason for the maintenance of their phobia might be that they never confronted themselves with the feared situation or object, and if they were courageous enough to do so occasionally they probably escaped at the peak of their fear, further strengthening the phobia. The therapist then explains the mechanisms of change. During exposure training the patient will stay in the feared situation as long as she/he recognizes that the fear will not increase to an inestimable point and that the fear ultimately will fade away. The patient will be instructed further that therapy is always teamwork and that the therapist never will do anything in treatment before describing it to the patient, modeling it, and getting the patient's permission.[6]
2. Direct exposure in vivo. During the exposure session, the therapist always first announces each exercise, models it, and then asks the patient to practice her/himself. The patient should approach the feared object from as close as possible and stay in this position until the fear completely disappears or is reduced by at least 50%. The average duration of such exposure sessions varies between 2 (for animal-type phobias) to 3 (for height phobia) hours.
3. Maintenance of treatment results. The patient is informed to continue to practice at home using self-exposure techniques. Moreover, the patient is instructed what to do in case of a setback.[7]

Exposure in Virtual Reality

With the increasing availability of virtual reality technology, treatment of specific phobias has used computer-generated interactive virtual environments. Exposure to the feared situation in a virtual reality especially was developed for treating flying phobia and height phobia,[8,9] where it is sometimes difficult to realize an environment for in vivo exposure.[10]

Efficacy of Exposure-based Therapies

In a recent meta-analysis, Wolitzky-Taylor and colleagues[11] conducted a literature search for treatment studies published between 1966 and 2007 and extracted 33 studies that fulfilled the criteria of using a randomized clinical trial with patients meeting full DSM criteria. The trials also reported phobia-specific outcome measures. Meeting these criteria were 33 studies, including 90 treatments administered to 1193 patients. Similarly, Choy and colleagues[12] did a literature search for treatment studies published between 1960 and 2005 and selected 31 studies that:

> Included at least two groups (without the criterion of being a randomized controlled trial [RCT])

Investigated clinically diagnosed phobia patients (excluding all studies with analog samples)

And reported behavioral or self report outcome measures

Although using comparable Internet search engines, there was only little correspondence (only seven studies were listed in both reviews) between the studies selected for both reviews. (One thousand twenty-six patients who had flight phobia were treated with the standardized cognitive behavior therapy [CBT] training program from 1994 to 1999 by the group at the University of Leiden in the Netherlands [Van Gerwen and colleagues, 2002].) The conclusions that can be drawn from the meta-analysis and the narrative review are very clear.

Exposure-based therapies result in significantly better outcome after treatment irrespective of whether assessed by verbal report measures or by behavioral avoidance test (BAT) relative to the wait list control condition.[11,12] The overall between-group effect size for this comparison is d = 1.05 and is comparable for behavioral measures and questionnaire data. In the group of patients who had specific phobia animal type, 92% of the patients treated with in vivo exposure compared with 0% of the wait list control were able to perform the terminal task in the BAT.[5,13,14] Comparable percentages were reported for patients with either height or driving phobia (87% of the treated patients completed the terminal task of the BAT) and claustrophobia (79% completers). Choy and colleagues[12] found 16 studies In their review, which investigated outcome measures in a follow-up period ranging from 6 to 14 months and found stable treatment effects for the treatment of animal phobia, height phobia, flight phobia, and claustrophobia. Some studies even found an increase in the treatment, while other studies did not find any further improvement compared with postmeasures. Overall one could state that exposure-based therapies are highly effective and produce stable improvement in self-reported fear and behavioral avoidance. What remains under debate is not the efficacy of such treatment but what are the active ingredients of the therapy and what are the mechanisms of change. Answering these questions has important implications for precisely tailoring exposure therapy to the individual case.

Active Ingredients of Exposure-based Therapies

Five studies compared in vivo exposure therapy with explicit placebo conditions. In these placebo treatments, patients were informed that these interventions would help them to overcome their phobia to explicitly induce positive expectations or a placebo effect. For example, patients were informed that messages would be presented subliminally to reduce their fears while they watched a nature film, or patients received pulsed audiophotic stimulation with the instruction that this device would relax them. Again, exposure therapy was overall more effective relative to such placebo interventions, although the effect sizes were lower for post-treatment measures compared with the wait list control condition but substantially increased for the comparisons of the follow-up assessments (average length of follow-up assessment was about 5 to 6 months in this meta-analysis). Several studies compared the efficacy of different modalities of exposure. It generally is assumed that exposure in vivo is more effective than systematic desensitization.[15] The empirical basis for this conclusion, however, is very sparse, because only two studies directly compared in vivo exposure versus systematic desensitization (methodological difficulties such as differences in duration or pace of exposure or other adjuvants might explain why there are only so few studies[16]) and found in vivo exposure to produce better outcome than systematic desensitization in patients who had animal type and situational type phobias.[13,17] On the other hand, if relaxation is omitted, imaginal exposure can be used effectively for treating specific phobias animal type.[18,19] These data show that exposure in sensu can be effective if it is possible to evoke the fear response during imagery, which might explain why exposure in sensu is less effective in patients who have agoraphobia.[20,21] In these patients, imagery of the most feared situation does not result in any substantial physiological fear response (despite strong verbal reports of fear experience), while patients who have specific animal type phobia exhibit a clear physiological fear response during imagery of their most feared situation.[22] I will come back to these findings when I discuss the possible mechanisms of change during exposure-based therapy.

Four studies compared in vivo exposure with exposure therapy in virtual reality. There is evidence that exposure therapies using virtual reality are more effective compared with the wait list control for treating height[23] and flying phobias.[9,24,25] Two studies compared virtual reality with in vivo exposure and found virtual reality to be equally effective irrespective of whether verbal report measures or behavioral tests (taking a graduation flight) were taken as outcome measures,[23,24] particularly at follow-up assessment.[11] Data from Mühlberger and colleagues, however, suggest that including in vivo exposure (eg, taking a graduation flight) increases the long-term effects of exposure therapy in virtual reality. Completion of the graduation flight was a strong predictor for long-term treatment efficacy.

Based on a review of 25 controlled treatment studies of specific phobias (with 800 patients and 150 control subjects), including many conducted at his own institution, Öst[26] concluded that one-session in vivo exposure is the treatment of choice for specific phobias. Across different types of phobias, such individual single-session treatment results in a clinically significant improvement (eg, an improvement of 2 SDs relative to the mean symptom score of the patient population) in 77% to 95% of the patients. What is also noteworthy is that the average duration of such treatment varies between 1.9 and 3.5 hours. **Table 1** gives an overview of these results.

These data would be in line with findings from exposure treatments of agoraphobia, where massed exposure (daily exposure) was found to be superior to spaced (one session per week) exposure sessions.[27,28] On the other hand, there are also studies that did not find any difference between massed (daily) and spaced (weekly) exposure.[29] More importantly, these studies did not evaluate long-term follow-up, where the benefit of spaced exposure sessions theoretically would be expected (see mechanisms of change). Accordingly, the more recent meta-analysis by Wolitzky-Taylor and colleagues[11] did not find a difference between single- and multiple-session exposure treatment of specific phobias after treatment but an overall larger effect size for multiple session exposure treatment at follow-up assessment at least for reported

Table 1
Duration of the exposure in vivo and proportion of patients who are clinically significantly improved

Type of Phobia	Treatment Method	Clinically Significantly Improved (%)	Mean Duration (Hours)
Snake phobia	Participant modeling	87	1.9
Spider phobia	Exposition in vivo	89	2.1
Blood injury phobia	Exposition in vivo + applied tension training	80	2.0
Claustrophobia	Exposition in vivo	80	3.0
Height phobia	Guided mastery	77	3.5
Flying phobia	Exposure in vivo	94	3.0

symptoms. This difference was not caused by return of fear for the single-session treatment but rather by continued improvement in the multiple session treatment. One should be cautious, however, to draw too strong conclusions, because the empirical basis for a clear decision for either single- of multiple-session treatment remains meager. Moreover, there are studies suggesting that exposure training might be more effective if exposure sessions are conducted in different contexts. Vansteenwegen and colleagues[30] compared physiological fear responses with video clips of spiders after viewing these clips either at the same or at different locations and found reduced renewal responses for those phobia patients who made the exposure experience at different locations. In the same vein, better treatment effects were found, if not only one (eg, a single animal) but variable phobic objects or situations were used for exposure treatment.[31,32] Again, more clinical studies are needed for systematically evaluating the effects of different modalities of exposure therapy.

Another important issue regarding the active ingredients of exposure-based therapies is the degree of therapist involvement. There is evidence mainly from research with agoraphobia patients that self-exposure is as effective (although the drop-out rate is higher) as therapist-aided exposure.[16,33] For treating specific phobias, however, pure self-exposure seems to be less effective than therapist-directed in vivo exposure. In a larger study, 103 patients who had spider phobia first were instructed to practice self-exposure using a self-help manual that was handed to them. Only 16 of the 103 patients showed a significant improvement after this stage of treatment; 38 patients dropped out. The remaining patients received a video clip of a successful exposure therapy and were instructed to proceed with their self-exposure as was demonstrated on the video. Five patients showed benefit from this intervention, and another patient dropped out. In the next step, therapist-directed exposure training was conducted in a group sessions (with four patients each). Twenty-six patients benefited from this intervention, and five patients dropped out at this stage. The remaining 12 patients received therapist-guided individual exposure therapy, and all patients showed a clinically significant improvement; not a single patient dropped out.[34] These data demonstrate that therapist-guided exposure cannot be replaced easily by more economic approaches like Internet-based interventions that are being discussed, at least not for the treatment of specific phobia. Although self-exposure might not be as effective as therapist-guided exposure to induce therapeutic changes, it might be important for maintaining acute treatment gains.[35] Most treatment studies report follow-up data from a period between 6 months and 1 year. Studies with a longer follow-up period are scarce. Two studies of dental phobia did follow up assessments after 5[36] and 10 years[37] and found that treatment gains were maintained across such a long period of time. In contrast, data from Lipsitz and colleagues[38] suggest that relapse rates are rather high for such long periods of time. Therefore, it remains important to better understand those factors that contribute to the stability of the treatment effects that can be achieved by exposure in vivo training.

PHARMACOTHERAPY

There is general consensus that medication provides little to no benefit for treating specific phobias.[39] Five studies investigated the effect of benzodiazepines or sedatives for treating dental and flying phobias and found that although benzodiazepines effectively reduced subjective fear before the flight or dental treatment, phobic fear even increased at the beginning of a second flight in the medicated group and returned to baseline for dental fear after 3 months.[40,41] Studies testing the effects of general anesthesia of nitrous oxide for treating dental fear also found that this medication can facilitate dental treatment, but avoidance rates for further dental treatment were significantly higher than for those patients treated with exposure therapy.[12] There is almost no research on the effect of antidepressants for treating specific phobias. There are, however, recent data from Ressler and colleagues[42] demonstrating that D-cycloserine (DCS), a partial agonist at the N-methyl-D-asparate (NMDA) glutaminergic receptor, can be used as a cognitive enhancer during exposure-based learning. Therefore, it can increase the effectiveness of exposure therapy. In this study, 28 participants who had clinically diagnosed height phobia were treated with two weekly sessions of 35 to 45 minutes exposure in a virtual reality environment. Seventeen patients received 50 or 500 mg DCS before exposure therapy, while 10 patients received identical placebo capsules. DCS significantly improved exposure treatment effects on all outcome measures. These facilitating effects of DCS for exposure-based therapies recently also were demonstrated for treating social phobia,[43] and several trials for testing the enhancing effect of DCS for treating agoraphobic avoidance are on their way. In an RCT of the effect of DCS on exposure therapy of spider fear in a sample of high spider fearful volunteers, DCS did not increase the effect of a single-session in vivo exposure.[44] Such an exposure therapy might, however, lead to a ceiling effect, especially in the subclinical group that was studied, preventing DCS from having any additional therapeutic impact.

COGNITIVE THERAPY

Although exposure therapies are the intervention of choice, there are some studies that have investigated cognitive therapies (eg, restructuring) as solo treatments and found comparable effects as exposure training for treating claustrophobia.[14,45] This does not come as a complete surprise, because claustrophobia particularly is characterized by cognitive symptoms and worries like being trapped or suffocating rather than increased sympathetic arousal like in animal phobia.[46] Accordingly, cognitive therapy was not helpful as an adjunctive treatment for exposure therapy of patients who had spider phobia.[47] Cognitive therapy also has been used for treating dental phobia and has been proven to be more effective than wait list control.[48] Studies investigating cognitive therapy for treating flying phobia have produced mixed results. Thus, cognitive therapies are effective for treating claustrophobia but are less effective than exposure therapy for treating animal, dental, and flying phobias.

THE INFLUENCE OF RELAXATION

According to the current status of scientific findings, isolated application of relaxation training (eg, as is done in a stress inoculation treatment) is not more effective than the wait list control condition for treating specific phobias. Therefore, relaxation training rarely has been used as an isolated treatment component but rather has been employed in combination with exposure therapy. Moreover, numerous studies have shown that the induction of relaxation is not a necessary condition for effective exposure treatment, especially during exposure in sensu.[49] Öst[50] developed a variant of a relaxation training that he called applied relaxation. In this approach, he trained patients to use their learned relaxation response as a coping skill during the exposure training in vivo. The additional effect of using this coping skill during exposure training, however, never really was tested systematically, probably also because relaxation training was not an element in the one-session treatment of specific phobia later developed by Öst and collegues.[6,51] As a consequence, another training, applied tension, later was developed and evaluated specifically for exposure treatment of blood injection phobia by this group. Here patients were trained to identify the earliest signs of bradycardia and drop in blood pressure (which are evoked during exposure in vivo) and then tensed the gross body muscles to increase blood pressure and prevent fainting. Two studies have shown that exposure in combination with applied tension is more effective than exposure training alone.[52,53] Thus, using techniques that help to better master the goal of exposure therapy might be more important for therapeutic success than reducing the fear by learning to relax. Thus the question remains: what is learned during exposure therapy? If one wants to improve treatment of specific phobias and other anxiety disorders, one needs to better understand not only the mechanisms underlying the etiology of phobias but also those processes responsible for reducing phobic fears and anxiety.

ETIOLOGY OF SPECIFIC PHOBIAS: NEW DEVELOPMENTS

Family studies suggest that there is an increased risk for specific phobias if a first-degree relative already is diagnosed with such disorder. Fyer and colleagues[54] interviewed 49 relatives of 15 patients who had specific phobia and found that 31% of these first-degree relatives also had a diagnosis of specific phobia. In a larger longitudinal study, Schreier and colleagues[55] interviewed 933 mother–child pairs. Children of those 154 mothers who were diagnosed as having a specific phobia had an elevated risk (hazard ratio was 1.3) for also developing a specific phobia. Gelernter and colleagues[56] interviewed 129 individuals from 14 families and found that 57 subjects were diagnosed as having a specific phobia. A genome-wide linkage scan suggested a region on chromosome 14 as a marker for specific phobia. The linked region contains among other things the somatostatin receptor 1 as a potential candidate for the behavioral phenotype. Results from twin studies also suggest a genetic predisposition for developing a specific phobia. The pair-wise twin concordance rate was 25% for monozygotic (MZ) twins compared with 11% for dizygotic (DZ) twins for animal phobia in the Virginia twin study.[57] Increasing reliability of the interview data by obtaining two assessments (8 years apart) of lifetime history of phobias, the heritability estimates increase to 47% for animal phobia, 59% for blood injection phobia, and 46% for situational phobia.[58] Specific phobia, however, also can be acquired by direct aversive experience with the feared object (like an intense panic-like fear response at the first contact with the feared object), clearly demonstrating the influence of the environment as a causal factor for developing specific phobias. As a result of such fear-conditioning experience, remnants of the threatening event will stick to the individual as components of the fear memories evoked by stimuli associated with the aversive event. Recent data from the author's laboratory suggest that there is not an impenetrable barrier between genes and environment but that there is a more dynamic relationship, suggesting that genes also may act through the environment. In this study, Lonsdorf and colleagues demonstrated that fear conditioning is facilitated in participants carrying the short allele of the serotonin transporter gene (5 HTTLPR) (reducing the 5-HTT expression and serotonin uptake by close to 50%[59]) while homozygosity for the met allele of the COMT gene (causing a higher dopamine level particularly in the prefrontal cortex) selectively impairs the ability to extinguish the previously conditioned fear.[60] These data suggest a dynamic interaction between genetic predisposition and the learning experience during lifetime in the development of specific phobia.

Moreover, much progress has been made to delineate the neural networks that mediate perception of phobic objects and the organization of the fear response, providing further insight in the etiology of specific phobia. Animal research and recent human brain imaging data have demonstrated that the amygdala, a limbic structure located in the anterior lobe, is the core structure involved in the learning and evocation of fear. It also orchestrates the organization of the fear response such as increase in blood pressure, tachycardia, increased vigilance and attention, and freezing and activation of the hypothalamic-pituitary-adrenal (HPA) axis.[61] Lesions of the amygdala block many measures of conditioned and unconditioned fear responses.[62] Neuroimaging researchers also consistently have found increased fMRI signal strength in the amygdala during processing of fear conditioned cues[63] and photographs of phobic objects in patients with specific phobia.[64,65] Besides the amygdala, the insular cortex is another integral part of the neural network, mediating fear relevant cues. In a recent meta-analysis of different brain imaging studies, Etkin and Wagner[66] found consistent hyperactivation in the amygdala and the anterior insula in patients who had specific phobia during processing of their phobia-related objects. Interestingly, these networks not only are activated during first-hand experience with an aversive event like in fear-conditioning situations, but also through social observation with no personal experience of the aversive event. In a study from Olsson and colleagues,[67] participants observed a movie displaying a male participant in fear-conditioning experiment. It could be demonstrated that observing the aversive learning experience of the model in the movie resulted in stronger activation of the amygdala and the anterior insula, as if the observer would make the aversive experience directly by himself or herself. Moreover, presenting the fear cues to the observer in a later test stage also evoked the same pattern of activation, demonstrating that the previous observation resulted in an acquisition of a fear response. These data clearly demonstrate that observational learning of fear relies on the same mechanisms like those involved in learning fear through direct experience. Thus phobias are not acquired only by direct aversive experience but also by observing what others have feared before, a phenomenon that has been demonstrated for the acquisition of snake phobia in primates.[68] Finally, fear also can be acquired by symbolic communication. Instructing individuals that an aversive event (eg, a painful stimulus) might follow a certain stimulus (eg, a blue square) results in robust fear responses to that stimulus.[69] Not surprisingly, the same neural network including the amygdala and the insular cortex is activated during such instructed fear[70] as during direct fear conditioning. These findings clearly demonstrate that specific phobias can be acquired either by direct experience, observing an intense fear response in others, and by communication that some objects or situations might be dangerous. These different learning experiences are mediated by the same neural network, including the amygdala and the insula, both being core elements of the fear network. Moreover, genetic predisposition seems to modulate how such learning experiences affect the neural network in the brain. Finally, epidemiological evidence from the Dunedin longitudinal study suggests that not only aversive learning experiences may shape the fear circuit in the brain, but that also early exposure to potentially fearful situations might help to immunize the fear networks in the brain. Examining the origin of fear of heights, Poulton and Menzies[71] found that individuals at age 11 or 18 who had height phobia did not experience serious falls during childhood but rather had less exposure to height stimuli early in life. These findings clearly demonstrate that learning experiences are not only relevant for the development of fears and phobias but that successful coping of such potentially fear-evoking situations might engage important learning processes for reducing phobic fear.

MECHANISMS OF CHANGE

Based on his findings from animal experimentation, Wolpe[3] postulated that the activation of an appetitive response that is antagonistic to the fear response (eg, evocation of a relaxation response in the presence of the feared cue) would engage an inhibitory learning process that he called conditioned inhibition. Because relaxation induction — as has been shown in numerous studies — is neither a sufficient nor a necessary condition for the efficacy of exposure therapy, habituation long has been considered to be the central mechanism for the effect of exposure therapy.[16,72] Habituation is a form of nonassociative learning in which a response to a stimulus that is presented repeatedly declines, because the stimulus is losing its significance to the organism with increasing repetition.[73,74] Traditionally, stimulus significance has been defined in cognitive terms such novelty or task relevance, and habituation has been explained by reduced selective attention to the repeated stimulus.[75,76] Bradley[77] recently presented a theoretical approach how stimulus significance might be conceptualized in the context of emotional cues that are used in exposure therapy. According to this view, significance of emotional stimuli can be defined in terms of valence and arousal. Although pleasant stimuli activate an appetitive motivational system favoring approach behaviors like ingestion, care giving, and others, unpleasant threatening cues (like phobic objects) activate an aversive motivational system, priming defensive behaviors like withdrawal or escape. Arousal refers to the intensity of the activation of the corresponding motivational system. Thus, defensive or appetitive motivation increases (increased energy mobilization) with increasing arousal level of the cue. Repetitive presentation of the stimulus reduces the arousal level of the emotional cue, thus decreasing the intensity of the defensive response mobilization. Indeed many studies have shown that autonomic responses evoked by the feared objects clearly decline both within but also between exposure sessions.[78,79] These findings were supported by more recent brain imaging studies that found significant reduction of the activation of the insular cortex and the anterior cingulate cortex (ACC)[80] after exposure therapy in patients who had animal phobia. Both areas are coupled with the fear-associated arousal level.[66,81] Although autonomic arousal or intensity of fear activation reliably declines during exposure therapy, there is only little evidence from clinical studies that the amount of habituation sessions within and between is related to outcome of exposure therapy.[82] Moreover, a return of fear symptoms has been noted in some patients[38,83] after complete habituation of the fear response, a phenomenon that questions the validity of habituation as the only mechanism of change. Fear renewal (in this case the fear returns if the previously feared object occurs in a new context) or reinstatement of fear (in this instance the fear response returns if the organism makes other aversive learning experiences independent of the phobia) clearly suggest an associative learning process — extinction — being an important mechanism of change during exposure therapy.[84] During extinction, the organism learns that a cue that previously has been associated with a threatening experience no longer is coupled with the painful or threatening event. During extinction learning, the organism, however, does not forget or erase the previously learned association from memory, but rather has to actively learn that the original fear stimulus no longer is coupled with the threatening event.[84] Thus, on a cognitive level, the organism has to learn new contingencies (ie, that the conditioned stimulus [CS] no longer predicts the occurrence of the unconditioned stimulus [US]), and accordingly, activation of prefrontal cortical areas (particularly the ventromedial prefrontal cortex) is observed reliably during extinction learning in brain imaging studies.[85–87] Thus, cognitive interventions during exposure therapy focusing on discussing the worst possible aversive consequences that might happen during confrontation with the feared object or situation might help to optimize extinction learning. Actively testing these predictions and violating the expectancies by the experiences made during exposure therapy might be an important ingredient of exposure-based learning. Although methodologically quite challenging, empirical studies systematically testing the effect of such interventions are very important. Moreover, patients do not learn only on a cognitive level, that the feared object no longer predicts the occurrence of an aversive experience. They also have strong feelings of relief if they master the feared situation and that the threatening event does not occur. As a consequence, these rewarding experiences change affective values of the previously feared situation or object. Interestingly, the ventromedial prefrontal cortex also shows increased activity in response to reward outcomes and in same way in response to omission of punishment.[88,89] Interestingly, increased activation in prefrontal cortical areas was observed during viewing of spider pictures in spider phobia patients showing positive long-term (6 months) improvements of exposure therapy.[90] No such increase in prefrontal activation has been found immediately at post-treatment assessment.[80] Thus, permanent changes in the affective signature of the originally feared object might take some time to develop and might activate systems in the brain that are associated with rewarding outcomes. Moreover, data from Lonsdorf and colleagues[60] suggest that extinction learning is modulated by genes that regulate the dopamine level in the prefrontal cortex. This line of research is only beginning, and future research in this area might help to better understand the mechanisms of change during exposure therapy and might finally advise clinicians how exposure therapy should be tailored to reach stable positive long-term outcome effects.

IMPLICATIONS FOR DIAGNOSTIC AND STATISTICAL MANUAL OF MENTAL DISORDERS, FIFTH EDITION

Traditionally, phobic disorders have been subdivided according to the feared objects and situations that were translated into Greek or Latin and preceded the word phobia, producing endless lists of over 500 different phobias reaching from arachnophobia to zoophobia. Although attractive for the public media who love to call on Friday the 13th to ask experts about patients who have paraskevidekatriaphobia, such lists are practically and scientifically useless. As a consequence of the *DSM-III-R*, phobias have been subdivided according clinical features such as differences in age of onset, sex ratio, symptom reports, and epidemiological differences into three groups, namely agoraphobia, social phobia, and so-called simple phobias. The definitions of agoraphobia and social phobia have changed little from the Mark's descriptions. Debate, however, has persisted whether the remaining phobias constitute a homogenous category. Comorbidity analyses of different fear profiles of the interview data from 8089 respondents of the National Comorbidity Study (NCS) suggested four different clusters of fear profiles.[91] *DSM-IV* not only changed the name of the diagnostic category from simple phobia, which has the connotation of being insignificant, to specific phobia to emphasize the focal character of the disorder but also subdivided specific phobias into four different subtypes:

   Animal type, including fears of spiders, snakes, rats, mice, worms, birds, and a fear response that is characterized by strong sympathetically dominated autonomic physiological pattern (including strong cardiac acceleration and blood pressure increase) probably preparing the organism for a vigor escape[14]
   Blood-injection-injury type, including fears of seeing blood, receiving an injection, or other invasive medical or dental procedures and a typically diphasic fear response, characterized by an initial sympathetically mediated increase in heart rate and blood pressure followed in by a vagally mediated rapid bradycardia and hypotension that my ultimately lead to a syncope,[92] probably preparing the organism for tonic immobility[93]

Situational type, including fears of being trapped in enclosed spaces like tunnels, elevators, airplanes, or buses with cognitive symptoms like the fear of losing control or going crazy being the most prominent features of the fear response pattern.[46]

Natural environment type, including fears of heights, thunderstorms, being on or in the water, with avoidance behavior being the most prominent symptom of this phobia subtype

Thus, *DSM-IV* makes the effort to abandon the original classification of phobias according to the feared objects and situations (although the different diagnostic categories remain named after the feared situations) and rather focus on the fear response. The *DSM-V* probably should pursue this effort, especially because the different patterns of fear responses might have important implications for tailoring effective therapeutic interventions to reduce the fear response. Thus treating fear responses that are characterized mainly by worries of losing control or suffocating might need more cognitive interventions than treating fear responses that are dominated by a surge of sympathetic arousal and the urge to escape (like in spider phobia). In the latter case, touching the feared object might be an important learning experience for extinguishing the fear response. Finally, because a key feature of phobias is that the fear response is elicited almost every time the individual encounters the phobia-related situation, increases in intensity with increasing proximity of the feared object, and subsides as soon as the contact with the object or situation is terminated, it should be considered whether social phobia and agoraphobia should be categorized as phobic disorders in the *DSM-V*. There is evidence that a subgroup of patients who had panic disorder and agoraphobia show a clear-cut fear response during imagery of their personally most threatening experience[94] or during presence in a narrow dark room, while other agoraphobic patients do not show any activation of the fear system in these situations although exhibiting persistent agoraphobic avoidance. In these cases, therapeutic interventions should be directed rather toward reducing these safety behaviors instead of focusing on the fear response. In the same vein, social phobia might not be a good example for a phobic disorder, because worries about one's own performance or embarrassment by being in the focus of attention by others are the core features of the disorder much more related to the emotion of shame than to the emotion of fear. Finally, it might be important to subdivide patients who have dental fear into those who are characterized mainly by the fear of pain and those who fear fainting. Both patient groups might need different interventions.

REFERENCES

1. Emmelkamp PMG, Wittchen H-U. Specific phobias. In: Andrews G, Charney DS, Sirovatka PJ, Regier DA, editors. Stress-induced and fear circuit disorders. Arlington (VA): American Psychiatric Publishing, Incorporated; 2009. p. 85–110.
2. Wittchen H-U, Jacobi F. Size and burden of mental disorder in Europe: a critical review and appraisal of 27 studies. Eur Neuropsychopharmacol 2005;15:357–76.
3. Wolpe J. Psychotherapy by reciprocal inhibtion. Stanford (CA): Stanford University Press; 1958.
4. Hellström K, Öst L-G. One-session therapist directed exposure vs. two forms of manual directed self-exposure in the treatment of spider phobia. Behav Res Ther 1995;33:959–65.
5. Williams SL, Turner SM, Peer DF. Guided mastery and performance desensitization treatments for severe acrophobia. J Consult Clin Psychol 1985;53:237–47.

6. Öst L-G. One session treatment for specific phobias. Behav Res Ther 1989;27: 1–7.
7. Öst L-G. A maintenance program for behavioral treatment of anxiety disorders. Behav Res Ther 1989;27:123–30.
8. Mühlberger A, Herrmann MJ, Wiedemann GC, et al. Repeated exposure of flight phobics to flights in virtual reality. Behav Res Ther 2001;39:1033–50.
9. Rothbaum BO, Hodges L, Smith S, et al. A controlled study of virtual reality exposure therapy for the fear of flying. J Consult Clin Psychol 2000;68:1020–6.
10. Van Gerwen LJ, Spinhoven P, Diekstra RFW, et al. Multicomponent standardized treatment program for fear of flying. Description and effectiveness. Cogn Behav Pract 2002;9:138–49.
11. Wolitzky-Taylor KB, Horowitz JD, Powers MB, et al. Psychological approaches in the treatment of specific phobias: a meta-analysis. Clin Psychol Rev 2008;28:1021–37.
12. Choy Y, Fyer AJ, Lipsitz JD. Treatment of specific phobia in adults. Clin Psychol Rev 2007;27:266–86.
13. Bandura A, Blahard EB, Ritter B. Relative efficacy of desensitization and modeling approaches for inducing behavioral, affective, and attitudinal changes. J Pers Soc Psychol 1969;13:177–99.
14. Öst L-G, Alm T, Brandberg M, et al. One vs. five sessions of exposure and five sessions of cognitive therapy in the treatment of claustrophobia. Behav Res Ther 2001;39:167–83.
15. Telch MJ. Pushing the envelope in treating clinical phobias. In: Maj M, Akiskal HS, Lopez-Ibor JJ, et al, editors. Phobias: WPA series—evidence and experience in psychiatry, vol. 7. Chichester (UK): Wiley; 2004.
16. Marks IM. Fears, phobias, and rituals. New York: Oxford; 1987.
17. Egan S. Reduction of anxiety in aquaphobics. Can J Appl Sport Sci 1981;6: 68–71.
18. Lang PJ, Melamed BG, Hart J. A psychophysiological analysis of fear modification using an automated desensitization procedure. J Abnorm Psychol 1970;76: 220–34.
19. Rentz TO, Powers MB, Smits JA, et al. Active–imaginal exposure: examination of a new behavioral treatment for cynophobia (dog phobia). Behav Res Ther 2003; 41:1337–53.
20. Emmelkamp PMG, Wessels H. Flooding in imagination vs. flooding in vivo in agoraphobics. Behav Res Ther 1975;13:7–15.
21. Mathews AM, Johnston DW, Lancashire M, et al. Imagnial flooding and exposure to real phobic situations: treatment outcome with agoraphobic patients. Br J Psychol 1976;129:361–71.
22. Cook EW III, Melamed BG, Cuthbert BN, et al. Emotional imagery and the differential diagnosis of anxiety. J Consult Clin Psychol 1988;56:734–40.
23. Emmelkamp PMG, Krijn M, Hulsbosch AM, et al. Virtual reality treatment versus exposure in vivo: a comparative evaluation in acrophobia. Behav Res Ther 2002;40:509–16.
24. Rothbaum BO, Hodges L, Anderson PL, et al. Twelve-month follow-up of virtual reality and standard exposure therapies for the fear of flying. J Consult Clin Psychol 2002;70:428–32.
25. Mühlberger A, Weik A, Pauli P, et al. One session virtual reality exposure treatment for fear of flying: one-year follow-up and graduation flight accompaniment effects. Psychother Res 2006;16:26–40.
26. Öst L-G. Rapid treatment of specific phobias. In: Davey GCL, editor. Phobias. Chichester (UK): Wiley; 1997. p. 227–46.

27. Stern RS, Marks IM. Brief and prolonged flooding: a comparison in agoraphobic patients. Arch Gen Psychiatry 1973;28:270–6.
28. Foa EB, Jameson JS, Turner RM, et al. Massed vs. spaced exposure sessions in the treatment of agoraphobia. Behav Res Ther 1980;18:333–8.
29. Chambless DL. Spacing of exposure sessions in treatment of agoraphobia and simple phobia. Behav Ther 1990;21:217–29.
30. Vansteenwegen D, Vervliet B, Iberico C, et al. The repeated confrontation with videotapes of spiders in multiple contexts attenuates renewal of fear in spider anxious students. Behav Res Ther 2007;46:1169–79.
31. Rowe MK, Craske M. Effects of varied stimulus exposure train on fear reduction and return of fear. Behav Res Ther 1998;36:719–34.
32. Lang AJ, Craske M. Manipulations of exposure-based therapy to reduce return of fear: a replication. Behav Res Ther 2000;38:1–12.
33. Marks IM, Kenwright M, Mc Donough M, et al. Saving clinicians' time by delegating routine aspects of therapy to a computer: a randomized controlled trial in phobia/panic disorder. Psychol Med 2004;34:9–18.
34. Öst L-G, Stridth B-M, Wolf M. A clinical study of spider phobia: prediction of outcome after self-help and therapist-directed treatments. Behav Res Ther 1998;36:17–35.
35. Hellström K, Fellenius J, Öst L-G. One versus five sessions of applied tension in the treatment of blood phobia. Behav Res Ther 1996;34:101–12.
36. Willumsen T, Vassend O. Effects of cognitive therapy, applied relaxation, and nitrous oxide sedation in the treatment of dental fear. Acta Odontol Scand 2003;61:93–9.
37. Hakeberg M, Berggren U, Carlsson SG, et al. Long-term effects on dental care behavior and dental health after treatments for dental fear. Anesth Prog 1993;40:72–7.
38. Lipsitz JD, Mannuzza S, Klein DF, et al. Specific phobia 10–16 years after treatment. Depress Anxiety 1999;10:105–11.
39. Baldwin DS, Anderson IM, Nutt DJ, et al. Evidence-based guidelines for the pharmacological treatment of anxiety disorders: recommendations from the British Association for Psychopharmacology. J Psychopharmacol 2005;19:567–96.
40. Thom A, Sartory G, Jöhren P. Comparison between one-session psychological treatment and benzodiazepine in dental phobia. J Consult Clin Psychol 2000; 68:378–87.
41. Wilhelm FH, Roth WT. Acute and delayed effects of alprazolam on flight phobics during exposure. Behav Res Ther 1997;35:831–41.
42. Ressler KJ, Rothbaum BO, Tannenbaum L, et al. Cognitive enhancers as adjuncts to psychotherapy: use of D-cycloserine in phobic individuals to facilitate extinction of fear. Arch Gen Psychiatry 2004;61:1136–44.
43. Hofmann SG, Meuret AE, Smits JA, et al. Augmentation of exposure therapy with D-cycloserine for social anxiety disorder. Arch Gen Psychiatry 2006;63:298–304.
44. Guastella AJ, Dadds MR, Lovibond P, et al. A randomized controlled trial of the effect of D-cycloserine on exposure therapy for spider fear. J Psychiatr Res 2007;41:466–71.
45. Booth R, Rachman S. The reduction of claustrophobia I. Behav Res Ther 1992;30: 207–21.
46. Craske MG, Sipas A. Animal phobias versus claustrophobias: exteroceptive versus interorceptive cues. Behav Res Ther 1992;30:569–81.
47. Koch E, Spates R, Himle J. Comparison of behavioral and cognitive-behavioral one-session exposure treatments for small animal phobias. Behav Res Ther 2004;42:1483–504.

48. De Jongh A, Muris P, ter Horst G, et al. One-session cognitive treatment of dental phobia: preparing dental phobics for treatment by restructuring negative cognitions. Behav Res Ther 1995;33:947–54.
49. Marks IM. Phobias and obsessions: clinical phenomena in search of a laboratory model. In: Maser J, Seligman M, editors. Psychopathology: experimental models. San Francisco (CA): Friedman; 1975. p. 174–213.
50. Öst L-G. Applied relaxation: description of a coping technique and review of controlled studies. Behav Res Ther 1987;25:397–409.
51. Öst L-G, Salkovskis PM, Hellström K. One session therapist-guided exposure vs. self-exposure in the treatment of spider phobia. Behav Ther 1991;22:407–22.
52. Öst L-G, Sterner U, Fellenius J. Applied tension, applied relaxation, and the combination of treatment of blood phobia. Behav Res Ther 1989;27:109–21.
53. Öst L-G, Fellenius J, Sterner U. Applied tension, exposure in vivo, and tension-only in the treatment of blood phobia. Behav Res Ther 1991;29:561–74.
54. Fyer AJ, Mannuzza S, Chapman TF, et al. Specificity and familial aggregation of phobic disorders. Arch Gen Psychiatry 1995;52:564–73.
55. Schreier A, Wittchen H-U, Hoefler M, et al. Anxiety disorders in mothers and their children: a prospective longitudinal community study. Br J Psychol 2008;192:308–9.
56. Gelernter J, Page GP, Bonvicini K, et al. A chromosome 14 risk locus for simple phobia: results form a genome-wide linkage scan. Mol Psychiatry 2003;8:71–82.
57. Kendler KS, Neale MC, Kessler RC, et al. The genetic eopidemiology of phobias in women. Arch Gen Psychiatry 1992;49:273–81.
58. Kendler KS, Karkowski LM, Prescott CA. Fears and phobias: reliability and heritability. Psychol Med 1999;29:539–53.
59. Lesch K-P, Bengel D, Heils A, et al. Association of anxiety-related traits with polymorphism in the serotonin transporter gene regulatory region. Science 1996;274: 1527–31.
60. Lonsdorf TB, Weike AI, Nikamo P, et al. Genetic gating of human fear learning and extinction- possible implications for gene-environment interaction in anxiety disorder. Psychol Sci 2009;20:198–206.
61. Davis M. The role of the amygdala in conditioned and unconditioned fear and anxiety. In: Aggleton JP, editor. The amygdala: a functional analysis. 2nd edition. Oxford (UK): Oxford University Press; 2000. p. 213–87.
62. LeDoux JE. The emotional brain. New York: Simon & Schuster; 1996.
63. Morris JS, Öhman A, Dolan RJ. Conscious and unconscious emotional learning in the human amygdala. Nation 1998;393:467–70.
64. Dilger S, Straube T, Mentzel H-J, et al. Brain activation to phobia-related pictures in spider phobic humans: an event-related functional magnetic resonance imaging study. Neurosci Lett 2003;348:29–32.
65. Wendt J, Lotze M, Weike AI, et al. Brain activation and defensive response mobilization during sustained exposure to phobia-related and other affective pictures in spider phobia. Psychophysiology 2007;45:205–15.
66. Etkin A, Wager TD. Functional neuroimaging of anxiety: a meta-analysis of emotional processing in PTSD, social anxiety disorder, and specific phobia. Am J Psychother 2007;164:1476–88.
67. Olsson A, Nearing KI, Phelps EA. Learning fears by observing others: the neural systems of social fear transmission. Soc Cogn Affect Neurosci 2007;2:3–12.
68. Mineka S, Cook M. Mechanisms underlying observational conditioning of snake fear in monkeys. J Exp Psychol Gen 1993;122:23–38.
69. Grillon C, Ameli R, Woods SW, et al. Fear potentiated startle in humans: effects of anticipatory anxiety on the acoustic blink reflex. Psychophysiology 1991;28:511–7.

70. Phelps EA, ÓConnor KJ, Gatenby JC, et al. Activation of the left amygdala to a cognitive representation of fear. Nat Neurosci 2001;4:437–41.
71. Poulton R, Menzies RG. Nonassociative fear acquisition: a review of the evidence from retrospective and longitudinal research. Behav Res Ther 2002;40:127–49.
72. Lader MH, Mathews AM. A physiological model of phobic anxiety and desensitization. Behav Res Ther 1968;6:411–21.
73. Maltzman I. Orienting reflexes and significance: a reply to ÓGorman. Psychophysiology 1979;16:274–82.
74. Sokolov EN. Perception and the conditioned reflex. New York: Macmillan; 1963.
75. Donchin E. Surprise! Surprise? Psychophysiology 1981;18:493–513.
76. Öhman A. The orienting response, attention, and learning: an information processing perspective. In: Kimmel HD, van Olst EH, Orlebeke JF, editors. The orienting reflex in humans. Hillsdale (NJ): Erlbaum; 1979. p. 443–71.
77. Bradley MM. Natural selective attention: orienting and emotion. Psychophysiology 2009;46:1–11.
78. Alpers GW, Wilhelm FH, Roth WT. Physiological assessment during exposure in driving phobic patients. J Abnorm Psychol 2005;114:126–39.
79. Watson JP, Gaind R, Marks IM. Physiological habituation to continuous phobic stimulation. Behav Res Ther 1972;10:269–78.
80. Straube T, Glauer M, Dilger S, et al. Effects of cognitive–behavioral therapy on brain activation in specific phobia. Neuroimage 2006;29:125–35.
81. Paulus MP, Stein MB. An insular view of anxiety. Biol Psychol 2006;60:383–7.
82. Craske MG, Kircanski K, Zelikowsky M, et al. Optimizing inhibitory learning during exposure therapy. Behav Res Ther 2008;46:5–27.
83. Craske MG. Anxiety disorders: psychological approaches to theory and treatment. Boulder (CO): Westwood Press; 1999.
84. Bouton ME. Context and behavioral processes in extinction. Learn Memory 2004; 11:485–94.
85. Milad MR, Quirk GJ. Neurons in the medial prefrontal cortex signal memory for fear extinction. Nation 2002,418:70–4.
86. Quirk GJ, Mueller D. Neural mechanisms of extinction learning and retrieval. Neuropsychopharmacology 2008;33:56–72.
87. Schiller D, Levy I, Niv J, et al. From fear to safety and back: reversal of fear in the human brain. J Neurosci 2008;28:11517–25.
88. ÓDoherty JP, Critchley H, Deichmann R, et al. Dissociating valence outcome from behavioral control in human orbital and ventral prefrontal cortices. J Neurosci 2003;23:7931–9.
89. Kim H, Shimojo S, ÓDoherty JP. Is avoiding an aversive outcome rewarding? Neural substrates of avoidance learning in the human brain. PLoS Biol 2006;4:e233.
90. Schienle A, Schaefer A, Stark R, et al. Long-term effects of cognitive behavior therapy on brain activation in spider phobia. Psychiatry Res 2009;172:99–102.
91. Curtis GC, Magee WJ, Eaton WW, et al. Specific fears and phobias. Br J Psychol 1998;173:212–7.
92. Friedman BH, Thayer JF, Borkovec TD, et al. Autonomic characteristics of nonclinical panic and blood phobia. Biol Psychol 1993;34:298–310.
93. Campbell BA, Wood G, McBride T. Origins of orienting and defensive responses: an evolutionary perspective. In: Lang PJ, Simons RF, Balaban M, editors. Attention and orienting. Mahwah (NJ): Erlbaum; 1997. p. 41–67.
94. Shuman J, McTeague L, Laplante M-C, et al. Response mobilization in panic disorder and the role of agoraphobia. Psychophysiology 2008;45(Suppl):S78.

Empirically Supported Treatments for Panic Disorder

R. Kathryn McHugh, MA[a],*, Jasper A.J. Smits, PhD[b],
Michael W. Otto, PhD[a]

KEYWORDS

- Panic disorder • Empirically-supported treatment
- Cognitive behavioral therapy
- Pharmacotherapy • Combination treatment

Panic disorder (PD) is characterized by recurrent panic attacks (including at least one unexpected attack) accompanied by significant apprehension and behavior change related to these attacks. In many cases, this behavior change is avoidance of the somatic sensations or the external situations associated with panic attacks. Indeed, many cases of PD are accompanied by a diagnosis of agoraphobia, the fear and avoidance of situations in which escape would be difficult in the case of onset of panic-like symptoms. PD with and without agoraphobia is associated with high levels of disability[1,2] and societal costs.[3,4] The efficacy of both pharmacologic and cognitive behavioral interventions for the treatment of PD has been well established, with large-scale comparative trials and meta-analytic reviews indicating comparable outcomes for the two modalities.[5–8] Hence, both therapies may serve as first-line treatments for PD.

PHARMACOTHERAPY FOR PANIC DISORDER

Pharmacologic agents with established efficacy for the treatment of PD with and without agoraphobia include benzodiazepines[9,10] and antidepressant agents, prominently including the selective serotonin reuptake inhibitors (SSRIs) and tricyclic antidepressants (TCAs).[5,11,12] Early studies supported the efficacy of TCAs[5,12] and benzodiazepines[13–15] as well as monoamine oxidase inhibitors.[15] More recently, SSRIs and serotonin norepinephrine reuptake inhibitors (SNRIs) have emerged as

Dr. Otto has served as a consultant and receives research support from Organon (Schering-Plough). Dr. Smits receives research support from Organon (Schering-Plough).
[a] Department of Psychology, 648 Beacon Street, 6th Floor, Boston University, Boston, MA 02215, USA
[b] Department of Psychology, Southern Methodist University, 6116 Central Expressway, St 1100, Dallas, TX 75206, USA
* Corresponding author.
E-mail address: rkmchugh@bu.edu (R.K. McHugh).

front-line pharmacologic treatments for PD and also are preferred treatments for other anxiety disorders.[16] For example, in a placebo-controlled investigation of paroxetine (an SSRI) and venlafaxine (an SNRI) for PD, both treatments were superior to placebo and demonstrated significant improvement in frequency of panic attacks and other disorder symptoms.[17] At posttreatment evaluation, 70% of patients treated with venlafaxine and almost 60% of the patients treated with paroxetine reported remission from full panic attacks, as compared with 48% in the placebo group. Meta-analytic reviews have suggested similar efficacy for SSRIs and other pharmacotherapies.[18,19] The results of such reviews have been inconclusive with regard to tolerability, however, with some suggesting no differences between SSRIs and older agents[18] and others finding superior tolerability for SSRIs.[19] Thus, although efficacy may be similar, factors related to tolerability (as reflected by treatment drop-out) may indicate advantages of SSRIs and SNRIs relative to older agents.

Although they may be better tolerated than older agents, SSRIs and SNRIs nonetheless are associated with potential side effects, such as headaches, sleep difficulty, fatigue, nausea, weight gain, and sexual dysfunction.

Pharmacotherapy for PD also has been associated with reductions in symptoms of comorbid conditions including unipolar depression[20] and personality disorders.[21] This reduction may be attributable to the efficacy of similar agents for PD and other Axis I disorders. Several studies suggest that comorbid psychological disorders, such as personality disorders,[22,23] predict poorer treatment outcome; however, studies examining the impact on treatment outcome of comorbid anxiety disorders[24–26] and major depression[24,27] have been inconsistent. As significant predictors, duration of illness and disorder severity have achieved mixed results.[28] Other predictors of response include greater phobic avoidance related to fears of blood, injury, or injection[29] and biological factors such as neurotransmitter receptor affinity (eg, beta-adrenoceptor affinity).[30]

A number of pharmacologic alternatives have demonstrated efficacy for treatment-refractory PD.[31] Combination medication strategies are used frequently. Despite the popularity of the strategy, however, there is evidence that the addition of benzodiazepines to SSRI treatment may lead to only short-term additional benefits.[32] Also, only limited open data support the efficacy of combining a TCA and SSRI for patients who have not responded to antidepressant monotherapy.[33] The addition of other classes of agents has shown some efficacy. For example, among anticonvulsants, efficacy for refractory panic has been suggested for valproic acid,[34] gabapentin,[35] and tiagabine.[36] A double-blind trial suggested efficacy for pindolol, a β-blocker with antagonist effects on the $5HT_{1A}$ autoreceptor.[37] Finally, an open trial of 31 patients supported the efficacy of the atypical antipsychotic, olanzapine, for refractory PD.[38] Patients who had not responded to SSRI treatment for PD received a fixed dose of olanzapine (5 mg/d) for 12 weeks. Sixteen percent of the patients dropped out, but 57.7% of the remainder met remission criteria. The specific role of olanzapine augmentation in this study is unclear, given findings that longer-term treatment with an SSRI (eg, a 24-week continuation phase) may lead to a similar response rate after a initial failure to respond to an SSRI, at least for the treatment of posttraumatic stress disorder.[39] Accordingly, continuation treatment should be considered an additional strategy for initial pharmacotherapy nonresponse.

Thus, based on the results of efficacy trials, although briefer duration of pharmacotherapy has demonstrated efficacy, continuation of medication for longer durations may be indicated in the absence of response or to facilitate maintenance of gains. In fact, recommendations suggest continuing medication treatment for at least 1 year after acute response to maintain gains.[40] Moreover, tapering medication is recommended to minimize withdrawal symptoms and re-emergence of the disorder. The onset of action of pharmacotherapy also varies and for some agents (eg, SSRIs), effects may take several weeks to be achieved, particularly given recommendations to build up to a therapeutic dose over the course of several weeks.

COGNITIVE BEHAVIORAL THERAPY FOR PANIC DISORDER

In contrast to pharmacotherapy, [cognitive behavioral therapy (CBT) is a learning-based approach that targets the relearning of safety in relation to the fears and avoidance characteristic of panic] (Fig. 1). CBT for PD typically consists of components of psychoeducation, cognitive restructuring/reappraisal, and behavioral interventions (eg, behavioral experiments and interoceptive and in vivo exposure). Contemporary cognitive behavioral models of PD emphasize the role of fear of anxiety symptoms in the maintenance of the disorder.[41,42] Instead of relying on direct arousal-attenuation strategies, such as relaxation and breathing techniques, CBT uses a combination of cognitive restructuring and exposure exercises to help patients establish a sense of safety in the context of feared internal and external events.[43] Cognitive restructuring exercises are designed to help patients identify and restructure panic-related threat appraisals (eg, "I might have a heart attack," "I will go crazy," "I am going to faint"). In treatment, patients are asked to monitor their cognitions and to learn to treat their thoughts as guesses about the world rather than facts. By reviewing evidence for their thoughts, patients learn to generate and use rational responses (eg, "Heart racing does not mean that I am going to have a heart attack") when faced with a fear-provoking situation. To facilitate this type of learning, the therapist and patient design exposure exercises that can yield disconfirming evidence and build tolerance of uncomfortable sensations without maladaptive behavioral responses (eg, avoidance). For example, if the patient fears the experience of rapid heart beat because of the concern that this symptom may lead to a panic attack and a heart attack, the patient may be instructed to run up several flights of stairs to provoke heart racing and to repeat this exercise until the fear has extinguished.

Similar to the evidence for other anxiety disorders,[44] CBT for PD has demonstrated acute efficacy[5,44–46] and strong maintenance of treatment gains over time (eg, 2 years posttreatment).[5,8,47,48] In addition to direct effects on PD, CBT also offers global

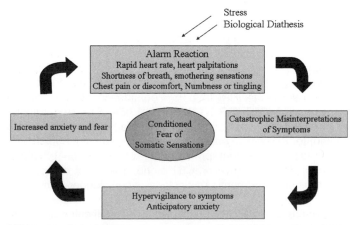

Fig. 1. Cognitive behavioral model of panic disorder. (*Adapted from* Otto MW, Pollack MH. Stopping anxiety medication, therapist guide, 2nd edition. New York: Oxford University Press; 2009. p. 9; with permission.)

improvements in quality of life and benefit for treating comorbid anxiety and depression.[49,50] CBT is a particularly cost-effective modality, in part because of the strong maintenance of treatment gains for this short-term treatment,[51,52] and has shown efficacy for group treatment of PD as well as in individual formats.[53–55] The typical duration of treatment is 12 to 15 sessions, but even briefer treatments have shown efficacy.[56,57] Brief treatments maintain the core elements of standard CBT, but administration involves a more intensive or efficient format with a particular emphasis on the importance of homework exercises.

PREDICTORS OF RESPONSE TO COGNITIVE BEHAVIORAL THERAPY

Comorbid conditions have received substantial attention in the literature as a potential moderator of treatment outcome, with mixed results. Several studies have suggested that severity of agoraphobia at baseline is a strong predictor of treatment outcome among patients who have PD, with those who have higher levels of agoraphobia exhibiting worse outcome.[58,59] Axis II disorders also have been associated with poorer treatment outcome among patients who have PD.[59,60]

Evaluations of comorbid major depression have suggested both worse outcome[58] and no attenuation of efficacy.[60,61] This inconsistency may be related to the degree to which comorbid conditions improve with treatment for PD. For example, Tsao and colleagues[61] found substantial improvement in other Axis I disorders, such as major depression and generalized anxiety disorder, with maintenance of gains for comorbid conditions at 6-month follow-up. In a study of CBT for PD compared with a more flexible CBT intervention in which treatment could shift to focus on comorbid disorders in 65 patients who had a principle diagnosis of PD, those who received treatment targeted at PD alone experienced greater improvement in both panic symptoms and comorbid conditions at posttreatment and 1-year follow-up.[62]

Other comorbidities, such as substance use disorders, have received relatively less attention in the literature and are an important area of inquiry, given the elevated rates of substance abuse among those who have PD.[63]

COMBINATION TREATMENT STRATEGIES

Despite the potential promise for improved outcomes with the concurrent combination of two efficacious monotherapies (pharmacotherapy and CBT), the success of this combination treatment strategy has been limited. Mirroring the results of large-scale trials,[5,9] the available evidence from empirical reviews of the literature suggests that combination treatment offers only limited benefits over monotherapy, particularly monotherapy with CBT. For example, in a meta-analysis of 21 trials (representing 1709 patients studied), combined therapy was found to be superior to antidepressant pharmacotherapy (relative risk [RR] 1.24, 95% confidence interval [CI] 1.02–1.52) and to psychotherapy (largely CBT) (RR 1.17, 95% CI 1.05–1.31).[7] Accordingly, Furukawa and colleagues[7] concluded that both combined therapy and psychotherapy serve as first-line treatment for PD with or without agoraphobia, with the choice between these treatments depending on patient preference rather than on efficacy. From the perspective of cost efficacy, however, CBT alone offers cost outcomes that are far superior to combined treatment, particularly when longer-term outcomes are considered.[51]

Combination treatment strategies also may introduce difficulties in treatment adherence. In general, meta-analytic reviews of acute pharmacotherapy and CBT trials indicate that CBT is equal to or more tolerable than pharmacologic alternatives across the anxiety disorders.[8] Given these data, the notion that pharmacotherapy may aid the retention of patients in CBT by reducing anxiety severity is challenged. Moreover, meta-analytic reviews of the PD literature[18] indicate that the dropout rate for combination treatment (22%) is more similar to that for treatment with TCAs or SSRIs (19.9%) than to that for CBT (5.6%); however, this trend was not evident in a multicenter trial of PD.[5] Given these mixed data, the authors tentatively conclude that combination treatment offers no reliable advantages to CBT alone in terms of the acute retention of patients.

In addition, there is some evidence that combination treatment may impair the longer-term maintenance of CBT when the medication is discontinued. For example, Barlow and colleagues[5] found that the combination of CBT with imipramine was associated with greater improvements in PD symptoms during ongoing maintenance treatment than seen with either treatment alone. In a 6-month no-treatment follow-up period (after discontinuation of medication use), however, only the CBT-alone and CBT-plus-placebo conditions continued to show an advantage over placebo treatment, a result consistent with the general loss of treatment gains observed for many patients after discontinuation of medication treatment.[8] Likewise, Marks and colleagues[9] evaluated the combination of alprazolam and exposure therapy and also found improved treatment effects acutely for this modality that decreased following medication taper, resulting in greater efficacy for exposure alone.

The observation that treatment gains are difficult to maintain once medications are discontinued is consistent with basic research indicating that the learning of safety that occurs with CBT may be context specific.[64,65] That is, during the acute phase of treatment, the patient learns safety with respect to the sensations and situations associated with panic attacks, but this learning may be specific to the contextual cues of being on medication. When the medication is discontinued, so might be aspects of the learned safety. Recent research also suggests that the increased rates of return of fear associated with combination treatments may be accounted for, in part, by a tendency for patients to make external attributions of gains.[66] Specifically, many patients who receive combination CBT and pharmacotherapy tend to attribute their gains to the medications[67] and therefore are susceptible to relapse when medication is discontinued.[66]

CBT and pharmacotherapy are not always added concurrently, and there is evidence from multiple small studies that adding CBT to patients previously treated with pharmacotherapy offers reliable benefits[68-71] that are long lasting.[70] The evidence regarding the cost of pre-existing medication treatment with respect to the longer-term outcome from CBT is mixed. However, in a naturalistic study of patients attending a specialty anxiety clinic offering both CBT and pharmacotherapy, Otto and associates[52] found higher relapse rates for combined treatment than for CBT alone, even when the medication treatment was continued. In examining the longer-term outcome of brief intensive group CBT for PD, however, Oei et al[55] found that CBT improved outcomes for patients who had been receiving pre-existing pharmacotherapy and for those who had not, with no differences between these two groups over follow-up periods ranging from 1.1 to 6.2 years. Notably, the large majority of patients treated without pre-existing medication (80%) remained medication-free at long-term follow-up.

One effective strategy for preventing relapse following medication discontinuation is starting CBT during the tapering phase. For example, in a study of 33 patients with PD receiving treatment with alprazolam or clonazepam, the addition of CBT to a slow taper was associated with substantially better rates of successful medication discontinuation (76% versus 25% in the taper-alone condition), which were maintained at 3-month follow-up.[72] Subsequent examination of this strategy has supported these initial findings,[73,74] and this intervention has been extended successfully to the discontinuation of SSRIs.[75,76]

MECHANISMS OF ACTION OF TREATMENTS

Hypothesized mechanisms of action of pharmacologic interventions for PD have focused primarily on restored function of neurotransmitter systems. Dysregulation of several neurotransmitters, such as norepinephrine, serotonin, and gamma-aminobutyric acid (GABA), may be important to the pathophysiology of PD.[77,78] Much remains to be understood about the specific mechanisms of action of pharmacologic agents for PD, however.

Consistent with the success of SSRIs and SNRIs in the treatment of PD, several studies have suggested a role of serotonin dysregulation in PD. Studies have found reductions in serotonin receptor binding in patients who have symptomatic PD relative to healthy controls[79] and in patients receiving pharmacotherapy for PD.[80] Regulation of this dysfunction may be achieved by agents acting on serotonin, such as SSRIs and SNRIs, which increase the availability of serotonin in the synaptic cleft. Several agents demonstrating efficacy for PD, such as benzodiazepines and certain antidepressants,[81,82] also impact noradrenergic systems. Studies of the role of norepinephrine in panic have focused on the importance of the locus coeruleus, which has been linked to increases in anxiety[83] and may be a mechanism for anxiogenic response to carbon dioxide challenge.[84]

GABAergic systems also may play a role in the mechanism of pharmacologic treatment for PD, given the efficacy of benzodiazepines, which increase GABA. Studies of receptor function in PD have found abnormalities in the binding of GABA receptors in patients who have PD relative to controls.[85,86] Moreover, lower GABA levels in the anterior cingulate cortex, basal ganglia, and occipital cortex have been noted in patients who have PD relative to controls.[87,88] At this time, further research on the role of these and other potential mechanisms for the pharmacologic treatment of PD is needed.

The mechanisms of action of CBT have received increased attention in recent years. In addition to cognitive restructuring, CBT for PD uses exposure to feared physiological sensations (eg, dizziness, shortness of breath; interoceptive exposure) and external cues (eg, crowds, public transportation; in vivo exposure) to provide patients with opportunities to extinguish the fear of fear. It is hypothesized that these reductions in fears of panic and related beliefs underlie the effects of CBT on PD symptoms.[89,90] Preliminary support for this hypothesis comes from two recent studies. Smits and colleagues[91] administered measures of fear of fear both before and after treatment to 140 adults who had PD who were assigned randomly to either CBT or wait-list. A series of regression analyses revealed that the changes in fear of fear partially mediated reductions in panic severity, anxiety, and avoidance and fully mediated improvements in quality of life. Hofmann and colleagues[92] recently extended these findings by demonstrating that this mediational process is specific to CBT. They found that changes in panic-related catastrophic cognitions that occurred from pretreatment to posttreatment to 6-month follow-up accounted for significant variance in the improvements seen in patients who received CBT (either alone or in combination with imipramine or placebo) but not among patients who received imipramine alone.

The necessity of facilitating concrete and clear tests of fears in exposure interventions is supported by research indicating the importance of emphasizing attending to the exposure objectively[93] and minimizing use of distraction strategies.[94]

Furthermore, the elimination of "safety behaviors" (eg, carrying medication "just in case," traveling only with a companion) or interfering coping behaviors (eg, listening to music as a distraction, engaging in relaxation exercises) facilitates successful exposure.[95,96] The use of safety behaviors, which often may be subtle and difficult to identify, may provide a context of conditional learning, in which the patient may attribute the outcome to the use of the coping strategy and thus undermine successful learning of safety. For example, carrying a medication bottle when traveling may fuel the belief that the patient "could not tolerate" the situation without this cue. In a sample of patients who had PD, Salkovskis and colleagues[95] reported greater reduction in anxiety in patients instructed to reduce safety behaviors than in those who used such behaviors. Likewise, despite their use in some CBT protocols, relaxation techniques such as breathing retraining may be detrimental to the effectiveness of exposure because they may attenuate extinction learning.[97]

Attempts to isolate the impact of cognitive restructuring relative to exposure interventions have been inconclusive, with some demonstrating similar efficacy when the interventions are use in isolation[98] but others demonstrating different efficacy for different symptoms (ie, agoraphobic avoidance versus panic symptoms)[99] and yet others suggesting that the addition of cognitive strategies to exposure does not improve outcome.[45]

Although treatment for PD has demonstrated significant success, there is much room for improvement. CBT has demonstrated high remission rates approaching 70% to 80%[5] and maintenance of gains;[100] however, rates of inadequate treatment response[6,48] and need for additional treatment remain high.[101] Thus, there remains a clear need for novel treatment strategies or combinations of existing strategies to increase the rates of treatment response, particularly among traditionally treatment-resistant patients.

OTHER PSYCHOSOCIAL TREATMENT APPROACHES

Compared with the wealth of evidence for CBT for PD,[8] there is little evidence to guide the application of alternative psychosocial treatments. Although the evidence suggesting that breathing retraining has no additive effects on outcomes has resulted in de-emphasis of this component in some applications of CBT, alternative treatments that target respiratory dysregulation (ie, hyperventilation) in PD have received recent support. For example, biometric feedback has shown efficacy for improving panic and agoraphobic symptoms.[102] A multicenter trial of emotion-focused psychotherapy emphasizing empathic listening and supportive strategies for managing painful emotions and stressors did not support its efficacy for PD.[103] In contrast, a recent trial of a manualized psychoanalytical psychotherapy showed significantly greater benefit than applied relaxation alone, with a 73% response rate relative to the 39% found for the relaxation condition.[104] This response rate is promising but was achieved across 24 sessions of treatment, roughly double the number offered in many CBT protocols. Also, it is unclear what elements of treatment were of importance to the manualized psychodynamic therapy. It shares a number of elements with emotion-focused approaches, including exploration of feelings surrounding panic onset and the meanings of panic symptoms. Additional elements of treatment focused on investigating transference and working through recurrent conflicts. In addition, according to an exploratory analysis, response in this trial seemed to be moderated by the presence of Cluster C personality symptoms,[105] raising questions regarding whether an additional focus on recurrent conflicts (eg, with treatment focused on problem-solving) may be of value with this subgroup of patients. Additional research is needed to clarify the reliability and strength of these effects and the elements of treatment most associated with differential responding.

The use of exercise as an intervention for psychological disorders has demonstrated efficacy of exercise for depression, with large effect sizes.[106] Growing evidence also supports the use of exercise for the treatment of PD. Specifically, several studies now have demonstrated that brief (2-week) programs of repeated short bouts (20 minutes) of exercise of moderate to vigorous intensity (brisk walking/running) yield large reductions in the fear of anxiety and related sensations.[107–109] More importantly, in a randomized, controlled trial involving 46 patients who had PD, Broocks and colleagues[110] found that a 10-week treatment protocol of regular aerobic exercise (running) outperformed placebo in reducing PD symptoms.

NOVEL STRATEGIES FOR COMBINED TREATMENT

As noted earlier in this article, combined pharmacologic and cognitive behavioral treatment strategies have shown only limited benefit over monotherapies. An alternative combination treatment strategy is not to use pharmacotherapy for additional anxiolysis but to promote the basic learning effects of CBT through memory enhancement. One such pharmacological strategy that seems promising for the treatment of anxiety disorders is the acute administration of the N-methyl-D-aspartic acid receptor partial agonist, D-cycloserine (DCS), during CBT. The aim is to facilitate therapeutic learning that occurs with CBT. In animal models, DCS seems to improve retention of extinction learning and is hypothesized to aid in the consolidation of learning following extinction trials.[111,112] In an important translation of this knowledge to the care of humans, Ressler and associates[113] showed that single-dose applications of DCS before exposure-based CBT enhanced efficacy of acrophobia treatment. Since this important early trial, similar positive results have been obtained for DCS augmentation of CBT for social phobia[114,115] and, with limited success, for obsessive-compulsive disorder.[116] Pilot work by the authors' group also has shown efficacy of DCS for augmenting CBT for PD.[117] As such, the use of memory enhancers (ie, agents that facilitate the consolidation of therapeutic learning) such as DCS may offer patients the opportunity for briefer treatment approaches (in which fewer sessions provide similar efficacy or gains are achieved more rapidly) or a new strategy should patients not respond to CBT alone. Indeed, if DCS is able to enhance extinction learning, it may make exposure sessions more effective, leading to more rapid or stronger gains.

ROUTINE CARE AND THE DISSEMINATION OF TREATMENTS

Both pharmacotherapy and CBT offer efficacious options for the treatment of panic and can provide alternatives to each other in the case of treatment nonresponse. As noted, there is evidence that CBT may be more cost effective [51,52,118] and more durable than pharmacotherapy, given the potential loss of efficacy upon medication discontinuation. Some evidence suggests that when a full course of CBT is not available to patients, the addition of cognitive behavioral strategies (eg, in vivo exposure) to medication may improve outcome[119–121] and thus may provide an alternative when CBT is not available. For example, patients who reported receiving at least one core component of CBT (eg, exposure, cognitive restructuring) had better outcomes than patients treated with medication alone.[119]

Despite support for the effectiveness and transportability of CBT for anxiety disorders into front-line clinical settings,[122–124] the availability of evidence-based care represents a continued problem in the treatment of PD. CBT often is less accessible than medication, particularly given the availability of pharmacotherapy through both specialty services (ie, psychiatrists) and primary care. Furthermore, both large-scale reports[125] and empirical studies[126,127] highlight the poor dissemination of evidence-based mental health care to service provision settings.

The improvement of the dissemination of these treatments has received increasing support in recent years. Specifically, the introduction of structured dissemination efforts and the consideration of novel treatments that may be disseminated more easily have been emphasized. For example, the use of brief treatment strategies has been suggested as a means to increase the efficiency of treatment episodes, particularly when resources are limited and patient retention is a barrier to the completion of a full course of treatment. Efficacy has been noted for treatments for PD only four or five sessions in length.[56,57] Moreover, group interventions provide an efficacious alternative for treating more patients.[53,68] The introduction of CBT for PD to primary care settings also has shown benefit for treatment outcome relative to treatment as usual and may increase access to care.[128] The addition of this care model to primary care also seems to be a particularly cost-effective treatment option.[129]

Another strategy that may improve the dissemination of psychosocial treatments is the use of computerized therapy packages. Computerized therapy for PD has demonstrated preliminary feasibility[130] and efficacy with therapist telephone support.[131,132] Computerized therapy may represent a particularly cost-effective modality that can be disseminated to areas where access to CBT is limited. Computerized therapy also has been used successfully as a component of collaborative care in primary care settings.[133] Little is known at this time about what the crucial elements of training in CBT for PD involve and what background may be necessary for achieving competence in the use of CBT. In the service of facilitating ongoing dissemination, future research in this area will be of particular importance.

SUMMARY AND IMPLICATIONS FOR THE *DIAGNOSTIC AND STATISTICAL MANUAL OF MENTAL DISORDERS*, EDITION V

Pharmacologic treatment with an SSRI or SNRI and CBT have demonstrated efficacy and cost efficacy for the treatment of PD and are the current first-line treatments for this disorder.[40] Remission rates are high for both modalities, and maintenance of gains has been supported over time. Moreover, quality-of-life improvements are noted in addition to symptom reduction for both pharmacologic and CBT interventions. With CBT, functional improvement in work, social, and family functioning has been observed both acutely and at follow-up periods.[49] Such functional improvement also is noted with medication treatment.[134,135]

Despite these successes, several areas for improvement remain. Of particular importance may be the development and evaluation of novel treatment strategies to increase rates of treatment response. Because access to evidence-based care, particularly CBT, remains limited, the development and dissemination of interventions that may increase the availability and accessibility of effective treatment for PD are of utmost importance. Brief or easily disseminated interventions, such as exercise, computerized CBT, and interventions administered through primary care settings, have demonstrated preliminary feasibility and efficacy and may be an important future direction in the treatment of PD.

As the field moves toward the introduction of the next iteration of the *Diagnostic and Statistical Manual of Mental Disorders* (DSM), there are several considerations relative to the classification of PD and agoraphobia. First, the hierarchical rules in *DSM-IV*[136] subsume agoraphobia under PD when these disorders co-occur. Given evidence for the existence of agoraphobia separate from PD, some have suggested reconsideration of this hierarchical rule in favor of a separate diagnosis for agoraphobia regardless of the presence of comorbid PD.[137] Indeed, evidence suggests that there may be a number of differences in onset and temporal stability between PD and agoraphobia.[137] Moreover, several studies suggest that in many cases agoraphobic avoidance may begin before the onset of panic attacks and PD.[138,139] Data suggest that lifetime rates of panic attacks are 28.3% (whereas only 3.7% of the population will meet criteria for PD, 1.1% will meet the criteria for PD with agoraphobia, and 0.8% will meet the criteria for agoraphobia without a history of panic) and that agoraphobia is associated with high levels of disability and distress even in the absence of PD.[140] Thus, converging evidence supports the independence of these diagnoses. Treatments for agoraphobia, for PD alone, and for PD with agoraphobia differ only minimally, however, with a focus on changing sensitivity to interoceptive and situational cues and with relative attention paid to in vivo or interoceptive exposures based on the specific presenting fears and avoidance areas.

Second, a potential innovation for *DSM-V* involves the addition of dimensional classification of disorders.[141] Evidence for the anxiety disorders in general, and for PD in particular, may support such a conceptual and practical shift.[142] Of particular importance to the classification of PD may be the role of anxiety sensitivity as a factor that may predispose individuals to PD, that predicts panic attacks, and that can be modified with treatment.[42] Moreover, anxiety sensitivity also is associated with agoraphobia without panic,[143] perhaps providing support for the linkage of these disorders in the *DSM* classification. In the classification of PD and agoraphobia, it would be particularly important to incorporate the two elements that are at the essence of these disorders—avoidance behaviors and sensitivity to physical sensations (anxiety sensitivity). At this time of potential shift in the way in which these disorders are classified, further research on their commonalities and distinguishing features is needed.

REFERENCES

1. Carrera M, Herran A, Ayuso-Mateos JL, et al. Quality of life in early phases of panic disorder: predictive factors. J Affect Disord 2006;94(1–3):127–34.
2. Cramer V, Torgersen S, Kringlen E. Quality of life and anxiety disorders: a population study. J Nerv Ment Dis 2005;193(3):196–202.
3. Hofmann SG, Barlow DH. The costs of anxiety disorders: implications for psychosocial interventions. In: Miller NE, Magruder KM, editors. Cost-effectiveness of psychotherapy: a guide for practitioners, researchers, and policymakers. New York: Oxford University Press; 1999.
4. Marciniak MD, Lage MJ, Dunayevich E, et al. The cost of treating anxiety: the medical and demographic correlates that impact total medical costs. Depress Anxiety 2005;21(4):178–84.
5. Barlow DH, Gorman JM, Shear MK, et al. Cognitive-behavioral therapy, imipramine, or their combination for panic disorder: a randomized controlled trial. JAMA 2000;283(19):2529–36.
6. Clark DM, Salkovskis PM, Hackmann A, et al. A comparison of cognitive therapy, applied relaxation and imipramine in the treatment of panic disorder. Br J Psychiatry 1994;164(6):759–69.
7. Furukawa TA, Watanabe N, Churchill R. Psychotherapy plus antidepressant for panic disorder with or without agoraphobia: systematic review. Br J Psychiatry 2006;188:305–12.

8. Gould RA, Otto MW, Pollack MH. A meta-analysis of treatment outcome for panic disorder. Clin Psychol Rev 1995;15:819 44.
9. Marks IM, Swinson RP, Basoglu M, et al. Alprazolam and exposure alone and combined in panic disorder with agoraphobia. A controlled study in London and Toronto. Br J Psychiatry 1993;162:776–87.
10. Tesar GE, Rosenbaum JF, Pollack MH, et al. Double-blind, placebo-controlled comparison of clonazepam and alprazolam for panic disorder. J Clin Psychiatry 1991;52(2):69–76.
11. Ballenger JC, Burrows GD, DuPont RL Jr, et al. Alprazolam in panic disorder and agoraphobia: results from a multicenter trial. I. Efficacy in short term treatment. Arch Gen Psychiatry 1988;45(5):413–22.
12. Mavissakalian MR, Perel JM. Long-term maintenance and discontinuation of imipramine therapy in panic disorder with agoraphobia. Arch Gen Psychiatry 1999;56(9):821–7.
13. Moroz G, Rosenbaum JF. Efficacy, safety, and gradual discontinuation of clonazepam in panic disorder: a placebo-controlled, multicenter study using optimized dosages. J Clin Psychiatry 1999;60(9):604–12.
14. Noyes R Jr, Burrows GD, Reich JH, et al. Diazepam versus alprazolam for the treatment of panic disorder. J Clin Psychiatry 1996;57(8):349–55.
15. van Vliet IM, Westenberg HG, Den Boer JA. MAO inhibitors in panic disorder: clinical effects of treatment with brofaromine. A double blind placebo controlled study. Psychopharmacology (Berl) 1993;112(4):483–9.
16. Hoffman EJ, Mathew SJ. Anxiety disorders: a comprehensive review of pharmacotherapies. Mt Sinai J Med 2008;75(3):248–62.
17. Pollack M, Mangano R, Entsuah R, et al. A randomized controlled trial of venlafaxine ER and paroxetine in the treatment of outpatients with panic disorder. Psychopharmacology (Berl) 2007;194(2):233–42.
18. Otto MW, Tuby KS, Gould RA, et al. An effect-size analysis of the relative efficacy and tolerability of serotonin selective reuptake inhibitors for panic disorder. Am J Psychiatry 2001;158(12):1989–92.
19. Bakker A, van Balkom AJ, Spinhoven P. SSRIs vs. TCAs in the treatment of panic disorder: a meta-analysis. Acta Psychiatr Scand 2002;106(3):163–7.
20. Lepola U, Arato M, Zhu Y, et al. Sertraline versus imipramine treatment of comorbid panic disorder and major depressive disorder. J Clin Psychiatry 2003;64(6):654–62.
21. Marchesi C, Cantoni A, Fonto S, et al. The effect of pharmacotherapy on personality disorders in panic disorder: a one year naturalistic study. J Affect Disord 2005;89(1–3):189–94.
22. Marchesi C, Cantoni A, Fonto S, et al. Predictors of symptom resolution in panic disorder after one year of pharmacological treatment: a naturalistic study. Pharmacopsychiatry 2006;39(2):60–5.
23. Mavissakalian M, Hamann MS. DSM-III personality disorder in agoraphobia. II. Changes with treatment. Compr Psychiatry 1987;28(4):356–61.
24. Pollack MH, Otto MW, Tesar GE, et al. Long-term outcome after acute treatment with alprazolam or clonazepam for panic disorder. J Clin Psychopharmacol 1993;13(4):257–63.
25. Scheibe G, Albus M. Predictors and outcome in panic disorder: a 2-year prospective follow-up study. Psychopathology 1997;30(3):177–84.
26. Pollack MH, Otto MW, Sachs GS, et al. Anxiety psychopathology predictive of outcome in patients with panic disorder and depression treated with imipramine, alprazolam and placebo. J Affect Disord 1994;30(4):273–81.

27. Noyes R Jr, Reich J, Christiansen J, et al. Outcome of panic disorder. Relationship to diagnostic subtypes and comorbidity. Arch Gen Psychiatry 1990;47(9): 809–18.

28. Slaap BR, den Boer JA. The prediction of nonresponse to pharmacotherapy in panic disorder: a review. Depress Anxiety 2001;14(2):112–22.

29. Overbeek T, Buchold H, Schruers K, et al. Blood-injury related phobic avoidance as predictor of nonresponse to pharmacotherapy in panic disorder with agoraphobia. J Affect Disord 2004;78(3):227–33.

30. Lee IS, Kim KJ, Kang EH, et al. Beta-adrenoceptor affinity as a biological predictor of treatment response to paroxetine in patients with acute panic disorder. J Affect Disord 2008;110(1–2):156–60.

31. Pollack MH, Otto MW, Roy-Byrne PP, et al. Novel treatment approaches for refractory anxiety disorders. Depress Anxiety 2008;25(6):467–76.

32. Pollack MH, Simon NM, Worthington JJ, et al. Combined paroxetine and clonazepam treatment strategies compared to paroxetine monotherapy for panic disorder. J Psychopharmacol 2003;17(3):276–82.

33. Tiffon L, Coplan JD, Papp LA, et al. Augmentation strategies with tricyclic or fluoxetine treatment in seven partially responsive panic disorder patients. J Clin Psychiatry 1994;55(2):66–9.

34. Ontiveros A, Fontaine R. Sodium valproate and clonazepam for treatment-resistant panic disorder. J Psychiatry Neurosci 1992;17(2):78–80.

35. Pollack MH, Matthews J, Scott EL. Gabapentin as a potential treatment for anxiety disorders. Am J Psychiatry 1998;155(7):992–3.

36. Zwanzger P, Baghai TC, Schule C, et al. Tiagabine improves panic and agoraphobia in panic disorder patients. J Clin Psychiatry 2001;62(8):656–7.

37. Hirschmann S, Dannon PN, Iancu I, et al. Pindolol augmentation in patients with treatment-resistant panic disorder: a double-blind, placebo-controlled trial. J Clin Psychopharmacol 2000;20(5):556–9.

38. Sepede G, De Berardis D, Gambi F, et al. Olanzapine augmentation in treatment-resistant panic disorder: a 12-week, fixed-dose, open-label trial. J Clin Psychopharmacol 2006;26(1):45–9.

39. Londborg PD, Hegel MT, Goldstein S, et al. Sertraline treatment of posttraumatic stress disorder: results of 24 weeks of open-label continuation treatment. J Clin Psychiatry 2001;62(5):325–31.

40. Workgroup on Panic Disorder. Practice guideline for the treatment of patients with panic disorder, second edition. Am J Psychiatry 2009;166(1)Suppl:1–48.

41. Bouton ME, Mineka S, Barlow DH. A modern learning theory perspective on the etiology of panic disorder. Psychol Rev 2001;108(1):4–32.

42. McNally RJ. Anxiety sensitivity and panic disorder. Biol Psychiatry 2002;52(10): 938–46.

43. Otto MW, Smits JA, Reese HE. Cognitive-behavioral therapy for the treatment of anxiety disorders. J Clin Psychiatry 2004;65(Suppl 5):34–41.

44. Hofmann SG, Smits JA. Cognitive-behavioral therapy for adult anxiety disorders: a meta-analysis of randomized placebo-controlled trials. J Clin Psychiatry 2008; 69(4):621–32.

45. Ost LG, Thulin U, Ramnero J. Cognitive behavior therapy vs exposure in vivo in the treatment of panic disorder with agoraphobia (corrected from agrophobia). Behav Res Ther 2004;42(10):1105–27.

46. Penava SJ, Otto MW, Maki KM, et al. Rate of improvement during cognitive-behavioral group treatment for panic disorder. Behav Res Ther 1998;36(7–8): 665–73.

47. Craske MG, Brown TA, Barlow DH. Behavioral treatment of panic: a two year follow-up. Behav Ther 1991;22:289–304.
48. Margraf J, Barlow DH, Clark DM, et al. Psychological treatment of panic: work in progress on outcome, active ingredients, and follow-up. Behav Res Ther 1993; 31(1):1–8.
49. Telch MJ, Schmidt NB, Jaimez TL, et al. Impact of cognitive-behavioral treatment on quality of life in panic disorder patients. J Consult Clin Psychol 1995;63(5): 823–30.
50. Tsao JC, Lewin MR, Craske MG. The effects of cognitive-behavior therapy for panic disorder on comorbid conditions. J Anxiety Disord 1998;12(4):357–71.
51. McHugh RK, Otto MW, Barlow DH, et al. Cost-efficacy of individual and combined treatments for panic disorder. J Clin Psychiatry 2007;68(7):1038–44.
52. Otto MW, Pollack MH, Maki KM. Empirically supported treatments for panic disorder: costs, benefits, and stepped care. J Consult Clin Psychol 2000; 68(4):556–63.
53. Telch MJ, Lucas JA, Schmidt NB, et al. Group cognitive behavioral treatment of panic disorder. Behav Res Ther 1993;31(3):279–87.
54. Heldt E, Blaya C, Isolan L, et al. Quality of life and treatment outcome in panic disorder: cognitive behavior group therapy effects in patients refractory to medication treatment. Psychother Psychosom 2006;75(3):183–6.
55. Oei TP, Llamas M, Evans L. Does concurrent drug intake affect the long-term outcome of group cognitive behaviour therapy in panic disorder with or without agoraphobia? Behav Res Ther 1997;35(9):851–7.
56. Clark DM, Salkovskis PM, Hackmann A, et al. Brief cognitive therapy for panic disorder: a randomized controlled trial. J Consult Clin Psychol 1999;67(4): 583–9.
57. Craske MG, Maidenberg E, Bystritsky A. Brief cognitive-behavioral versus nondirective therapy for panic disorder. J Behav Ther Exp Psychiatry 1995; 26(2):113–20.
58. Cowley DS, Flick SN, Roy-Byrne PP. Long-term course and outcome in panic disorder: a naturalistic follow-up study. Anxiety 1996;2(1):13–21.
59. Warshaw MG, Massion AO, Shea MT, et al. Predictors of remission in patients with panic with and without agoraphobia: prospective 5-year follow-up data. J Nerv Ment Dis 1997;185(8):517–9.
60. McLean PD, Woody S, Taylor S, et al. Comorbid panic disorder and major depression: implications for cognitive-behavioral therapy. J Consult Clin Psychol 1998;66(2):240–7.
61. Tsao JCI, Mystkowski JL, Zucker BG, et al. Effects of cognitive-behavioral therapy for panic disorder on comorbid conditions: replication and extension. Behav Ther 2002;33(4):493–509.
62. Craske MG, Farchione TJ, Allen LB, et al. Cognitive behavioral therapy for panic disorder and comorbidity: more of the same or less of more? Behav Res Ther 2007;45(6):1095–109.
63. Conway KP, Compton W, Stinson FS, et al. Lifetime comorbidity of DSM-IV mood and anxiety disorders and specific drug use disorders: results from the National Epidemiologic Survey on Alcohol and Related Conditions. J Clin Psychiatry 2006;67(2):247–57.
64. Bouton ME. Context, ambiguity, and unlearning: sources of relapse after behavioral extinction. Biol Psychiatry 2002;52(10):976–86.
65. Mystkowski JL, Mineka S, Vernon LL, et al. Changes in caffeine states enhance return of fear in spider phobia. J Consult Clin Psychol 2003;71(2):243–50.

66. Powers MB, Smits JA, Whitley D, et al. The effect of attributional processes concerning medication taking on return of fear. J Consult Clin Psychol 2008;76(3): 478–90.

67. Biondi M, Picardi A. Attribution of improvement to medication and increased risk of relapse of panic disorder with agoraphobia. Psychother Psychosom 2003; 72(2):110–1 [author reply 111].

68. Otto MW, Pollack MH, Penava SJ, et al. Group cognitive-behavior therapy for patients failing to respond to pharmacotherapy for panic disorder: a clinical case series. Behav Res Ther 1999;37(8):763–70.

69. Pollack MH, Otto MW, Kaspi SP, et al. Cognitive behavior therapy for treatment-refractory panic disorder. J Clin Psychiatry 1994;55(5):200–5.

70. Heldt E, Gus Manfro G, Kipper L, et al. One-year follow-up of pharmaco-therapy-resistant patients with panic disorder treated with cognitive-behavior therapy: outcome and predictors of remission. Behav Res Ther 2006;44(5): 657–65.

71. Heldt E, Manfro GG, Kipper L, et al. Treating medication-resistant panic disorder: predictors and outcome of cognitive-behavior therapy in a Brazilian public hospital. Psychother Psychosom 2003;72(1):43–8.

72. Otto MW, Pollack MH, Sachs GS, et al. Discontinuation of benzodiazepine treatment: efficacy of cognitive-behavioral therapy for patients with panic disorder. Am J Psychiatry 1993;150(10):1485–90.

73. Hegel MT, Ravaris CL, Ahles TA. Combined cognitive-behavioral and time-limited alprazolam treatment of panic disorder. Behav Ther 1994;25:183–95.

74. Spiegel DA, Bruce TJ, Gregg SF, et al. Does cognitive behavior therapy assist slow-taper alprazolam discontinuation in panic disorder? Am J Psychiatry 1994;151(6):876–81.

75. Schmidt NB, Wollaway-Bickel K, Trakowski JH, et al. Antidepressant discontinuation in the context of cognitive behavioral treatment for panic disorder. Behav Res Ther 2002;40(1):67–73.

76. Whittal ML, Otto MW, Hong JJ. Cognitive-behavior therapy for discontinuation of SSRI treatment of panic disorder: a case series. Behav Res Ther 2001;39(8): 939–45.

77. Pollack MH, Simon NM. Pharmacotherapy for panic disorder and agoraphobia. In: Antony MM, Stein MB, editors. Oxford handbook of anxiety and related disorders. New York: Oxford University Press; 2009.

78. Roy-Byrne PP, Craske MG, Stein MB. Panic disorder. Lancet 2006;368(9540): 1023–32.

79. Maron E, Kuikka JT, Shlik J, et al. Reduced brain serotonin transporter binding in patients with panic disorder. Psychiatry Res 2004;132(2):173–81.

80. Nash JR, Sargent PA, Rabiner EA, et al. Serotonin 5-HT1A receptor binding in people with panic disorder: positron emission tomography study. Br J Psychiatry 2008;193(3):229–34.

81. Bakker A, van Balkom AJ, Stein DJ. Evidence-based pharmacotherapy of panic disorder. Int J Neuropsychopharmacol 2005;8(3):473–82.

82. Szabo ST, de Montigny C, Blier P. Modulation of noradrenergic neuronal firing by selective serotonin reuptake blockers. Br J Pharmacol 1999;126(3):568–71.

83. Charney DS, Woods SW, Nagy LM, et al. Noradrenergic function in panic disorder. J Clin Psychiatry 1990;51(Suppl A):5–11.

84. Bailey JE, Argyropoulos SV, Lightman SL, et al. Does the brain noradrenaline network mediate the effects of the CO2 challenge? J Psychopharmacol 2003; 17(3):252–9.

85. Cameron OG, Huang GC, Nichols T, et al. Reduced gamma-aminobutyric acid(A)-benzodiazepine binding sites in insular cortex of individuals with panic disorder. Arch Gen Psychiatry 2007;64(7):793–800.
86. Hasler G, Nugent AC, Carlson PJ, et al. Altered cerebral gamma-aminobutyric acid type A-benzodiazepine receptor binding in panic disorder determined by [11C]flumazenil positron emission tomography. Arch Gen Psychiatry 2008; 65(10):1166–75.
87. Goddard AW, Mason GF, Almai A, et al. Reductions in occipital cortex GABA levels in panic disorder detected with 1h-magnetic resonance spectroscopy. Arch Gen Psychiatry 2001;58(6):556–61.
88. Ham BJ, Sung Y, Kim N, et al. Decreased GABA levels in anterior cingulate and basal ganglia in medicated subjects with panic disorder: a proton magnetic resonance spectroscopy (1H-MRS) study. Prog Neuropsychopharmacol Biol Psychiatry 2007;31(2):403 11.
89. Clark DM. A cognitive approach to panic. Behav Res Ther 1986;24(4):461–70.
90. Barlow DH. Anxiety and its disorders. the nature and treatment of anxiety and panic. 2nd edition. New York: Guilford Press; 2002.
91. Smits JA, Powers MB, Cho Y, et al. Mechanism of change in cognitive behavioral treatment of panic disorder: evidence for the fear of fear mediational hypothesis. J Consult Clin Psychol 2004;72(4):646–52.
92. Hofmann SG, Meuret AE, Rosenfield D, et al. Preliminary evidence for cognitive mediation during cognitive-behavioral therapy of panic disorder. J Consult Clin Psychol 2007;75(3):374–9.
93. Wells A, Papageorgious C. Social phobia: effects of external attention on anxiety, negative beliefs, and perspective taking. Behav Ther 1998;29:357–70.
94. Telch MJ, Jacquin K, Smits JAJ, et al. Emotional responding to hyperventilation as a predictor of agoraphobia status among individuals suffering from panic disorder. J Behav Ther Exp Psychiatry 2003;34(2):161–70.
95. Salkovskis PM, Clark DM, Hackmann A, et al. An experimental investigation of the role of safety-seeking behaviours in the maintenance of panic disorder with agoraphobia. Behav Res Ther 1999;37(6):559–74.
96. Wells A, Clark DM, Salkovskis PM, et al. Social phobia: the role of in-situation safety behaviors in maintaining anxiety and negative beliefs. Behav Ther 1995;26:153–61.
97. Schmidt NB, Woolaway-Bickel K, Trakowski J, et al. Dismantling cognitive-behavioral treatment for panic disorder: questioning the utility of breathing re-training. J Consult Clin Psychol 2000;68(3):417–24.
98. Bouchard S, Gauthier J, Laberge B, et al. Exposure versus cognitive restructuring in the treatment of panic disorder with agoraphobia. Behav Res Ther 1996; 34(3):213–24.
99. van den Hout M, Arntz A, Hoekstra R. Exposure reduced agoraphobia but not panic, and cognitive therapy reduced panic but not agoraphobia. Behav Res Ther 1994;32(4):447–51.
100. Addis ME, Hatgis C, Cardemil E, et al. Effectiveness of cognitive-behavioral treatment for panic disorder versus treatment as usual in a managed care setting: 2-year follow-up. J Consult Clin Psychol 2006;74(2):377–85.
101. Brown TA, Barlow DH. Long-term outcome in cognitive-behavioral treatment of panic disorder: clinical predictors and alternative strategies for assessment. J Consult Clin Psychol 1995;63(5):754–65.
102. Meuret AE, Wilhelm FH, Ritz T, et al. Feedback of end-tidal pCO2 as a therapeutic approach for panic disorder. J Psychiatr Res 2008;42(7):560–8.

103. Shear MK, Houck P, Greeno C, et al. Emotion-focused psychotherapy for patients with panic disorder. Am J Psychiatry 2001;158(12):1993–8.
104. Milrod BL, Leon AC, Busch F, et al. A randomized controlled trial of psychoanalytic psychotherapy for panic disorder. Am J Psychiatry 2007;164(2):265–72.
105. Milrod BL, Leon AC, Barber JP, et al. Do comorbid personality disorders moderate panic-focused psychotherapy? An exploratory examination of the American Psychiatric Association practice guideline. J Clin Psychiatry 2007; 68(6):885–91.
106. Stathopoulou G, Powers MB, Berry AC, et al. Exercise interventions for mental health: a quantitative and qualitative review. Br J Clin Psychol 2006;13(2): 179–93.
107. Broman-Fulks JJ, Berman ME, Rabian BA, et al. Effects of aerobic exercise on anxiety sensitivity. Behav Res Ther 2004;42(2):125–36.
108. Broman-Fulks JJ, Storey KM. Evaluation of a brief aerobic exercise intervention for high anxiety sensitivity. Anxiety Stress Coping 2008;21(2):117–28.
109. Smits JA, Berry AC, Rosenfield D, et al. Reducing anxiety sensitivity with exercise. Depress Anxiety 2008;25(8):689–99.
110. Broocks A, Bandelow B, Pekrun G, et al. Comparison of aerobic exercise, clomipramine, and placebo in the treatment of panic disorder. Am J Psychiatry 1998;155(5):603–9.
111. Davidson JR, Foa EB, Huppert JD, et al. Fluoxetine, comprehensive cognitive behavioral therapy, and placebo in generalized social phobia. Arch Gen Psychiatry 2004;61(10):1005–13.
112. Richardson R, Ledgerwood L, Cranney J. Facilitation of fear extinction by D-cycloserine: theoretical and clinical implications. Learn Mem 2004;11(5): 510–6.
113. Ressler KJ, Rothbaum BO, Tannenbaum L, et al. Cognitive enhancers as adjuncts to psychotherapy: use of D-cycloserine in phobic individuals to facilitate extinction of fear. Arch Gen Psychiatry 2004;61(11):1136–44.
114. Hofmann SG, Meuret AE, Smits JA, et al. Augmentation of exposure therapy with D-cycloserine for social anxiety disorder. Arch Gen Psychiatry 2006;63(3): 298–304.
115. Guastella AJ, Richardson R, Lovibond PF, et al. A randomized controlled trial of D-cycloserine enhancement of exposure therapy for social anxiety disorder. Biol Psychiatry 2008;63(6):544–9.
116. Kushner MG, Kim SW, Donahue C, et al. D-cycloserine augmented exposure therapy for obsessive-compulsive disorder. Biol Psychiatry 2007;62(8):835–8.
117. Norberg MM, Krystal JH, Tolin DF. A meta-analysis of D-cycloserine and the facilitation of fear extinction and exposure therapy. Biol Psychiatry 2008; 63(12):1118–26.
118. Heuzenroeder L, Donnelly M, Haby MM, et al. Cost-effectiveness of psychological and pharmacological interventions for generalized anxiety disorder and panic disorder. Aust N Z J Psychiatry 2004;38(8):602–12.
119. Craske MG, Golinelli D, Stein MB, et al. Does the addition of cognitive behavioral therapy improve panic disorder treatment outcome relative to medication alone in the primary-care setting? Psychol Med 2005;35(11):1645–54.
120. Mavissakalian M, Michelson L. Agoraphobia: relative and combined effectiveness of therapist-assisted in vivo exposure and imipramine. J Clin Psychiatry 1986;47(3):117–22.
121. Telch MJ, Agras WS, Taylor CB, et al. Combined pharmacological and behavioral treatment for agoraphobia. Behav Res Ther 1985;23(3):325–35.

122. Addis ME, Hatgis C, Krasnow AD, et al. Effectiveness of cognitive–behavioral treatment for panic disorder versus treatment as usual in a managed care setting. J Consult Clin Psychol 2004;72(4):625–35.

123. Stuart GL, Treat TA, Wade WA. Effectiveness of an empirically based treatment for panic disorder delivered in a service clinic setting: 1-year follow-up. J Consult Clin Psychol 2000;68(3):506–12.

124. Wade WA, Treat TA, Stuart GL. Transporting an empirically supported treatment for panic disorder to a service clinic setting: a benchmarking strategy. J Consult Clin Psychol 1998;66(2):231–9.

125. President's New Freedom Commission on Mental Health: report of the President's New Freedom Commission on Mental Health. Available at: http://www.mentalhealthcommission.gov/reports/FinalReport/toc.html; 2004. Accessed May 7, 2008.

126. Goisman RM, Warshaw MG, Keller MB. Psychosocial treatment prescriptions for generalized anxiety disorder, panic disorder, and social phobia, 1991-1996. Am J Psychiatry 1999;156(11):1819–21.

127. Stein MB, Sherbourne CD, Craske MG, et al. Quality of care for primary care patients with anxiety disorders. Am J Psychiatry 2004;161(12):2230–7.

128. Roy-Byrne PP, Craske MG, Stein MB, et al. A randomized effectiveness trial of cognitive-behavioral therapy and medication for primary care panic disorder. Arch Gen Psychiatry 2005;62(3):290–8.

129. Katon W, Russo J, Sherbourne C, et al. Incremental cost-effectiveness of a collaborative care intervention for panic disorder. Psychol Med 2006;36(3):353–63.

130. Kenwright M, Liness S, Marks I. Reducing demands on clinicians by offering computer-aided self-help for phobia/panic. Feasibility study. Br J Psychiatry 2001;179:456 9.

131. Kenwright M, Marks IM. Computer-aided self-help for phobia/panic via internet at home: a pilot study. Br J Psychiatry 2004;184:448–9.

132. Schneider AJ, Mataix-Cols D, Marks IM, et al. Internet-guided self-help with or without exposure therapy for phobic and panic disorders. Psychother Psychosom 2005;74(3):154–64.

133. Sullivan G, Craske MG, Sherbourne C, et al. Design of the Coordinated Anxiety Learning and Management (CALM) study: innovations in collaborative care for anxiety disorders. Gen Hosp Psychiatry 2007;29(5):379–87.

134. Jacobs RJ, Davidson JR, Gupta S, et al. The effects of clonazepam on quality of life and work productivity in panic disorder. Am J Manag Care 1997;3(8): 1187–96.

135. Rapaport MH, Pollack M, Wolkow R, et al. Is placebo response the same as drug response in panic disorder? Am J Psychiatry 2000;157(6):1014–6.

136. American Psychological Association. Diagnostic and statistical manual of mental disorders. Washington, DC: American Psychiatric Association; 1994.

137. Wittchen HU, Nocon A, Beesdo K, et al. Agoraphobia and panic. Prospective-longitudinal relations suggest a rethinking of diagnostic concepts. Psychother Psychosom 2008;77(3):147–57.

138. Fava GA, Grandi S, Canestrari R. Prodromal symptoms in panic disorder with agoraphobia. Am J Psychiatry 1988;145(12):1564–7.

139. Fava GA, Grandi S, Rafanelli C, et al. Prodromal symptoms in panic disorder with agoraphobia: a replication study. J Affect Disord 1992;26(2):85–8.

140. Kessler RC, Chiu WT, Jin R, et al. The epidemiology of panic attacks, panic disorder, and agoraphobia in the National Comorbidity Survey Replication. Arch Gen Psychiatry 2006;63(4):415–24.

141. Krueger RF, Watson D, Barlow DH. Introduction to the special section: toward a dimensionally based taxonomy of psychopathology. J Abnorm Psychol 2005;114(4):491–3.
142. Watson D. Rethinking the mood and anxiety disorders: a quantitative hierarchical model for DSM-V. J Abnorm Psychol 2005;114(4):522–36.
143. Hayward C, Wilson KA. Anxiety sensitivity: a missing piece to the agoraphobia-without-panic puzzle. Behav Modif 2007;31(2):162–73.

Generalized Anxiety Disorder: Between Now and DSM-V

Christer Allgulander, MD, PhD

KEYWORDS

- Anxiety disorders
- Classification • Anti-anxiety agents
- Antidepressive agents • Pharmacology
- Generalized anxiety disorder • GAD • DSM-V

Generalized anxiety disorder (GAD) differs from other anxiety disorders and from depression in terms of the pervasive cognitive dysfunction and associated prospective threat scenarios. It is accompanied by subjective tension, pain, sleep disturbance, fatiguability, and irritability, conducive to impaired performance in work, leisure, and family life. It is the most common anxiety disorder in medical treatment settings, and it increases the disease burden in cardiovascular and cerebrovascular disease, pulmonary disease, and diabetes mellitus. GAD is amenable to several pharmacotherapies and to cognitive behavioral therapy (see the article by Hoyer and Gloster in this issue).

This article presents the current evidence base for pharmacotherapy of GAD and an update on the phenomenology of GAD and its association with other psychiatric and somatic conditions. It discusses nosological issues and suggests ways to improve recognition, treatment, and care for patients who have GAD.

Patients who have GAD are excessively concerned with the safety and comfort of the immediate family and oneself.[1] Here are some examples of this kind of dysfunctional thinking:

> "What if Eva had breast cancer—would we have to move out of the house? Will junior be able to complete his studies, considering the problems his girlfriend are causing him? Why is Gertrude late from kindergarten; has there been an accident? I have double-checked the report, but I had still better go to the office on Sunday to make sure, considering the consequences if I have overlooked something. I cannot stop worrying all the time about the bills at the end of the month although I have always been able to pay them on time."

Department of Clinical Neuroscience, Karolinska Institutet, Section of Psychiatry at Karolinska University Hospital, SE 141 86 Huddinge, Sweden
E-mail address: christer.allgulander@ki.se

Psychiatr Clin N Am 32 (2009) 611–628
doi:10.1016/j.psc.2009.05.006
0193-953X/09/$ – see front matter © 2009 Elsevier Inc. All rights reserved.

Although these thoughts (talking to oneself) seem trivial at first glance, they preoccupy the subject's cognition, draw attention and energy, and cannot be put aside. They are future oriented and differ from depressive ruminations that deal with past failures and are associated with guilt feelings. In obsessive-compulsive disorder obsessions typically concern orderliness, contamination, and moral issues. Patients who have GAD often say that they have always worried excessively about minor matters to a degree that eventually impairs their social functioning. The worry serves to preempt episodes of exacerbated fear in an imaginary world with negative emotional affect. The somatic manifestations of GAD, particularly tension, evolve and finally lead to social consequences such as impaired work performance, reduced leisure activities, and a tense and irritable family atmosphere.

THE EVIDENCE FOR SPECIFIC FORMS OF PHARMACOTHERAPY FOR GENERALIZED ANXIETY DISORDER

The current regulatory climate determines how pharmacotherapies for GAD are made available to the public and encourages new measures, reproducibility of results, transparency, and accountability. The value of an anxiolytic for GAD now is measured in at least four domains: independent randomized, controlled trials in support of anxiolytic efficacy versus placebo and active compounds (always including the Hamilton Rating Scale for Anxiety, HAMA), an estimate of the risk of relapse into GAD upon treatment cessation after responding, self-ratings on restoration of social functioning, and clinical safety for up to 6 months of therapy. The recent regulatory request for noninferiority analyses in GAD studies stems from the increasing availability of medications for some disorders (eg, antibiotics, antihypertensives, and antidepressants/anxiolytics); noninferiority to a comparator drug should be demonstrated, based on predefined sets of statistical and clinical criteria.[2] In addition to satisfying these regulatory requirements in phase II to phase III studies, a wealth of data derived from secondary analyses ("data-mining") provide a basis for generating and testing new hypotheses, such as gender differences in symptom pattern and treatment response in cases of primary GAD, pharmacogenetic and clinical predictors of response and remission, and pharmacodynamic correlates to adverse drug reactions. Efficiency studies demonstrate the direct and off-set savings for the individual and for society that are realized by identifying and treating patients who have GAD.

Recent study programs of GAD anxiolytics have not been burdened with nonconclusive studies, contrary to the situation 10 years ago, when every other GAD study failed to distinguish active drug from placebo.[3] This improvement is a result of the improved training of clinicians in trials, the inclusion of patients with more psychopathology, and the use of sensitive objective and subjective rating instruments.

Although clomipramine, desipramine, and alprazolam were approved by regulatory bodies in the early 1980s for treating patients who have panic disorder, the first approval of a medication for GAD was given much later, with venlafaxine, in 1999. There was a need for new maintenance medications because benzodiazepine anxiolytic treatment had become restricted to short-term use.

Buspirone was approved for symptoms of GAD by the Food and Drug Administration in 1985, but most of the studies were performed in the 1970s in patients diagnosed with psychoneurosis, which, according to the criteria of the *Diagnostic and Statistical Manual of Mental Disorders,* edition 2 (DSM-II), could include substantial depressive symptoms. They then were re-diagnosed retrospectively with the GAD criteria specified in the third edition of the DSM (DSM-III).

A task force appointed by the World Federation of Societies of Biological Psychiatry recently updated the treatment recommendations for GAD.[4] The task force worked in the spirit of Cochrane methodology, rank-ordering treatments based on the quality of the evidence for efficacy as well as an assessment of the risk/benefit ratio. The strongest evidence was found for escitalopram, paroxetine, sertraline, venlafaxine, duloxetine, pregabalin, and quetiapine. Although the tricyclic imipramine is effective in GAD, its higher adverse effect burden and toxicity in overdose make it a secondary drug of choice. In treatment-resistant cases with no history of addiction, the benzodiazepines alprazolam and diazepam may be used. The benzodiazepines also are useful as adjuncts to attain immediate anxiolytic relief in the initiation of other treatments and in episodes of symptom exacerbation. The antihistamine hydroxyzine has been shown to be effective in GAD, but its utility is hampered by sedation. In cases refractory to first-line treatments, adjunct treatment with low doses of olanzapine and risperidone may be tried.

The first guideline for long-term and maintenance treatment of GAD was based on a total of 26 published controlled studies in 2001.[5] At that time, there were four published controlled trials of 6 months' duration in GAD. These trials showed sustained efficacy of venlafaxine and paroxetine compared with placebo. Clorazepate and buspirone showed sustained and comparable efficacy, but without a validating placebo study arm. No tolerance development to the anxiolytic effect was observed for clorazepate, but on rapid discontinuation of clorazepate most patients reported at least five new symptoms on the Physician Checklist of Withdrawal Symptoms. Escitalopram, duloxetine, and pregabalin were assessed subsequently in studies of at least 6 months' duration.[6–8] When patients who responded to treatment with the medications listed in **Table 1** were assigned randomly either to continued active drug or to placebo, there were substantially higher risks of relapse in GAD symptomatology in the group receiving placebo.

In clinical practice, remission rather than response is the goal in treating patients who have GAD.

In studies, remission is considered, by consensus, to be a score of 7 or less on the HAMA, accompanied by restoration of functioning.[9,10] Remission rates were analyzed in two 6-month studies of venlafaxine.[11] The remission rate on venlafaxine was 43%, compared with 19% on placebo ($P < .0001$). Most patients who had not responded after 2 months' treatment had remitted by 6 months, regardless of baseline severity, indicating that many patients require sustained treatment periods.

The efficacy of GAD medications was confirmed in a meta-analysis based on 21 studies between 1987 and 2003 that used criteria from the revised DSM-III (DSM-III-R), the fourth edition of the DSM (DSM-IV), or International Classification of Diseases (ICD)-10.[12] Two studies in children/adolescents were included. The primary

Table 1
Medications approved by regulatory authorities for treating patients who have GAD

Generic Name	Trade Names	Dosing for GAD (mg)
Venlafaxine	Effexor XR, Faxine, Effexor	75–375
Paroxetine	Seroxat, Eutimil, Paxil, Deroxat	20–50
Duloxetine	Cymbalta, Xeristar	(30–) 60–120
Pregabalin	Lyrica	150–600
Escitalopram	Cipralex, Sipralex, Lexapro, Entact	10–20

efficacy variable was the reduction in score on the HAMA rating scale after 8 to 24 weeks of treatment. In comparing all the drugs in **Table 2** versus placebo, the overall effect size of medications was 0.39 ± 0.06 ($P < .0001$). Treatment effects were higher in children and adolescents than in adults, perhaps because there was a shorter duration of illness in the young. Complementary/alternative compounds had a negative impact on symptom rating. The authors remarked that the effect size of medications in GAD was in keeping with those in posttraumatic stress disorder and were lower than seen in obsessive-compulsive disorder, panic disorder, and social anxiety disorder. The publication bias was regarded as negligible (23 additional studies would be required to overturn the findings).

THE EVIDENCE FOR COMBINED TREATMENTS FOR GENERALIZED ANXIETY DISORDER

There is no evidence base as yet for combining pharmacotherapy and psychotherapy in patients who have GAD. Good studies on combined treatments in GAD would entail large study populations and rigid assessment techniques to tease out the effective components. There is no consensus on how to combine such treatments in current practice. Psychodynamic therapists oppose concurrent anxiolytic medications, because the emotion of anxiety is assumed to stem from unconscious sources that are to be revealed and worked through in therapy.[13] Anxiety, according to the Freudian credo, is an essential emotion that is exacerbated in psychoanalysis and psychodynamic therapy at the peril of the patient's getting worse and even developing a secondary depression. Cognitive behavioral therapists, on the other hand, generally do not oppose anxiolytic medication, particularly if it enables the patient to develop coping skills and minimizes avoidance behavior. Medications and cognitive behavioral therapy thus may work hand in hand, and medications may empower the patient to confront his/her anxiety in exposing exercises. In clinical practice, the two treatments often are combined if the patient is motivated and can afford the treatments.

NEW DEVELOPMENTS IN TREATMENT

This section is a brief review of recent and ongoing clinical studies on various aspects of GAD that will provide useful insights and tools for treatment.

Table 2
Effect sizes versus placebo of different medications in GAD studies

Medication	Effect Size Versus Placebo	P-Value
Pregabalin	0.50	$P < .0001$
Hydroxyzine	0.45	$P < .0001$
Venlafaxine	0.42	$P < .0001$
Benzodiazepines	0.38	$P < .0001$
Selective serotonin-reuptake inhibitors	0.36	$P < .0001$
Buspirone	0.17	nonsignificant
Kava-kava, homeopathic preparation	−0.31	nonsignificant

Data from Hidalgo RB, Tupler LA, Davidson JRT. An effect-size analysis of pharmacologic treatments for generalized anxiety disorder. J Psychopharmacol 2007;21:870.

Insomnia in Generalized Anxiety Disorder

Sleep disturbance is a diagnostic criterion in GAD, causing impairment in daytime functioning that is different from the sleep pattern in depression.[14] It is reported by at least two thirds of patients who have GAD.[15] It is noteworthy that one study showed an increased and more rapid response rate in patients who have GAD who received a hypnotic as well as an anxiolytic.[1] The study included patients who had primary GAD (concurrent mild to moderate depression was allowed) and sleep latency of more than 30 minutes and who usually slept less than 6.5 hours per night. The participants initially were treated with escitalopram (10 mg/d) during run-in and then were assigned randomly to adjunct eszopiclone (3 mg) or to placebo at night. The primary efficacy variable was change in subjective sleep latency averaged during the double-blind study period of 8 weeks. Those taking adjunct eszopiclone had a mean improvement in sleep latency of 25 minutes, compared with 11 minutes in those taking adjunct placebo ($P < .001$). Total sleep time was subjectively increased by 61 minutes in the eszopiclone group and by 35 minutes in the placebo group ($P < .001$). The response rate in anxiety symptoms (ie, a reduction of > 50% in HAMA score) was 63% in the group receiving escitalopram plus eszopiclone, versus 49% in those receiving escitalopram plus placebo ($P = .001$). Reported daytime function also improved more in patients receiving escitalopram plus eszopiclone. There was no notable tolerance to eszopiclone or rebound insomnia. Men benefited from the combination more than women. A sub-hypnotic dose of eszopiclone per se had an anxiolytic effect in a recent report.[16] Also, pregabalin has been shown to enhance slow-wave sleep that frequently is reduced in GAD.[17] This effect is another indicator of the importance of addressing insomnia in GAD.

Quetiapine

Quetiapine is a dopamine (DA_2 receptor occupancy) modulator approved as an antipsychotic agent. Recent studies in GAD have exploited other pharmacodynamic effects: $5HT_{2A}$ receptor blockade and norepinephrine transporter occupancy.[18] A low dose range of 50 to 300 mg/d was compared with placebo, escitalopram, and paroxetine. in five controlled studies of quetiapine in adult and elderly patients who had GAD.[19–23] A 52-week relapse-prevention study showed a lower rate of symptom relapse in patients continuing with quetiapine treatment (10%) than in responders to quetiapine switched to placebo (39%).[24] Overall, these studies showed an anxiolytic effect over that of placebo, comparable with active comparators, and with a benign adverse effect burden. Remission rates were similar on quetiapine, escitalopram, and paroxetine, indicating that quetiapine may become a new therapeutic alternative in GAD, depending on a risk/benefit assessment of long-term safety.

Agomelatine

Agomelatine is an agonist at melatonin receptors and an antagonist at $5\text{-}HT_{2C}$ receptors. It is approved by the European Medicines Agency for the treatment of major depression. One controlled study indicating efficacy of agomelatine in patients who had GAD has been reported from Finland and South Africa.[25]

Tiagabine

Tiagabine is a selective γ-amino-butyric-acid reuptake inhibitor that has been assessed in three controlled GAD trials that did not demonstrate efficacy.[26]

Augmentation

Pilot studies have aimed at assessing the added benefit of olanzapine, risperidone, ziprasidone, and aripiprazole in patients who have anxiety disorder refractory to first-line treatments. Some results indicate benefit, and further augmentation studies are ongoing (www.clintrials.gov).

Muscle Relaxation

Muscle relaxation therapy, stemming from Jacobson's Progressive Muscle Relaxation postulated in 1934, has been shown to be effective in GAD, but its use now is questioned by both pharmacologists and leaders in cognitive behavioral therapy (see the article by Hoyer and Gloster in this issue).[27] Tension as a state of mind, however, remains a cardinal symptom in GAD that is highly responsive to treatment in controlled studies. According to one study, subjective tension, usually localized to the shoulders and neck, is the somatic component of GAD that is most strongly correlated with worry.[28]

A review of the concept of tension in GAD, however, concluded that it is ambiguous.[29] Multiple electromyographic studies did not find increased muscle tension in a study of 49 patients who had GAD, and muscle relaxation therapy failed to produce a response.[30] In phase III studies in Stockholm, the majority of the approximately 300 patients who had GAD spontaneously reported teeth grinding and bruxism at baseline (C. Allgulander, MD, PhD, unpublished data, 2007). Bite guards were prescribed so commonly by the patients' dentists that one might consider informing dentists of the study and suggesting a psychiatric referral of such patients. A recent study of escitalopram in patients who had GAD and temporomandibular disorders diagnosed by dentists indicated a therapeutic effect on this aspect.[31] This field deserves further research.

Patients who have GAD often are said to be in a constant state of increased vigilance and arousal. In an experiment, patients who had GAD failed to reduce sympathetic tone periodically, supporting the notion of constant vegetative arousal.[32]

Virtual Reality

Virtual reality is proposed as a method to enhance the ability of patients who have GAD to relax.[33] An ongoing study is using a virtual relaxing environment and audio-visual mobile narratives.

Internet-Based Services

Self-help by means of bibliotherapy and lay group activities is growing rapidly as a means for individuals to compare their symptoms with diagnostic criteria, to overcome stigma by associating with peers, and to try to develop coping skills. Universities and commercial vendors offer a range of such services. A meta-analytic study was performed on 13 studies of bibliotherapy and one self-help group study published before 2000, four of which pertained to anxiety disorders, nine to depression, and one to both.[34] The authors found a robust effect size for self-help treatments, significantly greater than that of the placebo or wait-list. They pointed out that the majority of patients in professional settings gain additional knowledge and may develop cognitive skills by bibliotherapy and by communicating with their peers. The Internet therefore may provide an important augmentation to manualized cognitive behavioral treatments for anxiety disorders as well as a range of other psychiatric disorders. It also may be useful in screening for patients with anxiety disorders.[35]

Computerized cognitive behavioral therapy for anxiety and depression was the subject of an effectiveness review by Kaltenthaler and colleagues,[36] who included 20 studies reported before 2004. To provide a basis for conclusions, the authors recommended more studies to tease out the specific benefits of computerized cognitive behavioral therapy (via the Internet) versus those of bibliotherapy.

MECHANISMS OF ACTION
Neuroimaging

Neuroimaging studies of anxiety have evolved since 1978.[37] The current focus is on amygdala hyperreactivity that has been demonstrated in anxiety disorders and in depression with functional magnetic resonance imaging (fMRI).[38,39]

An increased affective response to situations with uncertain outcomes (intolerance of uncertainty, IU) is a shared denominator in anxiety disorders.[40] fMRI has been used to find neurobiologic correlates to IU in models of affective ambiguity. One study showed insula activation bilaterally in a test of 14 college students.[39] An adolescent GAD/social anxiety study indicated activity in several frontal and limbic regions associated with IU.[41] Another adolescent GAD study reported right amygdala activation in exposure to angry faces and threat-related negative connectivity between the right ventrolateral prefrontal cortex and the amygdala, suggesting that the prefrontal cortex modulates the amygdala response to threat.[42] The neural circuitry dysfunction in adolescents who had GAD differed from that in adolescents who had social anxiety disorder and in controls.[43]

fMRI also has been used to predict individual response to treatment. One recent report in a controlled fMRI study of 14 subjects who had GAD found a correlation between high levels of pretreatment anterior cingulate cortex activity and reductions in anxiety and worry after 8 weeks' treatment with venlafaxine.[44] The subjects had been screened for major depression, and concurrent subclinical depressive scores were controlled for in the analysis to focus specifically on anticipatory anxiety. Interestingly, at baseline the subjects who had untreated GAD exhibited increased anticipatory response bilaterally in the dorsal amygdala to both neutral and aversive pictures, indicative of a trait emotional hyperresponsiveness. Such indiscriminate amygdala hyperreactivity points to the importance of anticipatory processes in the genesis of generalized anxiety. Similarly, persistent activations of the anterior cingulate and dorsal medial prefrontal cortex also were associated with worry during resting state scans.[45] Another study suggested that reactivity to fearful faces measured with fMRI is a predictor of response to pharmacotherapy in GAD.[46]

Neurotransmission

Vastly different pharmacodynamics without a shared common pathway (ie, opioids, alcohol, valerian, bromide, barbiturates, meprobamate, gluthetimide, clomethiazole, benzodiazepines, monoamine oxidase inhibitors, antipsychotics, buspirone, hydroxyzine, selective serotonin-reuptake inhibitors, selective norepinephrine-reuptake inhibitors, pregabalin, quetiapine, and agomelatine) modify clinical anxiety. The focus on serotonergic and noradrenergic transmission in anxiety has overshadowed other potential mechanisms in the central nervous system. Emerging studies of individual risk markers for depression and anxiety point partly to different underlying cognition pathways resulting from an interaction between the brain-derived neurotrophic factor (BDNF) *Val66Met* gene and early-life stress.[47]

Environmental Antecedents

The interaction between genetic vulnerability and environmental stressors in producing GAD has been elucidated in prospective studies. The Dunedin birth cohort study separated antecedents of 52 pure cases of GAD by age 32 years from those of

GAD with comorbid major depression and major depression alone.[48] The GAD diagnosis was based on DSM-IV criteria. Pure GAD cases differed significantly from healthy controls on certain baseline risk factors: maternal internalizing symptoms, low socioeconomic status, maltreatment, childhood internalizing symptoms, and conduct problems. They also had higher scores on inhibited temperament and greater negative affect. Patients who had comorbid GAD and major depression also had higher scores on most such antecedents but had a more episodic course than seen in cases of pure GAD. Pure cases of major depression had no such childhood risk factors but had a genetic and personality setup that predisposed the patients to react with depression to adult stressors. These results point to a set of early antecedents of GAD that may be both genetically and environmentally determined and that differ in part different from those for major depression.

HOW IS GENERALIZED ANXIETY DISORDER SIMILAR TO OTHER ANXIETY DISORDERS?

Work is on-going in the DSM-V expert committees to move beyond the "neo-Kraepelinian" basis of the current nosology. The committees are to consider dimensional, spectral, and developmental aspects, the influence of ethnicity and gender, and the concepts of severity, distress, and disability. The Axis II category is likely to be replaced by new headings. A joint DSM edition five (DSM-V)/ICD-11 task force has been charged with exploring the diagnostic validities of GAD and major depressive disorder.[49,50]

In June 2007, 25 experts were convened in London by the American Psychiatric Association, the World Health Organization, and the United States National Institutes of Health in a nosological conference focusing on GAD and depression. The purpose was to elucidate whether these concepts are different forms of the same disorder or are closely or distantly related and whether it is time to move from a descriptive to an etiologically based approach.[51] Several of the participants (Jack Hettema, Jules Angst, Myrna Weissman, Charles Nemeroff, Timothy Brown, Georg Brown, and Ronald Kessler) were in favor of retaining GAD as a disorder separate from affective disorders. Their arguments were based on the differences between GAD and major depression in time course in prospective studies, neuroendocrine and neuroimaging findings, sleep disturbance, and in the attentional bias to emotional stimuli. Johan Ormel summarized the reasons he regarded GAD and major depression to be related but not identical disorders: they co-occur beyond chance expectation; they share genetic susceptibility, they share some risk factors (eg, neuroticism or harm avoidance); they belong to the internalizing disorders domain; GAD often precedes MDD; and the disorders respond similarly to selective serotonin-reuptake inhibitors but differently to benzodiazepines. Terri Moffitt noted that, based on the Dunedin prospective cohort study, GAD and major depression are strongly related, but neither precedes the other or is milder than the other.[48] Martin Prince and others pointed to the large mixed category of anxiety depressive disorder that is found in primary care patients and that is associated with social dysfunction. David Goldberg proposed that major depression and GAD be made part of a dysphoric disorders group based on shared negative affect and separate from other anxiety disorders in a fear disorders category.

These issues deserve a brief historical note on how GAD first was conceptualized. A seminal paper was written in 1970 by Robins and Guze at Washington University in St. Louis.[52] They proposed establishing diagnostic validity in psychiatric illness based on clinical description, exclusion of other disorders, follow-up study, family study, and laboratory study. Such criteria-based diagnoses became the stem for the DSM-III in 1980 that was refined further in the DSM-III-R in 1987 and in the DSM-IV 1994. The initial 1980 set of GAD criteria was intended to substitute the psychodynamic concept of anxiety neurosis with panic disorder and a pervasive condition called "generalized anxiety." Subsequently, these criteria for GAD were found to overlap with those of major depressive disorder, and the criteria in the DSM-IV therefore were modified to focus on the cognitive dysfunction and a set of accompanying somatic symptoms with at least 6 months' duration.

There are other underpinnings for the diagnostic validity of GAD. The future-oriented worry in GAD differentiates the disorder from retrospective depressive ruminations and is fear related.[49,53] Worry in GAD also is qualitatively different from obsessions that deal with contamination, orderliness, and moral ambivalence.

The time courses of major depression and GAD differ in prospective studies. In samples of the United States adult population, risk factors were found to differ between major depression and GAD.[54] The Dunedin birth cohort study indicated partly separate etiological pathways.[48] The Zurich cohort study found that 75% of GAD cases had an onset before age 20 years, that 58% received professional treatment, and that 63% had had a remission (at least 12 months without GAD symptoms) by age 40 years.[55] Furthermore, only 7% in the cohort had a chronic unremitting course, and 22% had a comorbid major depression before age 40 years. Of note, 40% of the primary GAD cases were diagnosed subsequently with a bipolar disorder by age 40 years, indicating that GAD symptoms may be an early manifestation of bipolar disorder, particularly bipolar II. This report is in keeping with findings in Hungary.[56]

An interview study of Swedish twins found high genetic correlations between GAD and major depression in both men and women, indicating that the genetic substrates for the two disorders are interrelated.[57] A caveat when interpreting the results of such interview measures is that the wording and structure of different diagnostic interviews influence the results, thus compromising the phenotype.[58]

Will genetic research be the solution to a new nosology? The anxiety phenotypes that are based in the DSM definitions have performed poorly in applied genetic studies, but there also is a need for much larger data sets (using consortia), prospective cohorts, and the application of rapid technology such as the GeneChip. The strongest biological candidate yet, *5-HTTLPR* or the serotonin transporter gene, has been shown to be associated with a wide range of psychiatric and somatic conditions; this site is described ironically as "the source of all human suffering."[59]

Empiric support for the diagnostic validity of GAD also comes from phase II and phase III drug trials, for which "symptomatic volunteers" usually are recruited by advertising. For a subject's inclusion in a trial, a concurrent major depressive episode must be ruled out by both a formal diagnostic interview, such as the Mini International Neuropsychiatric Interview (MINI), and depressive symptom rating, usually a required score of 18 or lower on the Montgomery Åsberg Depression Rating Scale. Thus trial subjects who have a primary diagnosis of GAD are recruited, and those who have concurrent or recent depression are excluded. Perhaps some of the ambiguity about understanding the two conditions stems from selection bias, in that patients in routine health care settings usually present with a secondary depressive episode that is duly noted and treated as such, whereas patients who have non-comorbid GAD respond to advertisements at times of exacerbated worry, and are included in drug trials.

SYMPTOM COMPLEXITY IN PRIMARY CARE

Because most patients who have GAD present in primary care, it is noteworthy that several new studies point to the complexity of somatic and psychiatric symptoms in that setting. In a United States study of 2091 patients in 15 primary care clinics, different screening instruments were applied.[60] Comorbidity was found in the majority of cases between diagnoses of depression, GAD, and somatization. Nevertheless the three domains had important individual nonshared components. In the study, the odds ratio for GAD in patients who had one, two, or three gastrointestinal symptoms increased from 3.7 to 7.2.[61] Severe anxiety was almost four times more common among patients who had gastrointestinal symptoms than in those who did not. In another United States primary care study, patients reporting pain (headache, muscle pain, stomach pain) were likely to have GAD, panic disorder, or major depression.[62] A Swedish primary care study found that 38% of adult primary care patients had anxiety/depressive symptoms and/or alcohol problems.[63] In fact, GAD and/or depression is the largest patient category in Scandinavian primary care after musculoskeletal disorders.[64]

A complexity of symptoms similar to that in primary care is seen in general population surveys. In computer-assisted telephone interviews with 31,318 middle-aged twins in Sweden, pervasive pain, headaches, and fatigue were related to major depression or GAD.[65] The odds ratio of having both a pain disorder and GAD was found to be 16.0 in a community sample in Germany, independent of demographic factors and comorbid mental and physical disorders.[66] In an Israeli national health survey, correlates were found between GAD and bronchial asthma and osteoporosis but not between depression and these somatic conditions.[67]

WHAT NEEDS TO BE DONE TO IMPROVE TREATMENT?

These data point to the need for a broad-based psychiatric screening approach in addressing all diagnostic options and therapeutic needs of patients seeking primary care. Web-based self-screening before consultation or waiting room self-screening of psychiatric symptoms and alcohol/drug use that are computer-scored should be very cost efficient, because they offload the busy physician and provide immediate cues for a therapeutic alliance and a basis for clinical diagnoses and treatments. A recent screening tool developed in Quebec, The Worry and Anxiety Questionnaire (WAQ) focuses on excessive worry, its duration and severity, and its interference with daily functioning.[68] A WAQ scoring algorithm increased the probability of identifying GAD in a patient in primary care by 21 times compared with chance, thus providing the physician with a sensitive and specific tool. The GAD-7 self-rated questionnaire was validated with good results in a German general population study.[69] The Mental Health Inventory (MHI) also was useful as a screening tool in a Dutch study.[70]

The diagnosis then can be confirmed with the MINI 6.0 2009, and differential diagnoses can made based on the interview and clinical judgment (www.medical-outcomes.com). This process involves ruling out somatic conditions that may mimic GAD symptoms, such as caffeinism, alcohol dependence, hyperthyroidism, and adverse effects of corticosteroids.

A means of improving the care for primary care patients who have GAD or depression is to provide adjunct psychoeducation for the patient and key relatives, compliance monitoring, and feedback. A Pittsburgh-based study found telephone-based follow-up support to be effective in reducing symptom levels and sick leave.[71] Nurse-led patient groups were shown to improve compliance and symptom outcome in anxious/depressed patients in 46 primary care centers in Sweden.[72] Software is being developed to monitor patients in treatment by cellular telephone and interactive voice response.

THE CHALLENGES IN ROUTINE CARE AND OBSTACLES FOR DISSEMINATION

In managed medicine, the proportion of clinician time spent on entering data in electronic medical records and administrative databases has increased to a point that it is increasingly difficult to establish a therapeutic alliance with the patient.

Will this situation adversely affect the patient's willingness to confide and in the clinician's screening out soft data from the records? Such consequences may be noted over the next 5 to 10 years, in an effort to minimize the patient's risk of being denied life insurance and employment. A recent electronic record study found that anxiety or symptoms were not documented for most patients who had anxiety.[73] The quality of electronic health records depends on a number of factors.[74]

SPECIAL PATIENT POPULATIONS

GAD is associated with a number of somatic diseases.[75] Several modern studies have shown elevated risks of lethal and nonlethal cardiac events in patients, particularly men, who have cardiovascular disease and who also suffer from GAD/anxiety and/or depression and vice versa.[76–81] It is sensible to screen for anxiety syndromes to enable anxiolytic interventions in patients who have cardiovascular disease. Such interventions may prevent cardiac events and prolong life, as well as providing symptomatic relief. Regrettably, there are, to the author's knowledge, no published controlled trials to support this assumption.

Among the 41 000 patients in the United States diagnosed annually with primary brain tumors, as many as one half may develop GAD and/or depression.[82] Less than half these cases receive anxiolytic/antidepressant therapy. Psychiatric referral should be routine for such patients. About 1.5 to 2 million individuals annually in the United States have a traumatic brain injury (TBI). According to a literature review, 26% of patients who have a TBI have GAD, with a temporal onset that suggests causality.[83] GAD had a negative impact on recovery, although studies did not find neuroradiologic injuries that correlated with post-TBI GAD. This absence of findings does not rule out injuries to the brain anxiety circuits.

The association between type 1 and type 2 diabetes and anxiety was examined in a literature review.[84] Anxiety diagnoses derived from diagnostic interviews were associated with hyperglycemia. There thus is a need for controlled studies of diabetic patients who have anxiety disorders (or depression) to assess the utility of proper anxiolytic/antidepressant therapy, using HbA_{1c} as a primary outcome variable. A study of Vietnam veterans found an independent association between metabolic syndrome and GAD.[85]

Patients who have chronic obstructive pulmonary disease have increased rates of GAD and panic disorder.[86–88] Small studies of nortriptyline, buspirone, and sertraline as well as cognitive behavioral therapy in these patients indicate that anxiety levels can be reduced. Further studies are needed with sufficiently large populations and end points measuring effects on pulmonary function as well as anxiolytic effects.

LATE-LIFE GENERALIZED ANXIETY DISORDER

Anxiety in late life stems not only from inborn, childhood, and adult origins but also may be triggered by social isolation, migration, trauma (including crime), illness in the spouse, and bereavement. It is associated with stroke, cardiac arrhythmias, failure, and angina, chronic obstructive pulmonary disease, dementia, Parkinson's disease, malignancy, depression, malnutrition, and alcohol abuse. Suicide may be one consequence.[89] The mental health of caregivers for spouses who have dementia and other serious diseases seems largely overlooked. Anxiolytic drug trials generally also have precluded subjects older than 65 years from inclusion.

In his dissertation on 85-year-old residents in Gothenburg, Skoog[90] identified GAD in 21%, both in subjects who had dementia and those who did not. In comparing late-life GAD with major depression among 103 treated subjects, Lenze and colleagues[91] found support for both an adult-onset and late-onset GAD that was different from depression, and GAD preceded depression in most comorbid cases. Data from the longitudinal naturalistic cohort in New England indicate that older individuals who have GAD have a steeper decline in severity than younger patients.[92] In a study of late-life GAD, subjects had higher basal salivary cortisol levels than did non-anxious controls; these levels correlated positively with severity of anxiety, indicating hypothalamic-pituitary-adrenal axis dysfunction.[93]

Regulatory agencies advise caution in treating elderly patients with medications because of the risk of interaction with other medications and an impaired drug metabolism caused by kidney and hepatic disease. Drug-induced sedation, particularly by some benzodiazepines with a long half-life or active metabolites and by antihistamines, may increase the risk of falls and hip fractures. In Sweden, oxazepam is considered a primary drug of choice for elderly patients who have morbid anxiety, because it has a short half-life, no metabolites, a simple metabolic pathway by glucuronidation, and low sedation. Recent studies of pregabalin, quetiapine, duloxetine, and escitalopram in older adults who have GAD have yielded positive results and low rates of treatment termination caused by emerging adverse events.[7,94–96] Because of the complexity of all potential etiological factors for anxiety in late life, a dimensional approach is called for in clinical practice and in research to account for all of the competing hazards.[97] Diagnostic and symptom rating scales need to account for this complexity.[98] Worry management in late life, governed by prefrontal lobe executive function, needs to be addressed in research.[99]

Longevity is increasing in Europe and North America, changing the fundamental basics not only for economics but also for the provision of health care, including geriatric psychiatry. By social convention, retirement age is somewhere between 58 and 65 years of age, depending on the needs of the labor market and rising disability. From a neurobiologic viewpoint, there are vast differences in mental capacities across the late life span. The cognitive capacity is potentially jeopardized by concurrent cerebrovascular, pulmonary, and neurodegenerative disease, sensory loss, and adverse drug effects. With an optimal social support system, however, many 90-year-olds continue an independent lifestyle, as shown in the Kungsholmen longitudinal project in Stockholm.[100] There are several ongoing geriatric cohort studies that will produce important data for planning of public services in, for example, Australia, Canada, Germany, Holland, and the United Kingdom.

SUMMARY

GAD has evolved as a valid diagnostic entity characterized by a cognitive dysfunction that differs from that in depression and obsessive-compulsive disorder. Patients are vigilant in their attention to perceived threats. Recent neuroimaging studies identify this abnormality as higher trait activity in the bilateral dorsal amygdala and in the anterior cingulate cortex that is responsive to treatment. Prospective studies show a prognosis that is partly different from that in depression and is partly similar (eg, the association with subsequent bipolar disorder). Late-onset GAD may share criteria for early-onset GAD but may have different etiologies, such as stroke and social isolation. Anxiety, including GAD, is a risk factor for cardiovascular and pulmonary disease, diabetes, and brain injury.

Drugs of choice that have passed regulatory approval for GAD are venlafaxine, duloxetine, paroxetine, escitalopram, and pregabalin. Responders to all drug treatments usually remit in 6 to 12 months, and the symptom reduction is accompanied by a restored social function. The differences in pharmacodynamics among these medications indicate that there is no single common anxiolytic pathway. Studies indicate that it may be important to address the insomnia that accompanies GAD in most patients.

The move to electronic health records may adversely affect patients' willingness to seek treatment for anxiety disorders for fear of stigma and being denied employment and insurance. On the other hand, applying case-screening aids and structured diagnostic interviews may facilitate in uncovering this component in the patient's history. The Internet may become another means of case finding and outreach.

REFERENCES

1. Barlow DH. Anxiety and its disorders; the nature and treatment of anxiety and panic. New York: Guildford; 1988.
2. Nutt D, Allgulander C, Lecrubier Y, et al. Establishing noninferiority in treatment trials in psychiatry. Guidelines from an expert consensus meeting. J Psychopharmacol 2008;22:409–16.
3. Kahn A, Kolts RL, Rapaport MH, et al. Magnitude of placebo response and drug-placebo differences across psychiatric disorders. Psychol Med 2005;35:743–9.
4. Bandelow B, Zohar J, Hollander E, et al. WFSBP Task Force on Treatment Guidelines for Anxiety Obsessive-Compulsive Post-Traumatic Stress Disorders. World Federation of Societies of Biological Psychiatry (WFSBP) guidelines for the pharmacological treatment of anxiety, obsessive-compulsive and post-traumatic stress disorders–first revision. World J Biol Psychiatry 2008;9:248–312.
5. Allgulander C, Bandelow B, Hollander E, et al. WCA recommendations for the long-term treatment of generalized anxiety disorder. CNS Spectr 2003;8(Suppl 1): 53–61.
6. Allgulander C, Florea I, Trap Huusom AK. Prevention of relapse in generalized anxiety disorder by escitalopram treatment. Int J Neuropsychopharmacol 2006;9:495–505.
7. Davidson J, Allgulander C, Pollack MH, et al. Efficacy and tolerability of duloxetine in elderly patients with generalized anxiety disorder: a pooled analysis of four randomized double-blind, placebo-controlled studies. Hum Psychopharmacol 2008;23:519–26.
8. Feltner D, Wittchen H-U, Kavoussi R, et al. Long-term efficacy of pregabalin in generalized anxiety disorder. Int Clin Psychopharmacol 2008;23:18–28.
9. Allgulander C, Jörgensen T, Wade A, et al. Health-related quality of life (HRQOL) among patients with generalised anxiety disorder: evaluation conducted alongside an escitalopram relapse prevention trial. Curr Med Res Opin 2007;23: 2543–9.
10. Demyttenaere K, Friis Andersen H, Reines EH. Impact of escitalopram treatment on quality of life enjoyment and satisfaction questionnaire scores in major depressive disorder and generalized anxiety disorder. Int Clin Psychopharmacol 2008;23:276–88.
11. Montgomery SA, Sheehan DV, Meoni P, et al. Characterization of the longitudinal course of improvement in generalized anxiety disorder during long-term treatment with venlafaxine XR. J Psychiatr Res 2002;36:209–17.
12. Hidalgo RB, Tupler LA, Davidson JRT. An effect-size analysis of pharmacologic treatments for generalized anxiety disorder. J Psychopharmacol 2007;21: 864–72.
13. Klein DF. Anxiety reconceptualized. Compr Psychiatry 1980;21:411–27.

14. Nutt DJ. Neurobiological mechanisms in generalized anxiety disorder. J Clin Psychiatry 2001;62(Suppl 11):22–7.
15. Pollack M, Kinrys G, Krystal A, et al. Eszopiclone coadministered with escitalopram in patients with insomnia and comorbid generalized anxiety disorder. Arch Gen Psychiatry 2008;65:551–62.
16. Hopkins SC, Curry L, Dunn J, et al. Evaluation of low-dose eszopiclone on anxiolytic and sedative activity. Poster, ADAA, Albuquerque, NM; March 12–15, 2009.
17. Hindmarch I, Dawson J, Stanley N. A double-blind study in healthy volunteers to assess the effects on sleep of pregabalin compared with alprazolam and placebo. Sleep 2005;28:187–93.
18. McIntyre RS, Soczynska JK, Woldeyohannes HO, et al. A preclinical and clinical rationale for quetiapine in mood syndromes. Expert Opin Pharmacother 2007;8: 1211–9.
19. Khan A, Joyce M, Eggens I, et al. Extended release quetiapine fumarate (Quetiapine XR) monotherapy in the treatment of patients with generalized anxiety disorder (GAD). Poster, ADAA, Savannah, GA; March 6–9, 2008.
20. Chouinard G, Bandelow B, Ahokas A, et al. Once-daily extended release quetiapine fumarate (quetiapine XR) monotherapy in generalized anxiety disorder: a phase III double-blind, placebo-controlled study. Poster, ACNP, Boca Raton, FL; December 9–13, 2007.
21. Merideth C, Cutler A, Neijber A. Efficacy and tolerability of extended release quetiapine fumarate (quetiapine XR) monotherapy in the treatment of generalised anxiety disorder. Poster. ECNP, Barcelona, 2008.
22. Eriksson H, Mezhebovsky I, Mägi K, et al. Double-blind, randomised study of extended release quetiapine fumarate (quetiapine XR) monotherapy in elderly patients with generalised anxiety disorder (GAD). Poster, IFMAD, Vienna, Austria; November 12–14, 2008.
23. Chouinard G, Ahokas A, Bandelow B, et al. Once-daily extended release quetiapine fumarate (quetiapine XR) monotherapy in generalized anxiety disorder (GAD): a placebo-controlled study with active-comparator paroxetine. Poster, ADAA, Savannah, GA; August 30–September 3, 2008.
24. Katzman M, Brawman-Mintzer O, Reyes E, et al. Extended release quetiapine fumarate (quetiapine XR) monotherapy in maintenance treatment of generalized anxiety disorder (GAD): efficacy and tolerability results from a randomized, placebo-controlled trial. Poster, APA; Washington DC; May 3–8, 2008.
25. Stein DJ, Ahokas AA, de Bodinat C. Efficacy of agomelatine in generalized anxiety disorder. A randomized, double-blind, placebo-controlled study. J Clin Psychopharmacol 2008;28:561–6.
26. Pollack MH, Tiller J, Xie F, et al. Tiagabine in adult patients with generalized anxiety disorder. Results from 3 randomized, double-blind, placebo-controlled, parallel-group studies. J Clin Psychopharmacol 2008;28:308–16.
27. Conrad A, Isaac L, Roth WT. The psychophysiology of generalized anxiety disorder: 1. Pretreatment characteristics. Psychophysiology 2008;45:366–76.
28. Joorman J, Stöber J. Somatic symptoms from the DSM-IV: associations with pathological worry and depression symptoms in a nonclinical sample. J Anxiety Disord 1999;13:491–503.
29. Pluess M, Conrad A, Wilhelm FH. Muscle tension in generalized anxiety disorder: a critical review of the literature. J Anxiety Disord 2009;23:1–11.
30. Conrad A, Isaac L, Roth WT. The psychophysiology of generalized anxiety disorder: 2. Effects of applied relaxation. Psychophysiology 2008;45:377–88.

31. Lydiard B, Johnson RH, Emmanuel NP, et al. A pilot study of escitalopram treatment of GAD patients with temporomandibular disorders. Poster, ADAA, Albuquerque, NM; March 12–15, 2009.
32. Roth WT, Doberenz S, Dietel A, et al. Sympathetic activation in broadly defined generalized anxiety disorder. J Psychiatr Res 2008;42:205–12.
33. Gorini A, Riva G. The potential of virtual reality as anxiety management tool: a randomized controlled study in a sample of patients affected by generalized anxiety disorder. Available at: http://trialsjournal.com/content/9/1/25. Accessed June 16, 2009.
34. Den Boer PCAM, Wiersma D, van den Bosch RJ. Why is self-help neglected in the treatment of emotional disorders? A meta-analysis. Psychol Med 2004;34:1–13.
35. Van Ameringen M, Mancini C, Simpson W, et al. The potential use of internet-based screening for anxiety disorders. Poster, ADAA, Albuquerque, NM; March 12–15, 2009.
36. Kaltenthaler E, Brazier J, De Nigris E, et al. Computerised cognitive behaviour therapy for depression and anxiety update: a systematic review and economic evaluation. Health Technol Assess 2006;10.1–187.
37. Damsa C, Kosel M, Moussally J. Current status of brain imaging in anxiety disorders. Curr Opin Psychiatry 2008;22:96–110.
38. Carter CS, Krug MK. Editorial: the functional neuroanatomy of dread: functional magnetic resonance imaging insights into generalized anxiety disorder and its treatment. Am J Psychiatry 2009;166:263–5.
39. Beesdo K, Lau JYF, Guyer AE, et al. Common and distinct amygdala-function perturbations in depressed vs anxious adolescents. Arch Gen Psychiatry 2009;3:275–85.
40. Simmons A, Mathews SC, Paulus MP, et al. Intolerance of uncertainty correlates with insula activation during affective ambiguity. Neurosci Lett 2008;430:92–7.
41. Krain AL, Gotimer K, Ernst M, et al. A functional magnetic resonance imaging investigation of uncertainty in adolescents with anxiety disorders. Biol Psychiatry 2008;63:563–8.
42. Monk CS, Telzer EH, Mogg K, et al. Amygdala and ventrolateral prefrontal cortex activation to masked angry faces in children and adolescents with generalized anxiety disorder. Arch Gen Psychiatry 2008;65:568–76.
43. Blair K, Shaywitz J, Smith BW, et al. Response to emotional expressions in generalized social phobia and generalized anxiety disorder: evidence for separate disorders. Am J Psychiatry 2008;165:1193–202.
44. Nitschke JB, Sarinopoulos I, Oathes DJ, et al. Anticipatory activation in the amygdala and anterior cingulate in generalized anxiety disorder and prediction of treatment response. Am J Psychiatry 2009;166:302–10.
45. Paulesu E, Sambugaro E, Danelli TT, et al. Neural correlates of worry in generalized anxiety disorder and in normal controls: a functional MRI study. Psychol Med 2009 May 7:1–8. [Epub ahead of print].
46. Whalen PJ, Johnstone T, Somerville LH, et al. A functional magnetic resonance imaging predictor of treatment response to venlafaxine in generalized anxiety disorder. Biol Psychiatry 2008;63:858–63.
47. Gatt JM, Nemeroff CB, Dobson-Stone C, et al. Interactions between BDNF Val66Met polymorphism and early life stress predict brain and arousal pathway to syndromal depression and anxiety. Mol Psychiatry 2009;14(7):681–95.
48. Moffitt TE, Caspi A, Harrington H, et al. Generalized anxiety disorder and depression: childhood risk factors in a birth cohort followed to age 32. Psychol Med 2007;37:441–52.

49. Mennin DS, Heimberg RG, Fresco DM, et al. Is generalized anxiety disorder an anxiety or mood disorder? Considering multiple factors as we ponder the fate of GAD. Depress Anxiety 2008;25:289–99.
50. Hettema JM. The nosologic relationship between generalized anxiety disorder and major depression. Depress Anxiety 2008;25:300–16.
51. First MB. Summary of Conference on Comorbidity of Depression and Generalized Anxiety Disorder, June 20–22, 2007, London. Available at: http://www.psych.org/MainMenu/Research/DSMIV/DSMV/DSMRevisionActivities/ConferenceSummaries/ComorbidityofDepressionandGAD.aspx. Accessed June 16, 2009.
52. Robins E, Guze SB. Establishment of diagnostic validity in psychiatric illness: its application to schizophrenia. Am J Psychiatry 1970;126:983–7.
53. Brown TA. Temporal course and structural relationships among dimensions of temperament and DSM-IV anxiety and mood disorder constructs. J Abnorm Psychol 2007;116:313–28.
54. Kessler RC, Gruer M, Hettema JM, et al. Co-morbid major depression and generalized anxiety disorders in the National Comorbidity Survey follow-up. Psychol Med 2008;38:365–74.
55. Angst J, Gamma A, Baldwin DS, et al. The generalized anxiety spectrum: prevalence, onset, course and outcome. Eur Arch Psychiatry Clin Neurosci 2009;259:37–45.
56. Rihmer Z, Szádóczky E, Füredi J, et al. Anxiety disorders comorbidity in bipolar I, bipolar II and unipolar major depression: results from a population-based study in Hungary. J Affect Disord 2001;67:175–9.
57. Kendler KS, Gardner CO, Gatz M, et al. The source of co-morbidity between major depression and generalized anxiety disorder in a Swedish national twin sample. Psychol Med 2007;37:453–62.
58. Kubarych TS, Aggen SH, Hettema JM, et al. Assessment of generalized anxiety disorder diagnostic criteria in the National Comorbidity Survey and Virginia Adult Twin Study of Psychiatric and Substance Use Disorders. Psychol Assess 2008;20:206–16.
59. Smoller JW, Gardner-Schuster E, Misiaszek M. Genetics of anxiety: would the genome recognize the DSM? Depress Anxiety 2008;25:368–77.
60. Löwe B, Spitzer RL, Williams JBW, et al. Depression, anxiety and somatization in primary care: syndrome overlap and functional impairment. Gen Hosp Psychiatry 2008;30:191–9.
61. Mussell M, Kroenke K, Spitzer RL, et al. Gastrointestinal symptoms in primary care: prevalence and association with depression and anxiety. J Psychosom Res 2008;64:605–12.
62. Means-Christensen AJ, Roy-Byrne PP, Sherbourne CD, et al. Relationships among pain, anxiety, and depression in primary care. Depress Anxiety 2008;25:593–600.
63. Nordström A, Bodlund O. Every third patient in primary care suffers from depression, anxiety, or alcohol problems. Nord J Psychiatry 2008;62:250–5.
64. Munk-Jörgensen P, Allgulander C, Dahl AA, et al. Prevalence of generalized anxiety disorder in general practice in Denmark, Finland, Norway, and Sweden. Psychiatr Serv 2006;57:1738–44.
65. Kato K, Sullivan PF, Evengård B, et al. A population-based twin study of functional somatic syndromes. Psychol Med 2009;39:497–505.
66. Beesdo K, Hoyer J, Jacobi F, et al. Association between generalized anxiety levels and pain in a community sample: evidence for diagnostic specificity. J Anxiety Disord 2009;23:684–93.

67. Muhsen K, Lipsitz J, Garty-Sandalon N, et al. Correlates of generalized anxiety disorder: independent of co-morbidity with depression. Findings from the first Israeli National Health Interview Survey (2003–2004). Soc Psychiatry Psychiatr Epidemiol 2008;43:898–904.
68. Belleville G, Bélanger L, Ladouceur R, et al. Sensitivity and specificity of the worry and anxiety questionnaire (WAQ) in a sample of health-care users in the province of Quebec. Encephale 2008;34:240–8.
69. Löwe B, Decker O, Müller S, et al. Validation and standardization of the generalized anxiety disorder screener (GAD-7) in the general population. Med Care 2008b;46:266–74
70. Cuijpers P, Smits N, Doner T, et al. Screening for mood and anxiety disorders with the five-item, the three-item, and the two-item Mental Health Inventory. Psychiatry Res 2009;168(3):250–5.
71. Rollman BL, Belnap BH, Mazumdar S, et al. A randomized trial to improve the quality of treatment for panic and generalized anxiety disorders in primary care. Arch Gen Psychiatry 2005;62:1332–41.
72. Hansson M, Bodlund O, Choutai J. Patient education and group counselling to improve the treatment of depression in primary care: a randomized controlled trial. J Affect Disord 2008;105:235–40.
73. Calleo J, Stanley MA, Greisinger A, et al. Generalized anxiety disorder in older medical patients: diagnostic recognition, mental health management and service utilization. J Clin Psychol Med Settings 2009;16:178–85.
74. Häyrinen K, Saranto K, Nykänen P. Definition, structure, content, use and impacts of electronic health records: a review of the research literature. Int J Med Inf 2008;77:291–304.
75. Culpepper L. Generalized anxiety disorder and medical illness. J Clin Psychiatry 2009;70(Suppl 2):20–4.
76. Allgulander C. Suicide and mortality pattern in anxiety neurosis and depressive neurosis; a record-linkage study of 48,440 patients in Sweden. Arch Gen Psychiatry 1994;51:708–12.
77. Frasure-Smith N, Lespérance F. Depression and anxiety as predictors of 2-year cardiac events in patients with stable coronary artery disease. Arch Gen Psychiatry 2008;65:62–71.
78. Goodwin RD, Davidson KW, Keyes K. Mental disorders and cardiovascular disease among adults in the United States. J Psychiatr Res 2009;43:239–46.
79. Bankier B, Barajas J, Martinez-Rumayor A, et al. Association between C-reactive protein and generalized anxiety disorder in stable coronary heart disease patients. Eur Heart J 2008;29:2212–27.
80. Shen B-J, Avivi YE, Todaro JF, et al. Anxiety characteristics independently and prospectively predict myocardial infarction in men. The unique contribution of anxiety among psychologic factors. J Am Coll Cardiol 2008;51:113–9.
81. Phillips AC, Batty D, Gale CR, et al. Generalized anxiety disorder, major depressive disorder, and their comorbidity as predictors of all-cause and cardiovascular mortality: the Vietnam Experience Study. Psychosom Med 2009;71:395–403.
82. Arnold SD, Forman LM, Brigidi BD, et al. Evaluation and characterization of generalized anxiety and depression in patients with primary brain tumors. J Neurooncol 2008;10:171–81.
83. Rogers JM, Read CA. Psychiatric comorbidity following traumatic brain injury. Brain Inj 2007;21:1321–33.

84. Anderson RJ, Grigby AB, Freedland KE, et al. Anxiety and poor glycemic control: a meta-analytic review of the literature. Int J Psychiatry Med 2002;32: 235–47.
85. Carroll D, Phillips AC, Thomas GN, et al. Generalized anxiety disorder is associated with metabolic syndrome in the Vietnam Experience Study. Biol Psychiatry 2009;66:91–3.
86. Brenes GA. Anxiety and chronic obstructive pulmonary disease: prevalence, impact and treatment. Psychosom Med 2003;65:963–70.
87. Mikkelsen RL, Middelboe T, Pisinger C, et al. Anxiety and depression in patients with chronic obstructive pulmonary disease (COPD). A review. Nord J Psychiatry 2004;58:65–70.
88. Härter MC, Conway KP, Merikangas KR. Associations between anxiety disorders and physical illness. Eur Arch Psychiatry Clin Neurosci 2003;253:313–20.
89. Waern M, Rubenowitz E, Wilhelmson K. Predictors of suicide in the old elderly. Gerontology 2003;49:328–34.
90. Skoog I, Nilsson L, Landahl S, et al. Mental disorders and the use of psychotropic drugs in an 85-year-old urban population. Int Psychogeriatr 1993;5:33–48.
91. Lenze EJ, Mulsant BH, Mohlman J, et al. Generalized anxiety disorder in late life. Lifetime course and comorbidity with major depressive disorder. Am J Geriatr Psychiatry 2005;13:77–80.
92. Ramsawh HJ, Raffa SD, Orlando Edelen M, et al. Anxiety in middle adulthood: effects of age and time on the 14-year course of panic disorder, social phobia and generalized anxiety disorder. Psychol Med 2009;39:615–24.
93. Mantella RC, Butters MA, Amico JA, et al. Salivary cortisol is associated with diagnosis and severity of late-life generalized anxiety disorder. Psychoneuroendocrinology 2008;33:773–81.
94. Eriksson H, Mezhebovsky I, Mägi K, et al. Once-daily extended release quetiapine fumarate (quetiapine XR) monotherapy in elderly patients with generalized anxiety disorder (GAD): results from a double-blind, randomized, placebo-controlled study. Poster, ACNP, Scottsdale, AZ; December 7–11, 2008.
95. Lenze EJ, Rollman BL, Shear MK, et al. Escitalopram for older adults with generalized anxiety disorder. A randomized controlled trial. JAMA 2009;301:295–303.
96. Montgomery S, Chatamra K, Pauer L, et al. Efficacy and safety of pregabalin in elderly people with generalised anxiety disorder. Br J Psychiatry 2008;193: 389–94.
97. Bryant C, Jackson H, Ames D. The prevalence of anxiety in older adults: methodological issues and a review of the literature. J Affect Disord 2008;109: 233–50.
98. Beck JG, Stanley MA, Zebb BJ. Characteristics of generalized anxiety disorder in older adults: a descriptive study. Behav Res Ther 1996;34:225–34.
99. Mohlman J, Price R. Recognizing and treating late-life generalized anxiety disorder: distinguishing features and psychosocial treatment. Expert Rev Neurother 2006;6:1439–45.
100. Forsell Y, Winblad B. Feelings of anxiety and associated variables in a very elderly population. Int J Geriatr Psychiatry 1998;13:454–8.

Psychotherapy for Generalized Anxiety Disorder: Don't Worry, It Works!

Juergen Hoyer, PhD*, Andrew T. Gloster, PhD

KEYWORDS

• GAD • Worry • Psychotherapy • CBT • Exposure

As described by Allgulander in this issue and by others,[1] generalized anxiety disorder (GAD) differs from other anxiety disorders. Patients do not fear a specific external object or situation, as in the phobias. There is no distinct symptomatic reaction pattern, as in panic disorder. The feared scenarios are not bizarre, improbable, or inflexible, as they often are in obsessive compulsive disorder. Avoidance, although central, is less obvious and often is prominent only on the cognitive-emotional level.[2,3] Furthermore, the key component of GAD, uncontrollable and persistent worrying, is easily confused with the lay concept of worry,[4] and the frequently occurring comorbid disorders often make the recognition of GAD difficult.[5] These specifics highlight the challenge in treating patients suffering from GAD effectively with psychotherapy. On the other, research in the treatment of GAD has led to innovative, promising, and specific developments, such as massed worry exposure,[6] meta-cognitive therapy,[7,8] well-being therapy,[9] and combination treatments based on a cognitive behavioral therapy (CBT) platform,[10,11] all of which deserve specific attention.

EVIDENCE FOR THE EFFICACY AND EFFECTIVENESS OF PSYCHOTHERAPY IN GENERALIZED ANXIETY DISORDER

As mirrored by recent comprehensive meta-analyses,[12,13] the majority of psychotherapeutic treatment studies for GAD compared CBT with a wait-list or a treatment-as-usual control group. CBT was usually effective, with a mean between-group effect size (Hedges's g) of 0.82 for anxiety measures across all studies.[13] On the basis of 12 studies with 162 patients, Hunot and colleagues[12] found a standardized mean difference (SMD) between CBT and wait-list/treatment-as-usual of −1.00 (95%

This work was funded by the German Research Council (DFG; HO, 1900/1–3).
Klinische Psychologie und Psychotherapie, Technische Universität Dresden, Hohe Street 53, D-01187 Dresden, Germany
* Corresponding author.
E-mail address: hoyer@psychologie.tu-dresden.de (J. Hoyer).

Psychiatr Clin N Am 32 (2009) 629–640
doi:10.1016/j.psc.2009.05.002
0193-953X/09/$ – see front matter © 2009 Elsevier Inc. All rights reserved.

confidence interval [CI], −1.24 to −0.77). The standardized mean difference was large, ranging between 0.08 and 2.00, indicating that it is possible to achieve very favorable results but that such a response is not standard. Results for worry only, the core symptom of GAD, are similar, with an average SMD of −0.90 (see also[14]). Within-group effect sizes are clearly higher (> 2),[15] and it must be emphasized that, when GAD was the primary disorder, the majority of studies included comorbid mental disorders.

Hunot and colleagues[12] and Westen and Bradley[16] summarize that about 50% of the GAD treatment completers and about 40% of the intend-to-treat samples achieve high end-state functioning after CBT for GAD. Psychopharmacological treatment was similarly effective.[12,13] In sum, CBT has clearly proven effective in GAD, but its effects nevertheless have been characterized as lower than in other anxiety disorders (eg,[10,16,17]). It is unclear whether these skeptical evaluations are correct, because they do not take into account that the anxiety disorders differ in natural persistence and that GAD has been characterized as especially persistent.[18] Thus, the better improvement rates reported in other anxiety disorders may be attributable in part to a higher a priori probability of the disordered system to change (eg, in panic disorder). This possibility is also likely because everyone worries (ie, nonpathological worry is part of every person's psychological constellation), whereas this universality is not the case with panic attacks. As a result, typical outcome indices used in GAD studies may be less malleable than in other anxiety disorders. That said, a number of recently published randomized, controlled trials (RCTs) using CBT[10,11,15,19,20] reach clearly higher within-group effect sizes than reported in the cited meta-analyses, with within-group effect sizes greater than 2 for the main outcome measures.

Another problem in evaluating previous findings is that many older studies fail to describe which specific CBT interventions and techniques were used. Instead, they often simply refer to a classic overarching book on the treatment of anxiety.[21] In other trials, techniques were stipulated but were combined (eg, the trial by Borkovec and Costello[22] combined applied relaxation, self-control desensitization, and brief cognitive therapy). Other common elements encompass self-monitoring of worrying, stimulus control, cognitive restructuring, and different forms of anxiety management.[15,23] The finding of a global effect of such treatment mixtures makes it hard to understand which of the treatment elements contribute effectively to treatment success and should be optimized – and which do not.[24] Newer CBT approaches specifically designed for GAD are reviewed in more detail later in this article.

One specific CBT intervention, applied relaxation,[25] also reached favorable results without being combined with other CBT techniques.[6,25–28] In applied relaxation, patients learn relaxation procedures that reduce autonomic arousal and are taught to use these procedures to cope better with situations in which they previously experienced excessive tension or worrying. The importance of this finding is that the effects are achieved without the exposure techniques usually applied in CBT for anxiety, and no element from cognitive therapy is integrated.[6]

Only a few studies have systematically examined the efficacy of interventions for GAD from therapeutic orientations other than CBT (see[12] for a comprehensive review). Until recently, there was only one controlled study for psychodynamic treatment in GAD.[29] A new study by Leichsenring and colleagues[19] compared manualized short-term psychodynamic psychotherapy (STPP) and CBT for GAD. Both CBT and STPP yielded significant, large, and stable improvements in symptoms of anxiety and depression. Although no significant differences in outcome were found between treatments with respect to the primary outcome measure (anxiety symptoms as measured by the Hamilton Anxiety Rating Scale;[30] effect size = 2.62 for CBT, effect size = 2.14 for STPP), CBT was superior to STPP on measures of trait anxiety, worry, and depression. Additionally, a third RCT testing STPP demonstrated the efficacy of a modified version of STPP, affect-focused body therapy.[31]

To summarize, there is clear evidence that the collection of interventions consistent with CBT theory is efficacious for adult patients who have GAD. Nevertheless, only some adult studies achieved extensive rates of improvement or remission. Further, preliminary evidence suggests that STPP can be effective, although it currently seems to be inferior to CBT in its ability to reduce trait anxiety, worry, and depression.

The results presented in the previous paragraphs come from RTCs that used structured diagnostic interviews with independent assessors and explicit treatment manuals and incorporated fidelity checks of treatment (eg,[12]). The extent to which positive results derived under such conditions transfer to practitioners who may service a different patient population and have different supervision intensity remains to be investigated. Kehle[32] demonstrated that CBT for GAD was effective for completers of a treatment delivered in a "frontline service setting," with favorable effect size for the reduction of worrying and depression. Only 28% ($n = 8$) of those originally intending to receive treatment ($n = 29$) actually completed treatment, however. In this study, treatment consisted of only eight manualized, highly structured sessions. For noncompleters ($n = 21$), CBT was not or was only marginally effective. On the other hand, CBT for GAD was highly effective in the private practitioner setting when 15 to 25 sessions were used.[19,20] These trials yielded effect sizes at the upper bound of those published to date, thereby demonstrating that CBT also can work in the natural setting, at least when quality monitoring is implemented at the level used in a RCT and treatment is not too short.

GAD typically develops during childhood and adolescence, often reaching clinical levels of symptom expression during early adulthood.[33] Effective treatment for GAD in younger samples is therefore desirable, but RCTs are lacking in this specific age group. Two case series demonstrate that CBT might also be effective in youth[34,35] and point to the need to enhance efforts to investigate more intensely early treatment approaches to GAD.

GAD is also the anxiety disorder with the highest incidence in older age.[18] Six RCTs have examined CBT for GAD in elderly participants.[12,36] The trials showed that anxiety symptoms, worry, and depression could also be effectively reduced in the elderly, and also in a primary care setting,[36] but the magnitude of effects on anxiety and depression symptoms was smaller in the elderly than in adult participants. Accordingly, the attrition rate was higher in elderly participants.

Furthermore, it has been demonstrated that four sessions of CBT combined with four sessions specifically designed to maintain well-being (well-being therapy) successfully prevented relapse in patients who had GAD and who had undergone pharmacological treatment.[9] Finally, all trials that included follow-up assessments (of up to 1 year) indicated that treatment gains were maintained. Although maintenance of treatment gains thus has been better documented than in pharmacotherapy,[12,13] longer follow-up intervals are desirable, given the "waxing and waning" nature of GAD.[18]

Although all this evidence indicates that psychotherapy for GAD is efficacious in various forms, subgroups, and settings, major limitations in the present knowledge must be emphasized. First, long-term follow-up studies (with a follow-up interval of more than 1 year) are largely lacking (see[29] or[15] for exceptions), leaving the duration of treatment gains unclear. Second, it is unclear which treatment elements are most effective and what changes in current treatments could further improve response rates, treatment success, and transfer to specific populations and routine practice. Finally, because extant treatments based on different or even contradictory rationales achieve nearly equivalent outcomes, the mechanism(s) through which psychotherapy works remain unclear. This uncertainty signals the need for more theory-driven research.

NEW TREATMENT DEVELOPMENTS

Numerous efforts have been made in recent years to enhance symptom reduction and response rates in CBT. Efforts have centered either on targeting more directly the putative underlying core mechanisms of disorder[6,8] or on broadening the range of interventions toward dysfunctional aspects of the patients' lives that previously were ignored or at least not explicitly targeted.[10,11]

Massed Worry Exposure

Systematic exposure to worrisome thoughts operates on the assumption that worry functions as avoidant behavior. That is, worry is believed to prevent deeper, and often more aversive, emotional processing of thoughts and images, thus perpetuating worry via negative reinforcement.[2] To the extent that this assumption is correct, excessive worrisome thinking can be reduced by exposing the patient to the emotions and cognitions that are avoided during worrying episodes. This exposure traditionally is accomplished by first generating a fear hierarchy of worrisome thoughts, then having the client expose him-or herself to purposeful worry and corresponding images for an extended period (ie, 20–30 minutes). Gradually, the worry and images are increased in intensity. Conceptually, this procedure makes a great deal of sense, especially in light of the generally strong effects generated by exposure therapies in other disorders.[37] Recently, Hoyer and colleagues[6] refined worry exposure and applied it as a massed exposure in sensu. In other words, patients were motivated to confront their worst worry imagery right away and to try to experience the accompanying anxiety as intensely as possible until habituation occurred rather than proceeding gradually through the stimulus hierarchy. It was demonstrated that this treatment, which directly targets the avoidance described in the avoidance theory of worry,[2] could be deployed successfully as a stand-alone treatment of GAD (ie, without the additional use of cognitive or relaxation interventions). Patients treated with massed worry exposure achieved stable improvement equal to applied relaxation.[6] Furthermore, negative meta-cognitions about worry (ie, fearful cognitions that worrying could be debilitating) were reduced successfully. Although worry exposure was used as a singular treatment component to demonstrate that it is an active treatment ingredient, treatment efficacy might be increased by adding other empirically validated treatments components. It also is of theoretical importance that this treatment focused solely on worry and yet proved efficacious. This finding can be seen as strong evidence that clinical worry should continue to be regarded the core syndrome of GAD.

Meta-Cognitive Therapy

The psychological understanding of the clinically relevant forms of worrying is of vital importance for an adequate treatment planning in GAD.[7] The meta-cognitive model of GAD[7] asserts that individuals who have GAD, like most people, hold positive beliefs about worrying as an effective means to prevent negative things from happening (positive meta-cognitions). When worrying becomes inflexible and persistent, however, patients also begin to develop negative assumptions about worrying, most importantly beliefs and appraisals about the uncontrollability of worrying and about the dangerousness of its consequences for personal functioning (negative meta-cognitions). According to the self-regulatory executive function theory, meta-cognitions guide cognition, emotion, and behavior.[38] The negative meta-cognitions about worrying both lead to an elevation in distress and worry and motivate counterproductive efforts to control, stop, or prevent worrying. As a consequence, interventions aiming at cognitive restructuring in meta-cognitive therapy do not target the multiple fearful beliefs and assumptions that patients who have GAD may have; instead, these interventions focus on the negative meta-cognitions about worrying. Short episodes of worry exposure are among the behavior experiments suitable for challenging dysfunctional meta-cognitive beliefs about worrying.[7] In these episodes, patients learn that worrying is not harmful and that efforts to suppress worrying are superfluous. Because meta-cognitive therapy of GAD is based directly on a theory of disorder, this approach seems particularly elegant and promising, although independent validation is needed. Currently no controlled trials of meta-cognitive therapy in GAD exist, but an open trial with 10 patients achieved quite favorable results, including recovery rates of 87.5% at posttreatment and 75% at 6 and 12 months' follow-up.[8]

Interpersonal Aspects

Both applied relaxation and cognitive therapy, or a combination of both, led to significant changes in symptoms of anxiety and depression, but both procedures failed to improve interpersonal functioning.[15] Because of this finding and the need to improve the moderate rates of high end-state functioning following treatment, CBT has begun to target interpersonal problems in addition to GAD symptoms. The additive interpersonal features concentrate on four areas: (1) current relationships, (2) origins of current interpersonal problems, (3) the therapeutic relationship, and (4) avoidance of emotion.[2] The authors suggest that these areas should be targeted strategically based on a functional analysis of the contingencies that shape and maintain the client's interpersonal problems. The theoretical rationale for targeting these factors is based on the assumption that a client's worry is associated with the tendency to avoid negative emotions and reactions from others. This avoidance, in turn, leads to protective behaviors that have the effect of shutting others out and keeping the patients from expressing their feelings and opinions. Recent data from an open trial[10] demonstrate the overall efficacy of the approach of integrating CBT with elements from interpersonal therapy and emotional processing and the incremental contribution of interpersonal emotional processing therapy (see also[39]).

Acceptance and Mindfulness Techniques

Because worry is primarily verbal behavior, Roemer and Orsillo[40] hypothesize that procedures derived from theories of verbal behavior and stimulus equivalence (ie, mindfulness and acceptance and commitment therapy [ACT]),[41] might increase the efficacy of treatment targeting chronic worriers. Some of the procedures used are found also in other CBT packages, including early cue detection, self-monitoring, and reduction of avoidance behaviors. ACT differs in its promotion of mindfulness and personal values and in the acceptance of problems rather than striving for direct change, which itself is conceptualized as a form of emotional avoidance. Mindfulness may be effective precisely because it brings worriers into the present as opposed to the future, where they spend so much time and where refutable evidence is not obtainable.[42] Current data using ACT and mindfulness is preliminary but encouraging. Beyond a series of case studies[40] and a small open trial ($n = 11$),[43] an RCT[11] demonstrated very favorable effect sizes even in the intent-to-treat analyses: 86.7% of the completers reached high end-state functioning at 9-month follow-up, and 76.5% no longer met diagnostic criteria for GAD.

Although these newer developments seem promising, direct comparison of these treatments and their effects is not possible because of differences in inclusion criteria, experience of therapists, and other differences that make it hard to identify which treatment is the best for a particular patient.[44] The active or even the indispensable ingredients in the treatment packages remain unknown—a quagmire addressed in the next section.

EVIDENCE FOR ACTIVE INGREDIENTS AND MECHANISMS

Given that GAD is a condition that involves interacting cognitive, emotional, and somatic components,[3] a comprehensive package of CBT interventions can be expected to yield the highest therapeutic impact; however, comparison between a full CBT package and some if its components (ie, cognitive therapy alone; applied relaxation with self-control desensitization) failed to find clear superiority of the complex program and found no differences between the components.[15] Until additional methodologically rigorous component-control studies are funded and conducted that allow clear delineation of which techniques are active components and which are inactive or even iatrogenic,[24] the search for the most potent specific ingredients of CBT therapy will remain a matter of theorizing. Clear understanding of the mechanisms of therapeutic action is further frustrated by the different levels of abstraction and constructs that are used across studies. The different levels of target variables range from neurotransmitters and neurons to thoughts and meta-cognitions. When different terms are used to describe the same phenomenon, nonproductive debates can develop. In addition to more precise definitions, research is charged with the task of providing a clearer understanding of how each level of analysis adds explanatory and predictive value, thereby providing practitioners concrete information on which to base clinical decisions.

At the phenomenological level, patients who have GAD behave as if negative events should never happen in their lives unless they know ahead of time exactly what will occur. This attitude has been referred to as an intolerance of uncertainty, which has proven to be an important vulnerability factor for GAD.[45,46] But how can what these patients fear be better understood? What is at the core of their avoidance? Why do they find it necessary to avoid strong negative emotions and resort to using the subtle strategy of worrying? The answer to these questions is seldom clear for patients when they begin treatment,[6,47] as evidenced by patients' common description that they "fear something indescribable." When therapy begins, patients often state that they believe that they are incapable of coping with or even imagining their feared outcomes (eg, imagining the death of a loved one) and that such situations exceed their limits. They fear they might go insane when imagining these scenes. Such statements suggest that the apprehension centers around the anxiety about feeling "overwhelmed" in surprising situations characterized by negative outcomes with the likelihood of strong emotions. Because negative surprises are always possible, a state referred to as "anxious apprehension" ensues and can be present most of the time (more than 6 hours a day[4,48]). It follows, then, that treatments work by counteracting anxious apprehension, be it by developing familiarity and tolerance of the feared emotions (eg, worry exposure), by restructuring assumptions about their feared consequences (eg, meta-cognitive therapy), by combinations of these mechanisms (eg, ACT; interpersonal and emotional processing therapy), or by teaching the patient skills to manage upcoming unintended apprehension directly (eg, applied relaxation).

Direct comparisons of these diverse efficacious techniques are needed to optimize future offers of treatment not only in terms of effect sizes but also in terms of attrition and applicability in practice.

Clues for understanding the mechanism of action can also be derived at the procedural level of analysis (eg, what a therapist does) and at the process level (eg, what interventions are thought to change). Procedures include nonspecific factors, such as talking, listening, and encouraging, that cut across treatment approaches and very specific factors, including the application of techniques previously described (eg, worry exposure, counteracting the tendency to avoid emotionally aversive, cognitive reframing, relaxation, and other techniques). Arguably, however, process analysis generates the most interesting debates, the resolution of which offers the greatest promise for improving current therapies. For instance, one theory of verbal behavior posits that therapeutic change occurs because the relational networks that exist between verbal stimuli have been altered so that the patient is more flexible to engage in value-laden behaviors while simultaneously abandoning inflexible value-inconsistent behaviors (eg, uncontrollable worry is replaced by the ability to stop and start worrying when doing so serves the patient's chosen values).[49] Testing these assumptions, however, requires complex mediational analyses: it must be demonstrated that the relational frameworks change first and that other positive changes follow. Similarly, in meta-cognitive theory it is assumed that the change of meta-cognition is the central element that precedes further change (eg, in the tendency to worry), an assumption that awaits empirical confirmation.[50]

In summary, based on the present empirical evidence, it can be argued only that patients' subjective deficit—anxious apprehension surrounding a perceived inability to cope with ambiguous and catastrophized outcomes and the emotions associated with them—can be reduced by diverse strategies and that multiple pathways seem to reach the same end point.[17] Or, as Borkovec and colleagues[15] put it (p. 296): "targeting some response processes in therapy for a sufficiently long period of time might ... affect all the other processes involved in the therapy of anxiety." At the same time, there is no psychological therapy of GAD, including the STPP approach, that does not include an element which makes patients (at least subjectively) more competent to cope with strong emotions and feared negative outcomes.

SIMILARITY TO OTHER ANXIETY DISORDERS

The phenomenological characteristics of GAD may mislead researchers and clinicians alike. Among the factors that differentiate GAD from other anxiety disorders is the fact that observable avoidant behavior is less frequent and, when present, is more difficult to detect (eg, not reading the newspaper, not opening letters). As such, the status of GAD as an independent anxiety disorder has been questioned. Evidence for this position has included the fact that the diagnostic category of GAD is less reliable than other anxiety disorders,[51] largely because of the difficulty of rating "uncontrollable" (as opposed to everyday) worry. Worry also is mistaken as simply a symptom of depression because its topographical characteristic of repetitive negative thinking[52] is not easily discernible from depressive rumination. Thus, when repetitive negative thinking is combined with the absence of clearly observable avoidance, it is easy to assume erroneously that GAD is simply a prodromal stage of depression, especially because patients who have GAD often develop subsequent depression.[53]

In contrast to these assumptions, evidence has accumulated that worrying can well be distinguished from depressive rumination.[54,55] Furthermore, the fact that GAD often precedes depression is similar to other anxiety disorders[56] and can be explained by the high and persistent impairment that is associated with GAD even when no other comorbid mental disorders exist.[57] Longitudinal epidemiological studies also show that the pattern of symptom development in GAD is more similar to other anxiety disorders than to depressive disorders.[58] Based on current evidence, the authors believe that GAD should be characterized primarily as a disorder of dysfunctional avoidance and remain subsumed under the category of anxiety disorders.

The categorization of GAD as an anxiety disorder is supported further by the approaches used to treat it. Although the effectiveness of a treatment alone cannot logically be used to understand the etiology of a disorder, it is clear that all treatments reviewed earlier in this article are basically treatments for anxiety (and not, for example, for negative mood). The targeted fear in GAD is less concrete than that seen in other anxiety disorders, but the experience or notion that this fear is not justified is part of all treatments described earlier.

WHAT NEEDS TO BE DONE TO MAKE IT BETTER?

It is generally agreed that therapy works better in some patients than in others. To find out which variables determine these different responses to treatment is more than complicated, however. To improve the treatment of GAD outcomes, prediction research needs to test hypotheses about the underlying mechanisms of change and the factors that influence these processes.[50] This knowledge could directly inform treatment planning and increase the responder rates for those who complete treatment. But what are the moderators and mediators of change? Ideally, an examination of interventions for GAD would examine which intervention works best for a particular level of worry (eg, high versus medium versus low), with which comorbidities (either with other diagnoses or common dimensions), in which cluster of symptoms (eg, full-fledged GAD, subclinical GAD, or another primary diagnosis), in which situations and time frames (eg, proximal or distant threat), and with which therapeutic goals (eg, interpersonal conflicts, indecision, or poor performance). Furthermore, therapy time, format, and setting also must be taken into account. This list of response-modifying factors could easily be continued (see[50]).

Unfortunately, little information exists at this level of analysis, and only a few studies have systematically analyzed the predictors of change in GAD. In his review, Durham[50] summarized that beyond the possible exception of symptom severity (which may predict not only treatment responsiveness but also the natural course), no other predictor of treatment change could be confirmed across studies. Only very few studies on the prediction of treatment success in GAD exist, and those that do indicate that homework adherence was associated positively with outcome as well as, contradictory to expectations, symptom severity and number of comorbid diagnoses.[59] Although based on pooled data from three trials of older adults, the results from this study nevertheless may not be robust as defined by consistent replication across multiple independent studies. Therefore one possibility for improving knowledge about treatment is increased coordination in prediction research across studies. Unfortunately, in the present research practice of psychotherapy for GAD, such coordinated research efforts do not exist.

One final critical consideration is that outcome prediction research often focuses primarily on outcome defined as the reduction of symptoms in those who complete therapy. Because efficacious treatments exist, such research should focus more on what is necessary to attract patients to treatment and to keep them in treatment and on whether the treatment is acceptable to therapists and patients.

ROUTINE CARE AND OBSTACLES FOR DISSEMINATION

Although GAD is common, patients who have GAD are less often seen in specialty anxiety clinics.[60] Instead, patients who have GAD regularly seek help from general practitioners; their complaints may focus on the bodily symptoms associated with disorder, and the disorder itself may easily go undetected.[5] Few patients are diagnosed correctly, and even fewer are referred to psychiatric or psychotherapeutic treatment. This failure in diagnosis and referral is especially common in older adults who have GAD.[61] One necessary improvement, therefore, is to get more patients into the ideally suited treatment, and optimized screening tools may be part of this avenue.[5]

As outlined in this article, the problems with the reliability of the diagnosis of GAD[51] may result in part from the less pronounced and less discernible nature of the disorder. Nevertheless, the forthcoming revision of the *Diagnostic and Statistical Manual of Mental Disorders* (DSM), the DSM-V, may help make GAD criteria more reliable and less complicated and make the use of this diagnosis easier in practice. Once the patient is referred to a psychotherapist, it still is not clear whether a modern and efficacious psychotherapeutic treatment will be offered. The data by Kehle[32] indicate that patients in routine practice do not necessarily adhere to a CBT treatment, at least not when it is highly structured and condensed. The most efficacious treatments have been published only recently, and it makes sense to increase efforts to transfer them into practice as soon as possible.

SUMMARY

Although room for improvement exists, the psychological treatment of GAD should not be viewed pessimistically. Especially more recent innovative refinements of CBT methods[8,11] yielded highly favorable recovery rates of up to 70% or 80% (depending on point of assessment). Treatment effects achieved using extant treatments therefore are no longer substantially worse than those for most other anxiety disorders. Nevertheless, future research is strongly encouraged to investigate assumed underlying mechanisms of action, mediators of change, and the length of therapy necessary to achieve change. Along this road, GAD, previously also described as "the basic anxiety disorder" (eg,[62]), may serve as a paradigm for the intriguing study of what really makes "the worried mind"[63] more calm.

REFERENCES

1. Mennin DS, Heimberg RG, Turk CL. Clinical presentation and diagnostic features. In: Heimberg RG, Turk CL, Mennin DS, editors. Generalized anxiety disorder: advances in research and practice. New York: The Guilford Press; 2004. p. 3–28.
2. Newman MG, Castonguay LG, Borkovec TD, et al. Integrative therapy for generalized anxiety disorder. In: Heimberg R, Turk CL, Mennin DS, editors. Generalized anxiety disorder: advances in research and practice. New York: Guilford; 2004. p. 320–50.
3. Borkovec TD, Ray WJ, Stöber J. Worry: a cognitive phenomenon intimately linked to affective, physiological, and interpersonal behavioral processes. Cognit Ther Res 1998;22(6):561–76.
4. Hoyer J, Becker ES, Roth WT. Subjective features of worry in GAD patients, social phobics and controls. Depress Anxiety 2001;13(2):89–96.

5. Wittchen H-U, Kessler RC, Beesdo K, et al. Generalized anxiety and depression in primary care: prevalence, recognition and management. J Clin Psychiatry 2002;63(Suppl 8):24–34.

6. Hoyer J, Beesdo K, Gloster AT, et al. Worry exposure versus applied relaxation in the treatment of generalized anxiety disorder. Psychother Psychosom 2009;78(2): 106–15.

7. Wells A. A metacognitive model and therapy for generalized anxiety disorder. Clin Psychol Psychother 1999;6(2):86–95.

8. Wells A, King P. Metacognitive therapy for generalized anxiety disorder: an open trial. J Behav Ther Exp Psychiatry 2006;37(3):206–12.

9. Fava G, Ruini C, Rafanelli C. Well-being therapy for generalized anxiety disorder. Psychother Psychosom 2005;74(1):26–30.

10. Newman MG, Castonguay LG, Borkovec TD, et al. An open trial of integrative therapy for generalized anxiety disorder. Psychother Theor Res Pract Train 2008;45(2):135–47.

11. Roemer L, Orsillo SM. Efficacy of an acceptance-based behaviour therapy for generalized anxiety disorder: evaluation in a randomized controlled trial. J Consult Clin Psychol 2008;76(6):1083–9.

12. Hunot V, Churchill R, Silva de Lima M, et al. Psychological therapies for generalised anxiety disorder. (Review). Cochrane Database Syst Rev 2007;(1): (CD001848).

13. Mitte K. Meta-analysis of cognitive-behavioral treatments for generalized anxiety disorder: a comparison with pharmacotherapy. Psychol Bull 2005;131(5):785–95.

14. Covin R, Quimet AJ, Seeds PM, et al. A meta-analysis of CBT for pathological worry among clients with GAD. J Anxiety Disord 2008;22(1):108–16.

15. Borkovec M, Newman MG, Pincus AL, et al. A component analysis of cognitive-behavioral therapy for generalized anxiety disorder and the role of interpersonal problems. J Consult Clin Psychol 2002;70(2):288–98.

16. Westen D, Bradley R. Empirically supported complexity. Rethinking evidence-based practice in psychotherapy. Curr Dir Psychol Sci 2005;14(5):266–71.

17. Fisher PL, Durham RC. Recovery rates in generalised anxiety disorder following psychological therapy: an analysis of clinical significant change in the STAI-T across outcome studies since 1990. Psychol Med 1999;29(6):1425–34.

18. Wittchen HU, Hoyer J. Generalized anxiety disorder: nature and course. J Clin Psychiatry 2001;62(Suppl 11):15–9.

19. Leichsenring F, Salzer S, Jaeger U, et al. Short-term psychodynamic psycho-therapy and cognitive-behavioral therapy in generalized anxiety disorder: a randomized controlled trial. Am J Psychiatry, in press.

20. Linden M, Zubrägel D, Bär T, et al. Efficacy of cognitive behaviour therapy in generalized anxiety disorders. Psychother Psychosom 2005;74(1):36–42.

21. Beck AT, Emery G, Greenberg RL. Anxiety disorders and phobias: a cognitive perspective. New York: Basic Books; 1985.

22. Borkovec TD, Costello E. Efficacy of applied relaxation and cognitive-behavioral therapy in the treatment of generalized anxiety disorder. Behav Res Ther 1993; 61(4):611–9.

23. Hazlett-Stevens H. Psychological approaches to generalized anxiety disorder: a clinician's guide to assessment and treatment. New York: Springer; 2008.

24. Borkovec TD, Castonguay LG. What is the scientific meaning of empirically supported therapy. J Consult Clin Psychol 1998;66(1):136–42.

25. Öst LG. Applied relaxation: description of a coping technique and review of controlled studies. Behav Res Ther 1987;25(5):397–409.

26. Arntz A. Cognitive therapy versus applied relaxation as treatment of generalized anxiety disorder. Behav Res Ther 2003;41(6):633–46.
27. Öst LG, Breitholtz E. Applied relaxation vs. cognitive therapy in the treatment of generalized anxiety disorder. Behav Res Ther 2000;38(8):777–90.
28. Siev J, Chambless DL. Specificity of treatment effects: cognitive therapy and relaxation for generalized anxiety and panic disorders. J Consult Clin Psychol 2007;75(4):513–22.
29. Durham RC, Murphy T, Allan T, et al. Cognitive therapy, analytic psychotherapy and anxiety management training for generalised anxiety disorder. Br J Psychiatry 1994;165(3):315–23.
30. Hamilton M. The assessment of anxiety states by rating. Br J Med Psychol 1959; 32(1):50–5.
31. Levy Berg A, Sandell R, Sandahl C. Affect-focused body psychotherapy in patients with generalized anxiety disorder: evaluation of an integrative method. J Psychother Integrat 2009;19(1):67–85.
32. Kehle S. The effectiveness of cognitive behavioral therapy for generalized anxiety disorder in a frontline service setting. Cogn Behav Ther 2008;37(3): 192–8.
33. Hoyer J, Becker ES, Margraf J. Generalized anxiety disorder and clinical worry episodes in young women. Psychol Med 2002;32(7):1227–37.
34. Leger E, Ladouceur R, Dugas MJ, et al. Cognitive behavioral treatment of generalized anxiety disorder among adolescents: a case series. J Am Acad Child Adolesc Psychiatry 2003;42(3):327–30.
35. Waters AM, Donaldson J, Zimmer-Gembeck MJ. Cognitive-behavioural therapy combined with an interpersonal skills component in the treatment of generalized anxiety disorder in adolescent females: a case series. Behav Change 2008;25(1): 35–43.
36. Stanley MA, Wilson NL, Novy DM, et al. Cognitive behavior therapy for generalized anxiety disorder among older adults in primary care: a randomized clinical trial. JAMA 2009;301:1460–7.
37. Richard DCS, Lauterbach D, Gloster AT. Description, mechanisms of action, and assessment. In: Richard DCS, Lauterbach D, editors. Handbook of exposure therapies. Burlington (NC): Academic Press; 2007. p. 1–28.
38. Wells A. Emotional disorders and metacognition. Innovative cognitive therapy. Chichester (UK): Wiley; 2000.
39. Mennin DS. Emotion regulation therapy for generalized anxiety disorder. Clin Psychol Psychother 2004;11:17–29.
40. Roemer L, Orsillo SM. Expanding our conceptualization of and treatment for generalized anxiety disorder: integrating mindfulness/acceptance-based approaches with existing cognitive-behavioral models. Clin Psychol Sci Pract 2002;9(1):54–68.
41. Hayes SC, Strosahl KD, Wilson KG. Acceptance and commitment therapy: an experiential approach to behavior change. New York: Guilford Press; 1999.
42. Borkovec M. Life in the future versus life in the present. Clin Psychol Sci Pract 2002;9(1):76–80.
43. Evans S, Ferrando S, Findler M, et al. Mindfulness-based cognitive therapy for generalized anxiety disorder. J Anxiety Disord 2008;22(4):716–21.
44. Höfler M, Gloster AT, Hoyer J. Causal effects in psychotherapy: a new conceptualisation based on counterfactuals. (submitted).
45. Ladouceur R, Talbot F, Dugas MJ. Behavioral expressions of intolerance of uncertainty in worry - experimental findings. Behav Modif 1997;21(3):355–71.

46. Dugas MJ, Ladouceur R. Treatment of GAD: targeting intolerance of uncertainty in two types of worries. Behav Modif 2000;24(5):635–57.
47. Hoyer J, Gloster AT. Massed worry exposure: clinical and practical refinements. (submitted).
48. Dupuy J-B, Beaudoin S, Rhéaume J, et al. Worry: daily self-report in clinical and non-clinical populations. Behav Res Ther 2001;39:1249–55.
49. Hayes SC, Barnes-Holmes D, Roche B. Relational frame theory: a post-Skinnerian account of human language and cognition. New York: Kluwer; 2001.
50. Durham RC. Predictors of treatment outcome. In: Davey G, Wells A, editors. Worry and its psychological disorders: theory, assessment and treatment. Chichester (UK): Wiley; 2006. p. 379–98.
51. Slade T, Andrews C. DSM-IV and ICD-10 generalized anxiety disorder: discrepant diagnoses and associated disability. Soc Psychiatry Psychiatr Epidemiol 2001;36(1):45–51.
52. Watkins E. Constructive and unconstructive repetitive thought. Psychol Bull 2008; 134:163–206.
53. Wittchen HU, Hoyer J, Friis R. Generalized anxiety disorder: a risk factor for depression? Int J Methods Psychiatr Res 2001;10:52–7.
54. Goring HJ, Papageorgiou C. Rumination and worry: factor analysis of self-report measures in depressed participants. Cognit Ther Res 2008;32:554–66.
55. Hong RY. Worry and rumination: differential associations with anxious and depressive symptoms and coping behaviour. Behav Res Ther 2007;45:277–90.
56. Sartorius N, Üstün TB, Lecrubier Y, et al. Depression comorbid with anxiety: results from the WHO study on psychological disorders in primary health care. Br J Psychiatry 1996;168(Suppl 30):29–34.
57. Hoffmann DL, Dukes EM, Wittchen HU. Human and economic burden of generalized anxiety disorder. Depress Anxiety 2008;25(1):72–90.
58. Beesdo K, Pine DS, Lieb R, et al. Similarities and differences in incidence and risk patterns of anxiety and depressive disorders: the position of generalized anxiety disorder. Arch Gen Psychiatry, in press.
59. Wetherell JL, Hopko DR, Diefenbach GJ, et al. Cognitive-behavioral therapy for late-life generalized anxiety disorder: who gets better? Behav Ther 2005;36(2): 147–56.
60. Barlow DH. Anxiety and its disorders. 2nd edition. New York: Guilford; 2002.
61. Gloster AT, Rhoades HM, Novy D, et al. Psychometric properties of the Depression Anxiety and Stress Scale-21 in older primary care patients. J Affect Disord 2008;110(3):248–59.
62. Brown TA, Barlow DH, Liebowitz MR. The empirical basis of generalized anxiety disorder. Am J Psychiatry 1994;151(9):1272–80.
63. Hofmann SG, Moscovitch DA, Litz BT, et al. The worried mind: autonomic and prefrontal activation during worrying. Emotion 2005;5(4):464–75.

Social Phobia: An Update on Treatment

Ellen C. Jørstad-Stein, MSc, Richard G. Heimberg, PhD*

KEYWORDS

- Social phobia • Social anxiety disorder
- Cognitive-behavioral treatment • Pharmacotherapy
- Efficacy • Effectiveness

SOCIAL PHOBIA

Social phobia, also known as social anxiety disorder, is a commonly occurring anxiety disorder[1,2] characterized by a fear of being embarrassed or humiliated by one's own behavior or anxiety symptoms in social or performance situations that may involve scrutiny by others.[3] People who have social phobia may experience anxiety in one or a few specific situations (eg, speaking in public, taking tests), or they may experience anxiety in most social or performance situations they encounter (the latter is referred to as the generalized subtype of social phobia).[4] As a result of their anxiety, they may suffer impairment in several life domains such as social functioning, educational attainment, and vocational productivity, and they are at increased risk for mood and substance use disorders as well (eg,[5-7]).

EVIDENCE FOR THE EFFICACY OF TREATMENTS FOR SOCIAL PHOBIA

Recent years have seen an increasing number of randomized, controlled trials (RCTs) and meta-analyses of the pharmacological and psychological treatment of social phobia. These studies have provided researchers and clinicians with evidence of treatment efficacy, which will now be considered. It should be noted that most RCTs, for social phobia or any other disorder, implement specific inclusion and exclusion criteria that may render the study population different from patients encountered in the clinician's office. In studies of pharmacotherapy, the most frequent exclusions are of (1) patients who have a comorbid diagnosis of major depressive disorder, because it is important to determine that medications used to treat social phobia are not simply demonstrating an antidepressant effect, and (2) patients who have comorbid alcohol or substance use disorders, who are likely to be noncompliant with treatment or whose uncontrolled use of alcohol or substances may make it difficult or dangerous

Adult Anxiety Clinic of Temple, Department of Psychology, Temple University, 1701 North 13th Street, Philadelphia, PA 19122-6085, USA
* Corresponding author.
E-mail address: heimberg@temple.edu (R.G. Heimberg).

Psychiatr Clin N Am 32 (2009) 641–663
doi:10.1016/j.psc.2009.05.003
0193-953X/09/$ – see front matter © 2009 Elsevier Inc. All rights reserved.

for them to participate in medication studies. In all RCTs, patients must be willing to accept randomly determined assignment to the experimental treatment or to a placebo or other control condition.

Pharmacotherapy

Two classes of drugs in particular are considered first-line pharmacological treatments for social phobia because they have demonstrated efficacy in placebo-controlled trials and because their potential side-effect profiles are more benign than those of other available medications. These drugs of choice are selective serotonin-reuptake inhibitors (SSRIs) including fluvoxamine, sertraline, paroxetine, citalopram, escitalopram, and fluoxetine, and the serotonin-norepinephrine reuptake inhibitor (SNRI) venlafaxine.[8–10] Mixed results in controlled trials have been reported for fluoxetine, however: only one of three studies found it to be superior to placebo.[11–13]

Benzodiazepines, such as clonazepam and alprazolam, also are used frequently to treat anxiety disorders. The results regarding their efficacy are mixed, however. Clonazepam seems to be an efficacious treatment for social phobia,[14,15] but in the only placebo-controlled study of alprazolam, it was not superior to placebo.[16] When considering benzodiazepine treatment, clinicians need to be aware that these drugs may be less effective or contraindicated for patients who have comorbid mood disorders. There is also potential for anxiety to return following withdrawal from the medication, although much of this concern may be mitigated with a gradual tapering program.[17] Benzodiazepines have abuse potential and are not recommended for people who have a history of substance use disorders. These drugs also may interfere with exposure to feared situations that often is a part of cognitive behavioral therapy (CBT) for social phobia. Benzodiazepines are known to inhibit the experience of anxiety during exposure to feared situations,[18] and it has been found in the treatment of other anxiety disorders that patients who receive the combination of benzodiazepines and exposure and who attribute their improvement to the medication rather than their own efforts are more likely to relapse (eg,[19]).

Monoamine oxidase inhibitors (MAOIs), such as phenelzine sulfate, are among the most efficacious treatments for social phobia.[11] Traditional MAOIs are a less-preferred treatment choice, however, because they may cause rapidly intensified blood pressure and increased the risk for heart attack and stroke unless dietary restrictions are followed strictly. Reversible inhibitors of monoamine oxidase-A have not been shown to be an efficacious alternative and are rarely used. Other classes of drugs that have been used to treat social phobia include anticonvulsants (eg, gabapentin) and β-adrenergic blockers (eg, atenolol). Gabapentin seems to be effective only at higher doses.[20] β-adrenergic blockers do not seem to be efficacious for social phobia when administered on a regular dosing schedule, but they may have a role in the management of anxiety experienced occasionally in performance situations.

Few studies have compared medications with one another, and the small number of studies limits conclusions. In one study, different doses of escitalopram were compared with paroxetine and placebo. There were no differences between the active treatments after 12 weeks, but after 24 weeks the highest dose of escitalopram (20 mg) generated improved outcomes on measures of social anxiety compared with paroxetine (20 mg[21]). Another study compared venlafaxine and paroxetine. Both were superior to placebo, but neither one was superior to the other.[22]

Empirical data also are scarce with respect to the maintenance of gains accomplished with pharmacotherapy. Two double-blind studies[23,24] have investigated discontinuation of paroxetine and sertraline for social phobia, respectively. Patients who continued treatment with paroxetine were significantly less likely to relapse than patients who had been switched to placebo.[23] Among patients who had improved with sertraline, those who continued treatment with sertraline were significantly less likely to relapse than those who were switched to placebo or who had continued on placebo because of a response during the treatment phase.[24]

Psychotherapy

Individual and group cognitive behavioral therapy

CBT is the most studied form of psychotherapy for social phobia. It is described most accurately as a family of techniques derived from the behavioral and cognitive traditions. The largest number of studies has been devoted to the development and evaluation of treatments that combine psychoeducation, in-session and in vivo exposure to feared situations, and techniques intended to modify maladaptive or irrational thinking patterns common among persons who have social phobia (ie, cognitive restructuring). Other techniques commonly included under the CBT umbrella are applied relaxation and social skills training. These techniques have been the focus of fewer trials. In one study, applied relaxation was more efficacious than a waiting-list control but was less efficacious than the combination of psychoeducation, cognitive restructuring, and exposure.[25] Social skills training has demonstrated efficacy in uncontrolled trials, but it is not possible to state with confidence that it is sufficient as a stand-alone treatment for social phobia.[26] One study compared a CBT package (ie, psychoeducation, cognitive restructuring, and exposure) with an additional social skills training module versus CBT without this module for patients who had generalized social phobia. Both treatments were efficacious, but the combination group demonstrated significantly greater gains.[27]

Several published meta-analyses have examined CBT for social phobia. Feske and Chambless[28] compared exposure plus cognitive restructuring versus exposure-only treatments for social phobia in a meta-analysis of 12 studies with a total of 208 participants. Studies involving only cognitive restructuring were excluded. In this meta-analysis, the two types of CBT were similarly efficacious, but a higher number of exposure sessions was related to better outcome. The most recent meta-analysis[29] of CBT for social phobia included 32 RCTs with a pooled total of 1479 participants. Unsurprisingly, the authors found that CBT produced better posttreatment outcomes on a range of measures than wait-list, psychological placebo, or pill placebo. Importantly, the gains from treatment were maintained at follow-up. The authors also investigated whether the type of treatment (ie, combined exposure and cognitive restructuring, exposure therapy only, cognitive restructuring only), the mode of delivery (ie, individual therapy, group therapy), or the number of hours times the number of sessions in treatment (ie, dose–response relationship) affected treatment outcome, but none did. Other factors that were not included in the meta-analysis may affect treatment outcome (eg, severity of social phobia symptoms or impairment, comorbidity, other treatment-related variables).

There may be numerous reasons for the findings of no difference between the various forms of CBT. For example, the meta-analyses may be based on a small number of trials, may not weight studies according to their quality, or may eliminate studies from the analysis in idiosyncratic fashion. In addition, different control conditions may be associated with different between-group effect sizes, a possibility that is not always taken into consideration. For example, exposure alone has been compared typically to a waiting-list condition. Conversely, exposure combined with cognitive restructuring more often has been compared with more stringent psychological or pill placebo conditions. Thus exposure with cognitive restructuring may artifactually generate lower mean effect sizes than exposure alone. Although meta-analyses provide a wealth of information in a synthesized manner, there also is important information that usually is not reported because it is not included in the majority of the source articles (eg, information about long-term maintenance of gains accomplished during treatment). Review of individual studies therefore may be helpful, and one set of studies is reviewed briefly here.

Cognitive behavioral group therapy for social phobia (CBGT)[30] is a well-investigated protocol that includes psychoeducation, structured cognitive exercises, exposures to simulated anxiety-evoking events in session, cognitive restructuring before, during, and after exposures, and behavioral and cognitive homework assignments. CBGT has been compared with educational-supportive group therapy, a highly credible psychological placebo condition.[31] Compared with educational-supportive group therapy, CBGT generated significant improvements in clinician ratings of severity, percent responders, and subjective anxiety ratings before and during behavioral performance at posttreatment that were maintained at follow-up assessments both 6 months and 5 years later.[32] CBGT and similar treatment packages have been compared with medication treatments, and those studies are reviewed in later sections.

Interpersonal therapy

Interpersonal therapy (IPT) is based on the assumption that psychiatric disorders occur and are maintained within an interpersonal context. IPT is a time-limited 12- to 16-week therapy that is efficacious in the treatment of acute depression,[33] dysthymic disorder,[34] and other disorders with an interpersonal component such as binge eating disorder.[35] Lipsitz and colleagues[36] modified IPT for social phobia. In this treatment, core interpersonal problem areas rather than social interaction and performance situations are identified and then are examined through multiple techniques (eg, exploration of feelings and thoughts related to the problem area, encouragement of affective expression, clarification of feelings, communication and decision analysis, and role playing of target situations but without a focus on exposure).

In the initial, uncontrolled study of IPT for social phobia, seven of nine individuals (78%) were classified as responders,[36] but a randomized trial that compared IPT to a supportive therapy control failed to replicate these initial findings.[37] Both groups demonstrated improvement in social anxiety, but they did not differ on the majority of measures or in the proportion of responders. Another recent study, however, did provide some support for the efficacy of IPT for social phobia.[38] Conducted in an inpatient setting, this study compared 10 weeks of IPT and CBT. Patients in each condition received four group sessions and one individual session per week. Treatments were modified to include individual and group components to fit an inpatient setting better. Both groups demonstrated improvements on measures of social anxiety, and these gains were maintained at 1-year follow-up. Definitive conclusions about the efficacy of IPT for social phobia cannot be made, however, because there were few differences between inpatient IPT and CBT (CBT was superior on a single secondary measure), and no control condition was included.

Psychodynamic therapy

Although no controlled trials of psychodynamic therapy for social phobia have been published, case studies have been presented (eg,[39]). The rationale for the focus of psychodynamic therapy is found in Gabbard's[40,41] work. Within this framework, people who have social phobia experience shame because of an unconscious need to be the center of attention, guilt related to an unconscious need to eradicate social competition, doubt concerning the ability to eradicate social competition, separation anxiety because of an unconscious need for autonomy, and loss of love from a caregiver because of autonomy. Representations of others, particularly caregivers, may have been internalized as critical, shaming, or abandoning. These internalized representations then are projected onto others, bringing about a need to avoid social situations. Recently, a short-term treatment manual has been developed for social phobia based on Luborsky's psychodynamically oriented supportive-expressive therapy.[42] The treatment includes several elements, such as a focus on the core conflictual relationship theme that influences the patient's primary symptoms, goal setting, enhancing insight, and understanding the role of shame and unrealistic demands. In addition, there is a component similar to exposure in which patients are encouraged to confront feared social situations. This treatment manual currently is being used in a large-scale investigation comparing psychodynamic therapy and CBT for social phobia.

Comparison and Combination of Pharmacotherapy and Cognitive Behavioral Therapy

One of the first meta-analyses to compare CBT and pharmacotherapy for social phobia[43] included 24 controlled trials. Both types of treatment were more efficacious than control conditions, and there were no significant differences between them. A later, larger meta-analysis[44] compared CBT and pharmacotherapy across 108 trials. Benzodiazepines and SSRIs were equally efficacious at posttreatment and were more efficacious than control conditions and applied relaxation. Benzodiazepines (based on a limited number of trials), but not SSRIs, were superior to MAOIs and other forms of CBT at posttreatment. Maintenance of gains could not be examined for pharmacotherapies because of insufficient follow-up data, a recurrent problem in most trials of the efficacy of pharmacotherapy. In another meta-analysis, patients treated with CBT demonstrated additional gains after follow-up periods averaging 3 months.[45] Additional light may be shed on the relative maintenance of gains in CBT versus pharmacotherapy by examination of individual trials.

CBGT, the MAOI phenelzine, educational-supportive group psychotherapy (ie, an attention-placebo treatment of equal credibility to CBGT), and pill placebo were compared in a trial of 133 patients who participated in 12 weeks of acute treatment, 6 months of maintenance treatment for responders to CGBT and phenelzine, and 6 months of naturalistic follow-up.[46] More patients responded to CBGT or phenelzine than to the control conditions, and patients treated with phenelzine tended to respond more quickly, after 6 weeks of active treatment, whereas the patients treated with CBGT more often demonstrated treatment response after 12 weeks. After 12 weeks, patients treated with phenelzine surpassed patients treated with CBGT on some dimensional measures, although both were superior to controls. During the maintenance and follow-up phases, however, 50% of phenelzine responders relapsed, compared with only 17% of CBGT responders, suggesting that CBGT provided better protection against relapse than phenelzine.[47] Another trial that compared CBT and fluoxetine[12] demonstrated the superiority of CBT. CBT continued to outperform fluoxetine between posttreatment and 12-month follow-up. Fluoxetine did not surpass placebo in this trial, however.

Very few trials have examined CBT and pharmacotherapy in combination for social phobia. One recent trial examined the combination of CBGT and phenelzine, in comparison with the monotherapies and pill placebo, in a sample of 128 patients.[48] After 24 weeks, combined treatment outperformed phenelzine, which was superior to CBGT, which was superior to placebo. Another trial[11] compared group CBT to fluoxetine, the combination of CBT plus fluoxetine, the combination of CBT plus placebo, and placebo alone. All active treatments surpassed placebo after 14 weeks, with no differences among them. Another study examining sertraline, exposure, and combined treatment found all active treatments to be superior to placebo after 12 weeks.[49] At 24 weeks, active treatments did not differ from each other, but only sertraline (alone or in combination with exposure) was superior to placebo. At 1-year follow-up, however, only patients who received exposure continued to improve, whereas patients who received sertraline alone or combined treatment showed a degree of deterioration.[50]

NEW TREATMENT DEVELOPMENTS
D-Cycloserine

D-cycloserine (DCS), a partial agonist of the N-methyl-D-aspartate receptor, has been shown to augment learning and memory, and doses of DCS received shortly after exposure facilitate extinction to feared stimuli in animals. Two double-blind RCTs have examined the use of DCS to augment the exposure treatment of social phobia involving public speaking.[51,52] The results of the trials are promising. Short-term dosing of DCS was found to be more effective than placebo in enhancing the effect of exposures. Patients who received DCS before exposures reported less social anxiety than patients who received placebo.[52] Patients who received DCS also reported improvement in their perception of their speech performance and were rated as more improved on the Global Assessment of Functioning Scale and on a measure of social phobia symptoms.[51]

Motivational Interviewing

Although CBT has substantial empirical support for the treatment of social phobia, a number of people do not respond adequately or drop out of treatment prematurely. It has been suggested that the people who fail to benefit from CBT may be ambivalent about change.[53] Westra and Dozois[53] hypothesized that it would be possible to increase compliance and decrease the risk of drop-out with a pretreatment intervention framed around motivational interviewing, which has been defined (p. 25) as "a client-centered, directive method for enhancing intrinsic motivation to change by exploring and resolving ambivalence."[54] The therapist helps the client explore his or her thoughts and feelings regarding change to enhance motivation for change. The client then becomes an advocate for his or her own change. This process differs from traditional CBT in which the therapist often assumes more of a leadership role. Fifty-five clients who had a variety of anxiety disorders (about one third of whom had social phobia) were assigned randomly to receive three weekly sessions of motivational interviewing or no intervention before CBT for their anxiety disorder, and the impact of CBT on homework compliance, treatment completion, and symptom change then was examined. Following CBT, the group who received pretreatment motivational interviewing reported significantly higher expectancies for anxiety control and was more compliant with homework assignments than the group that received no pretreatment intervention. Both groups exhibited significant symptomatic improvements, but clients in the motivational interviewing group were more likely to be classified as responders. There were improvements in the group that received CBT without pretreatment intervention, and both groups maintained their gains at follow-up, but motivational interviewing showed promise for increasing compliance and treatment response among potentially difficult clients.

Mindfulness/Meditation-Based Stress Reduction

Mindfulness and meditation originated in Eastern cultures centuries ago, but they have been incorporated increasingly into Western psychotherapeutic practice. Mindfulness is "the awareness that emerges through paying attention on purpose, in the present moment, and nonjudgmentally to the unfolding of experience moment by moment"[55] (p. 145). Meditation-based stress reduction has demonstrated efficacy in improving the well-being of patients who have medical disorders with or without a comorbid anxiety disorder and in reducing the stress of healthy people.[56,57] One recent randomized trial[58] compared eight weekly group sessions in meditation-based stress reduction and a full-day meditation retreat versus 12 weekly sessions of CBGT for social phobia. There were improvements in both groups on measures of depression, disability, and quality of life. Those who had received CBGT, however, demonstrated greater reductions on clinician- and patient-rated measures of social anxiety, and CBGT had a better response rate (66%) than meditation-based stress reduction (38.5%) in the intent-to-treat sample. Although the evidence suggests that CBGT is more efficacious than meditation-based stress reduction across the spectrum of symptoms of social phobia, meditation-based stress reduction also was an efficacious treatment for social phobia. Thus, meditation-based stress reduction may be helpful to some patients who have social phobia. Future research should examine whether there are specific patients who may be more likely to benefit from meditation-based stress reduction than CBT. Furthermore, it may be helpful to integrate mindfulness and meditation techniques into CBT for social phobia, because promising results have been demonstrated for other anxiety disorders (eg,[59]).

Acceptance and Commitment Therapy

Acceptance and commitment therapy (ACT) recently has been applied to the treatment of social phobia with promising results in two uncontrolled trials.[60,61] Dalrymple and Herbert[60] investigated the efficacy of a 12-week treatment integrating exposure therapy and ACT. Several measures were administered to assess social anxiety symptoms, experiential avoidance (ie, the attempt to alter the form, frequency, or situational sensitivity of private events even when doing so causes behavioral harm[62]), and general quality of life. Nineteen participants received 12 weekly 1-hour sessions that included presentation of the four main components of ACT. The first stage (sessions 1 and 2) involved "creative helplessness" in which participants come to understand the futility of their past efforts to control anxiety. The next phase (starting with session 3) presented the concept of "willingness" to have unwanted or distressing thoughts while being exposed to difficult social situations. Mindfulness techniques were presented in the third stage (beginning in session 4) to help teach nonjudgmental experience and appraisal of anxious thoughts and to move toward cognitive defusion, the exercise of distancing the self from internal experiences. The final stage (beginning in session 7) facilitated participation in experiences that reflect the participant's valued choices. These ACT concepts were demonstrated using metaphors and experiential exercises. The treatment also incorporated traditional behavior therapy techniques such as in-session role-plays, in vivo exposure, and social skills training. Patients displayed significant decreases in social anxiety, fear of negative evaluation, experiential avoidance, and a significant increase in quality of life at posttreatment and 3-month follow-up. A mid-treatment decrease in experiential avoidance predicted a posttreatment decrease in anxiety. Similar results were reported in a small uncontrolled trial of ACT-based group therapy.[61]

EVIDENCE FOR ACTIVE INGREDIENTS AND MECHANISMS
Brain Regions Active in Social Phobia and Response to Treatment

Recent studies using neuroimaging techniques such as functional MRI or positron emission tomography have started to identify various brain regions related to social phobia and the action of pharmacotherapy and CBT. One study[63] demonstrated that patients who had generalized social phobia showed greater activity in the amygdala, uncus, and parahippocampal gyrus than healthy controls in response to angry and contemptuous faces. An RCT[64] examined sites of action in the brain of social phobic patients who received the SSRI citalopram, CBGT, or wait-list for 9 weeks. Imaging of regional cerebral blood flow was assessed using positron emission tomography with oxygen 15-labeled water pre- and posttreatment or the wait-list period. Significant improvements were found in both treatment groups. Sites of action were observed, particularly in the right hemisphere, in the amygdala, hippocampus, and adjacent brain regions involved in defensive reactions to threat (ie, periamygdaloid, rhinal, and parahippocampal cortices). Blood flow to the identified regions was reduced significantly in patients in either treatment group who had been classified as responders. It is noteworthy that both citalopram and CBGT may cause changes in the activation of brain regions known to be associated with response to threatening stimuli. The mechanisms involved in these changes have not yet been explored.

Mediators of Change

Little is known about mediators of change in CBT in social phobia. Hofmann[65] hypothesized that negative cognitive appraisal (estimated social costs, or how bad negative social outcomes are perceived to be), perceived self-efficacy (perceived social skill), and perceived emotional control may be important mediators of change, but few studies actually have tested these hypotheses. In a study comparing group CBT, exposure group therapy, and wait-list control conditions, Hofmann[66] examined whether changes in estimated social cost mediated pretreatment to posttreatment changes in both active treatment groups. Only the group receiving group CBT showed continued improvement from posttreatment to the 6-month follow-up. Continued benefit was associated with an overall reduction in estimated social cost, suggesting that the cognitive behavioral intervention was associated with greater treatment gains that are mediated through changes in estimated social cost.

Moscovitch and colleagues[67] examined a different mediational pathway, namely whether changes in social anxiety mediated changes in depression among socially anxious patients who had depressed mood. Changes in depression were fully mediated by changes in social anxiety (accounting for 91% of the variance in depression scores), whereas changes in social anxiety were only partially mediated by changes in depression (accounting for only 6% of the variance in social anxiety scores). These findings suggest that, in this group of patients, improvements in the symptoms of depression tend to track improvements in the symptoms of social anxiety.

Predictors of Treatment Outcome

Treatment-related predictors of outcome also may be important active ingredients in CBT for social phobia. Several studies have examined the importance of homework compliance for treatment outcome. One study[68] found that more compliant patients reported less fear of negative evaluation posttreatment. Gains also were maintained at 6-month follow-up when patients reported less anxiety during a speech. Another study[69] also found homework compliance in CBGT to be important. Overall, greater compliance with homework significantly predicted reductions in social anxiety after pretreatment levels had been controlled. Additional results specific to phases of treatment were reported also. Greater compliance with homework actually was associated with higher levels of anxiety and fear of negative evaluation during the second phase of treatment, when in-session exposures were introduced. During the third phase of treatment, however, when in-session exposures were continued and in vivo exposures were introduced, greater homework compliance was related to reductions in anxiety. One other study[70] did not find evidence for a relationship between homework compliance and treatment outcome.

Recently, the therapeutic alliance has been considered as a predictor of outcome in CBT for social phobia, again with mixed results. Woody and Adessky[70] did not find the alliance to be a predictor of treatment outcome. A more recent study[71] examined the relationship between working alliance, session helpfulness, and measures of emotional processing in 18 clients undergoing CBT for social phobia. There was a positive correlation between client-rated working alliance and session helpfulness. Overall, a strong alliance was associated with clients engaging with the session and finding the session helpful. A moderate alliance, however, was most productive when the measure was the amount of anxiety reduction experienced during in-session exposures to feared situations. Speculatively, an alliance that is too weak may not provide a sufficient sense of safety for some patients, whereas a very strong alliance may suppress patients' anxiety experience and indirectly interfere with their ability to overcome it.

Expectancies about treatment have been considered an important factor in the treatment of several mental health problems. Studies examining this potential predictor have generated consistent results. In one study,[72] a treatment expectancy questionnaire was administered after the first and fourth sessions of CBGT. Expectancy ratings significantly predicted outcome as measured by various interviewer-administered and self-report measures of social anxiety, even after accounting for pretreatment severity. A second study[73] also found expectancy to be significantly correlated with a composite anxiety outcome measure at the posttreatment assessment. Expectancy also was a predictor of outcome at the follow-up assessment.

Another treatment-related predictor of CBT outcome to consider is group cohesion. Group cohesion was studied first by Woody and Adessky,[70] who did not find an effect. Another study,[74] however, found that better group cohesion ratings across sessions were related to better outcome. It is important to note that group cohesion was not measured until the midpoint of treatment, and it is possible that patient improvements predicted greater cohesion rather than the other way around. Finally, group participation in sessions was examined in one study.[68] Patients who had been rated by observers as engaging in high group participation were rated as more skillful in the delivery of speeches at 6-month follow-up.

ELEMENTS OF SOCIAL PHOBIA SIMILAR TO ELEMENTS OF OTHER DISORDERS

Several anxiety disorders and other disorders have elements similar to social phobia. Patients who have social phobia demonstrate many of the cognitive characteristics of patients who have other anxiety disorders, for example, biased interpretation of neutral or mildly negative cues as catastrophic,[75] hypervigilance for threat cues and avoidance of feared stimuli (for a review see[76]), and (although the evidence is somewhat equivocal) biased memory for anxiety-evoking events.[77] Additionally, individuals who have social phobia are known to engage in post-event processing,[78] which involves brooding over selectively retrieved negative information about oneself and others from a previously experienced social situation. This process may appear similar to worrying in generalized anxiety disorder or rumination in depression, but these cognitive styles focus on possible future events and on the consequences of stressful life events in general, respectively (eg,[79,80]).

Social phobia is similar to depression on a number of other dimensions. Whereas all of the anxiety disorders have a high level of negative affect, only social phobia is similar to depression in its association with low levels of positive affect.[81,82] This association is especially robust when considering social interaction anxiety,[83] a finding that may stem from the relationship between positive affect and interpersonal engagement[84] that typically is impaired in both depressed and socially anxious individuals.[82] Individuals who have social phobia, like individuals who have depression, also have demonstrated diminished positive experiences and curiosity.[85] Depressive disorders often are comorbid with social phobia, and it is curious that when depression co-occurs with social phobia, the hypervigilance for social threat noted earlier seems to be suppressed.[86,87]

The effects of comorbid anxiety and mood disorders on the efficacy of CBT for social phobia have been investigated. In one study,[88] individuals who had social phobia alone were compared with those who had comorbid anxiety disorders and those who had comorbid mood disorders. Patients who had comorbid mood disorders tended to have more severe symptoms both before and following 12 weeks of CBGT. Those who had comorbid anxiety disorders fared as well as those who had social phobia alone. This pattern remained evident at 1-year follow-up. In another study, higher self-reported depression at pretreatment was related to decreased reduction in anxious anticipation of a behavioral test, although this same pattern was not found for clinician ratings of depression.[73] In a recent placebo-controlled study, higher levels of depressive symptoms were related to more severe social anxiety and less change in social anxiety symptoms. Individuals who had greater depressive symptoms also were more likely to terminate treatment prematurely.[89] One additional study[90] found that socially anxious individuals who had comorbid depression attained the same treatment gains as individuals who had no comorbid disorders or those who had comorbid anxiety disorders (similar to[88]). After a 1-year follow-up period, however, individuals who had comorbid depression showed greater social anxiety than the other participants in the study. Collectively, these studies suggest that individuals who have comorbid depression may benefit from inclusion of a depression-specific component of treatment (eg, use of behavioral activation strategies[91]), additional monitoring and/or booster treatments after the acute course of treatment is concluded, or combining CBT for social phobia with antidepressant medication.

Avoidant personality disorder occurs as a comorbid diagnosis in 22.1% to 70% of people who have a primary diagnosis of social phobia.[92–95] It is diagnosed more commonly among patients who have generalized social phobia than among those who have the non-generalized subtype,[96] suggesting that avoidant personality disorder may be diagnosed more frequently among those who have more severe social phobia. In fact, avoidant personality disorder may best be considered as part of the continuum of severity of social phobia,[93] and this assertion is supported by two recent studies.[97,98] There is disagreement, however, as to whether the presence of avoidant personality disorder adversely affects the outcome of CBT for social phobia: some studies showed little effect,[98,99] and at least one other showed poorer outcome.[100] Persons who have avoidant personality disorder may avoid intense positive and negative emotions as well as experiencing a broad fear of new situations,[101] and these tendencies may suggest additional targets for future treatment research.

FUTURE EFFORTS TO IMPROVE TREATMENTS FOR SOCIAL PHOBIA
Integration of New Treatment Developments into Current Approaches to Cognitive Behavioral Therapy

The recent years have seen an increased interest in transdiagnostic approaches to the treatment of anxiety disorder.[102] Transdiagnostic models of emotional disorders (including anxiety and mood disorders) theorize that there is a common underlying core pathological construct that maintains the disorders, and recently negative affect has been proposed as a candidate construct.[103] Persons who have high negative affect may experience several learning situations that result in various types of fears or other emotional states that subsequently are seen as comorbid. A quantitative review[103] of the available transdiagnostic protocols found large effect sizes of pre- to posttreatment change that were comparable to effect sizes of CBT for social phobia.[28,29] Gains also were maintained through follow-up of up to 6 months. These types of treatments seem promising, and it may be feasible to transport them to community and private practice settings because the treatment protocols may be used with a range of anxiety disorders. More research is needed to gain understanding of the optimal transdiagnostic treatment approach, however, because there are differences between transdiagnostic treatment protocols. Additionally, all transdiagnostic treatment protocols reviewed were compared either with a wait-list control or with no control group at all. Thus far, none of the protocols have been compared with each other or with CBT for specific anxiety disorders. Therefore the efficacy of individual transdiagnostic treatment protocols relative to each other and to established treatment protocols for specific anxiety disorders is unknown.

Motivational Interviewing and Cognitive Behavioral Therapy for Social Phobia with Comorbid Alcohol or Substance Use Disorders

The rate of comorbid alcohol use disorders among patients who have social phobia is high,[104] but treatment studies targeting this specific population are scarce, and these patients are excluded from many controlled trials of both CBT and medications. One pilot case study[105] of a 33-year-old Caucasian man who had comorbid generalized social anxiety disorder and alcohol abuse examined the effectiveness of conducting motivational interviewing directed at drinking behavior (three sessions) before commencing CBT for social phobia (16 sessions). Motivational interviewing and CBT reduced both alcohol-related problems and social anxiety. The first three sessions focused on the relationship between alcohol use and social anxiety. The patient reported he was stuck in a cycle of using alcohol to cope with anxiety brought on by social situations. In turn, his alcohol use subsequently increased his anxiety in later social situations. Motivational interviewing helped the patient contemplate changing his alcohol-use behaviors. After the patient reported not consuming alcohol during a social event, something that was less challenging than he imagined, daily monitoring of alcohol use was initiated. The patient set a goal of not drinking primarily to manage social anxiety. Alcohol-use behaviors were monitored throughout CBT and were reviewed with regards to his treatment goal. A few sessions into exposures, the patient suggested conducting a "no drinking" social anxiety exposure. The exposure was successful, and additional "no drinking" exposures were conducted. The patient reported that he did not use alcohol to manage anxiety in social situations between the first "no drinking" exposure and the final session. He also reported clinically significant improvement in his fear of negative evaluation. At the final session, positive outcomes also were reported on a measure of change in social anxiety between sessions and a measure of symptoms of alcohol use disorders. The results provided by this pilot study suggest that CBT and motivational interviewing may be incorporated successfully into treatments for patients who have social phobia and alcohol use disorders. Controlled trials are needed, however.

Situational Panic Attacks

There is little research about situationally bound panic attacks in people who have social phobia. Persons who have social phobia often experience panic attacks that are related to social and/or performance situations. Compared with persons who have social phobia but do not have panic attacks, persons who have social phobia and who experience situationally bound panic attacks have exhibited greater fear and avoidance of social situations. They also have reported more distress and impairment related to their social phobia, higher levels of anxiety sensitivity, and greater hopelessness.[106] Another preliminary study[107] compared the expression of panic symptoms in social situations in patients who had a primary diagnosis of social phobia with that of patients who had a primary diagnosis of generalized anxiety disorder. In addition to the 13 primary symptoms of panic attacks, patients were asked whether they experienced six additional symptoms (ie, blushing, tics/muscle spasms, dry mouth, fear of being unable to speak, fear of their mind going blank, fear of doing or saying something embarrassing) hypothesized to characterize panic attacks in social situations. For the most recent and the worst experience of panic, socially anxious patients endorsed blushing, fear of being unable to speak, fear of their mind going blank, and fear of doing or saying something embarrassing significantly more than did the patients who had generalized anxiety disorder. Similarly, they endorsed experiencing heart palpitations, sweating, shaking, and chills or hot flushes during situationally bound panic attacks more often than did the patients who had generalized anxiety disorder. It appears that individuals who have primary social phobia and who experience panic attacks bound to social anxiety–evoking situations experience a unique set of panic symptoms compared with individuals who have generalized anxiety who experience panic attacks. Clinicians should be alert to the possible presence and configuration of symptoms in these attacks. Consequently, panic attacks may require attention during treatment for social anxiety disorder, and it may be necessary to incorporate procedures directed at panic symptoms (eg, interoceptive exposure, that is, exposure to evoked symptoms of panic) into more traditional CBT approaches to social phobia.

Prevention

Few studies have examined ways of preventing social phobia, but there is strong evidence for familial and environmental influences. Because parents may reinforce the avoidant choices anxious children make,[108] it is important to consider including parents in treatment to provide them with strategies to help their child manage social phobia. Parents who have social phobia may benefit from treatment as well.

Treatment of children and adolescents may prevent chronicity of social phobia because the disorder has an early age of onset, with the highest standardized incidence rates per person-year between 10 and 19 years of age.[109] Promising avenues for prevention may be found in school-based prevention programs or in prevention programs that target children at risk for developing social phobia or other anxiety disorders. Demonstration prevention programs have been integrated into schools to provide children and parents with coping skills (eg, cognitive restructuring, relaxation) and instruction for conducting exposures to feared situations. There was significant improvement in the intervention group compared with children who did not receive the intervention.[110] In addition, prevention programs targeting youth at risk of developing anxiety disorders have been found to reduce anxiety symptoms and rates of anxiety disorders compared with control groups.[111]

What May Be in Store for Social Phobia in the Diagnostic and Statistical Manual of Mental Disorders-V and Are There Implications for Treatment?

The process of revising the *Diagnostic and Statistical Manual of Mental Disorders* (DSM) is well underway, and the DSM-V will be completed in the next few years. These revisions may bring about several changes in the diagnostic criteria for social phobia. Some of the possible changes that may arise from this process are discussed here, with comments regarding how the possible changes may affect clinicians and researchers. What follows is the opinion of the authors and does not reflect the deliberations of any DSM committee or decisions arising there from.

First, the name "social anxiety disorder" was introduced as an alternative to "social phobia" in the DSM-IV, but there is reason to consider social anxiety disorder the better label because it more accurately reflects the severity and pervasiveness of symptoms and impairment associated with the disorder.[112] Second, the current exclusion criterion H regarding general medical conditions (ie, if a general medical condition or another mental disorder is present, the fear must be unrelated to it) is highly restrictive. There are several medical conditions that may bring about social anxiety, for example, physically visible congenital or acquired differences, such as cleft lip and palate, port wine stains, effects of surgery following various cancers, or burns. Visible behavioral differences also can result from a medical disorder, as would be the case for stuttering or for tremors related to Parkinson's disease. It may be more useful to consider revising the current language to allow diagnosis of social phobia (or social anxiety disorder) if the fear is substantially greater than would be expected or normative for persons who have a particular medical condition that produces visible symptoms that may be evaluated by others. A person who will not engage in social interaction for fear of negative evaluation of a physical difference or behavioral symptom may be seriously impaired, and at least one case series[113] suggests that persons in this circumstance do respond to cognitive behavioral and pharmacological treatments for social phobia. Allowing the diagnosis to be applied to these individuals should help reduce their suffering.

The literature suggests that it may make sense to reconsider the current subtyping scheme, which currently describes individuals who fear most social situations as having "generalized" social phobia. Although there are some differences between generalized and non-generalized social phobia (eg, generalized social phobia is associated with greater severity and impairment and is more likely to run in families[114]), this approach to subtyping is, in effect, a dichotimization of a continuously distributed variable, the number of feared situations.[115] In the study by Vriends and colleagues,[115] the number of feared social situations was distributed continuously without any clear demarcation between subtypes, and a greater number of feared situations was significantly related to increased functional impairment, comorbidity, treatment seeking, dysfunctional attitudes, and decreased social support and mental health. A specifier indicating the number of feared situations may be a useful means by which to index severity of the disorder in the individual case, but at the present time, the best indication from the available data is that a greater number of feared situations is related to severity, and severity may be related to treatment outcome or the dose of treatment required for a positive outcome. The current dichotomous system has not lived up to its promise.

An additional concern that should be addressed is the relationship between social phobia and avoidant personality disorder. It has been argued, here and elsewhere,[96–98] that (1) avoidant personality disorder rarely occurs unless the person diagnosed also meets criteria for generalized social phobia as currently defined, and (2) the criteria for generalized social phobia and avoidant personality disorder are simply too similar and do not described two independent disorders. It seems unwise to give two diagnoses on two different axes to the same set of symptoms.

Finally, it is somewhat curious that for persons over 18 years of age, there is no specification of a minimum duration of symptoms required for a diagnosis of social phobia. For those under 18 years of age, the required duration is 6 months, and it seems reasonable to consider the same duration of symptoms for those who are older.

These are some of the issues that may be considered in the DSM revision process. Of course, any changes will have implications for researchers and clinicians alike. Researchers may find that some criterion changes may restrict the inclusion of participants to their studies (eg, if the duration criteria of 6 months is adopted), whereas changes to other criteria may allow the inclusion of participants who previously were excluded from clinical trials or psychopathology studies (eg, participants who have excessive anxiety about the visible symptoms of medical conditions). Inclusion of previously excluded participant groups could bring about new challenges to empirically supported treatment manuals that were developed in studies that did not address these individuals' specific concerns. Although clinicians working in the community do not have to adhere to the strict boundaries of an empirically supported treatment manual, they also may find that they must be more creative in working with different client groups. In both psychotherapy and pharmacotherapy, many studies have been conducted using samples of persons who have generalized social phobia. Although it is likely that persons who have fewer fears would be responsive to these same treatments, the empirical basis for this assertion is lacking.

What Differentiates Cognitive Behavioral Therapy and Pharmacotherapy for Social Phobia from Treatment for Other Anxiety Disorders?

For pharmacotherapy, the response to the question posed in the heading may be, "Not much." For CBT, the answer is a bit different. The basic form of treatment procedures tend to cut across the anxiety disorders, but the substance and content of the procedures tend to be specific to the anxiety disorder, the initial attempts at transdiagnostic treatments notwithstanding. In fact, Butler[116,117] first discussed these issues more than 20 years ago, and a complete discussion is beyond the scope of this issue. Social phobia presents significant challenges in CBT, because patients may have made isolationist choices so that their lives include few easily available opportunities for exposure, because they may be too afraid to make big steps (eg, to join a health club or take a class to have an opportunity to talk to another human being), because some social situations occur so quickly that there is little time available to implement cognitive or behavioral coping skills before the situation is over, because social situations do have real consequences that need to be managed or contained, because at least a modicum of skillful social behavior is required and executing skillful social behavior requires attentional capacity that may be devoted to thinking catastrophic thoughts about oneself or the situation, and because the responses of the other person(s) in the situation may be unpredictable or anti-therapeutic.

The reader is referred to manuals for the treatment of social phobia, which address these issues and many others.[30,118,119]

ROUTINE CARE AND OBSTACLES FOR DISSEMINATION

As previously covered in this article, there is abundant literature providing evidence of the efficacy of pharmacotherapy and CBT for social phobia. The evidence supporting the use of CBT for social phobia, however, usually comes from RCTs conducted in university or other specialty settings in which a structured treatment manual requiring strict adherence is followed, and study participants are carefully screened. Patients who have comorbid major depression, comorbid alcohol or substance abuse or dependence, light to moderate impairment, prior treatment, or who fall outside a certain age range often are excluded.[120] Thus, it has been argued that patients who receive treatments in non-research settings may not achieve outcomes comparable to the outcomes obtained in a research setting (eg,[121]).

Therefore, studies examining the generalizability and transportability of empirically supported treatments for social phobia to outpatient community or private practice settings are needed. Only a small handful of these studies has been conducted, but the results are quite encouraging. The first benchmarking study (ie, a study that compares the effectiveness of a treatment as administered in the community with its efficacy as administered in the laboratory) included 217 patients in four outpatient clinics in Germany.[120] Patients were unselected, and all had a primary diagnosis of social phobia. There were significant reductions in social anxiety and avoidance 6 weeks following the end of treatment, as well as significant reductions in general anxiety and depression. There were no differences in outcome between the four outpatient clinics. Interestingly, effect sizes were comparable to the average effect sizes reported in published meta-analyses. Another benchmarking study[122] compared the outcome of CBGT for 58 clients who had social phobia treated in a university research clinic with the outcomes for 54 patients treated in a private practice clinic. There were no significant differences in outcome posttreatment. In addition, both groups maintained their gains 3 months after treatment had been completed. The most recent benchmarking study[123] investigated CBGT for 153 clients who had social phobia seen in a community mental health clinic. Again, effect sizes were comparable to those reported in previously published efficacy and effectiveness studies on group and individual treatment for social phobia. Thus far the evidence suggests that CBT for social phobia is transportable to and effective in outpatient, private practice, and community mental health clinics. It will be important for researchers and clinicians in the community to connect to conduct studies of the generalizability and transportability of social phobia treatments to the community as well as to facilitate dissemination of treatment.

SUMMARY

Social phobia is a commonly occurring anxiety disorder. Persons living with this disorder experience interference across various life domains including social life, school, work, or daily activities. The difficulties associated with living with social phobia may cause the person to seek treatment, and both pharmacotherapy and psychotherapy have proved efficacious in clinical trials. The SSRIs and the SNRI venlafaxine are the first-line pharmacological treatments for social phobia. In terms of psychotherapy, CBT is the treatment of choice. There is no conclusive evidence whether pharmacotherapy or CBT is more effective for the treatment of social phobia. The evidence in favor of the combination of pharmacotherapy and CBT is limited as well, but new developments in treatment are taking place. For example, studies are underway to examine the utility of D-cycloserine to enhance exposures in CBT. There also is interest in integrating motivational interviewing with CBT and in taking advantage of the recent mindfulness- and acceptance-based approaches. As these recent developments are subjected to further study, it would be valuable to include cost-benefit analyses of long-term outcome and cost effectiveness in trials.

Few studies have investigated the active ingredients and mechanisms of action in treatments for social phobia. Treatment with an SSRI or CBT revealed activity in the amygdala, hippocampus, and adjacent brain regions including the periamygdaloid, rhinal, and parahippocampal cortices. Greater gains in CBT may be mediated through changes in estimated social cost. Further it seems that improvements in symptoms of depression tend to follow improvements in social phobia symptoms among socially phobic patients who have depressed mood. Some evidence suggests that homework compliance, therapeutic alliance, and group cohesion may moderate CBT outcome. Stronger evidence exists for the moderating role of group participation and expectancies about treatment. Social phobia shares common elements with other disorders, and the disorders that seem most relevant often are comorbid with social phobia. Thus, elements of these other disorders may affect the efficacy of treatment and require specific consideration in treatment.

Efforts to improve treatments for social phobia are ongoing. There is interest in streamlining treatments for anxiety disorders in general. Transdiagnostic theory and therapy spanning the anxiety disorders as well as the mood disorders by targeting underlying core pathological processes is an example of this recent development. There also is a pull for developing treatments specific to patients who have social phobia and comorbid alcohol use disorder because this particular comorbid combination is so common. A recent case study integrated motivational interviewing with CBT to successfully treat a patient who had this diagnostic picture, but clinical trials are needed. There also may be a need to incorporate interoceptive exposure into CBT for patients who have social phobia who also experience situationally bound panic attacks. This particular group of patients has exhibited greater fear and avoidance of social situations in addition to reporting more distress and impairment related to their social phobia, higher levels of anxiety sensitivity, and greater hopelessness. They may require additional, different treatment strategies to achieve gains in treatment equivalent to those seen in patients who do not have panic attacks. There also is room for prevention efforts with children and adolescents, an area that has not been well studied. Despite concerns regarding the transportability and generalizability of psychological treatments studied in laboratory settings to community settings and a relative lack of studies investigating this issue, the evidence thus far suggests that CBT for social phobia is transportable to and effective in outpatient, private practice, and community mental health clinics.

REFERENCES

1. Kessler RC, Berglund P, Demler O, et al. Lifetime prevalence and age-onset distributions of DSM-IV disorders in the National Comorbidity Survey Replication. Arch Gen Psychiatry 2005;62(6):593–602.
2. Kessler RC, Chiu WT, Demler O, et al. Prevalence, severity, and comorbidity of 12 month DSM-IV disorders in the National Comorbidity Survey Replication. Arch Gen Psychiatry 2005;62(6):617–27.
3. American Psychiatric Association. Diagnostic and statistical manual of mental disorders. 4th edition. Washington, DC: American Psychiatric Association; 1994.
4. Heimberg RG, Holt CS, Schneier FR, et al. The issues of subtypes in the diagnosis of social phobia. J Anxiety Disord 1993;7(3):249–69.

5. Schneier FR, Heckelman LR, Garfinkel R, et al. Functional impairment in social phobia. J Clin Psychiatry 1994;55(8):322–31.
6. Stein MB, Kean YM. Disability and quality of life in social phobia: epidemiologic findings. Am J Psychiatry 2000;157(10):1606–13.
7. Wittchen HU, Fuetsch M, Sonntag H, et al. Disability and quality of life in pure and comorbid social phobia: findings from a controlled study. Eur Psychiatry 1999;14(3):118–31.
8. Blackmore MA, Erwin BA, Heimberg RG, et al. Social anxiety disorder and specific phobias. In: Gelder M, Andreasen N, Lopez-Ibor J, Geddes J, editors. The new Oxford textbook of psychiatry. 2nd edition. London: Oxford University Press; 2009. p. 739–50.
9. Blanco C, Schneier FR, Schmidt A, et al. Pharmacological treatment of social anxiety disorder: a meta-analysis. Depress Anxiety 2003;18(1):29–40.
10. Ledley DR, Heimberg RG. Social anxiety disorder. In: Antony MM, Ledley DR, Heimberg RG, editors. Improving outcomes and preventing relapse in cognitive-behavioral therapy. New York: Guilford Press; 2005. p. 38–76.
11. Davidson JR, Foa EB, Huppert JD, et al. Fluoxetine, comprehensive cognitive behavioral therapy, and placebo in generalized social phobia. Arch Gen Psychiatry 2004;61(10):1005–13.
12. Clark DM, Ehlers A, McManus F, et al. Cognitive therapy vs. fluoxetine in generalized social phobia: a randomized placebo-controlled trial. J Consult Clin Psychol 2003;71(6):1058–67.
13. Kobak KA, Greist JH, Jefferson JW, et al. Fluoxetine in social phobia: a double-blind, placebo-controlled pilot study. J Clin Psychopharmacol 2002;22(3):257–62.
14. Davidson JRT, Potts N, Richichi E, et al. Treatment of social phobia with clonazepam and placebo. J Clin Psychopharmacol 1993;13(6):423–8.
15. Otto MW, Pollack MH, Gould RA, et al. A comparison of the efficacy of clonazepam and cognitive-behavioral group therapy for the treatment of social phobia. J Anxiety Disord 2000;14(4):345–58.
16. Gerlernter CS, Uhde TW, Cimbolic P, et al. Cognitive-behavioral and pharmacological treatments of social phobia: a controlled study. Arch Gen Psychiatry 1991;48(10):938–45.
17. Connor KM, Davidson JRT, Potts NLS, et al. Discontinuation of clonazepam in the treatment of social phobia. J Clin Psychopharmacol 1998;18(5):373–8.
18. Sartory G. Benzodiazepines and behavioral treatment of phobic anxiety. Behavioural Psychotherapy 1983;11:204–17.
19. Basoglu M, Marks IM, Kilic C, et al. Alprazolam and exposure for panic disorder with agoraphobia: attribution of improvement to medication predicts subsequent relapse. Br J Psychiatry 1994;164(5):652–9.
20. Pande AC, Davidson JRT, Jefferson JW, et al. Treatment of social phobia with gabapentin: a placebo-controlled study. J Clin Psychopharmacol 1999;19(4):341–8.
21. Lader M, Stender K, Burger V, et al. Efficacy and tolerability of escitalopram in 12- and 24-week treatment of social anxiety disorder: randomized, double-blind, placebo-controlled, fixed-dose study. Depress Anxiety 2004;19(4):241–8.
22. Liebowitz MR, Gelenberg AJ, Munjack D. Venlafaxine extended release vs placebo and paroxetine in social anxiety disorder. Arch Gen Psychiatry 2005;62(2):190–8.
23. Stein DJ, Versiani M, Hair T, et al. Efficacy of paroxetine for relapse prevention in social anxiety disorder. Arch Gen Psychiatry 2002;59(12):1111–8.

24. Walker JR, van Ameringen MA, Swinson R, et al. Prevention of relapse in gener-
    alized social phobia: results of a 24-week study in responders to 20 weeks of
    sertraline treatment. J Clin Psychopharmacol 2000;20(6):636–44.
25. Clark DM, Ehlers A, Hackmann A, et al. Cognitive therapy versus exposure and
    applied relaxation in social phobia: a randomized controlled trial. J Consult Clin
    Psychol 2006;74(3):568–78.
26. Ponniah K, Hollon SD. Empirically supported psychological interventions for
    social phobia in adults: a qualitative review of randomized controlled trials.
    Psychol Med 2008;38(1):3–14.
27. Herbert JD, Gaudiano BA, Rheingold AA, et al. Social skills training augments
    the effectiveness of cognitive behavioral group therapy for social anxiety
    disorder. Behav Ther 2005;36(2):125–38.
28. Feske U, Chambless DL. Cognitive behavioral versus exposure only treatment
    for social phobia: a meta-analysis. Behav Ther 1995;26(4):695–720.
29. Powers MB, Sigmarsson SR, Emmelkamp PMG. A meta-analytic review of
    psychological treatments for social anxiety disorder. International Journal of
    Cognitive Therapy 2008;1(2):94–113.
30. Heimberg RG, Becker RE. Cognitive behavioral group therapy for social phobia:
    basic mechanisms and clinical applications. New York: Guilford Press; 2002.
31. Heimberg RG, Dodge CS, Hope DA, et al. Cognitive-behavioral group treatment
    for social phobia: comparison to a credible placebo control. Cognit Ther Res
    1990;14(1):1–23.
32. Heimberg RG, Salzman DG, Holt CS, et al. Cognitive-behavioral group treatment
    for social phobia: effectiveness at five-year follow-up. Cognit Ther Res 1993;
    17(4):325–39.
33. De Mello MF, de Jesus Mari J, Bacaltchuk J, et al. A systematic review of
    research findings on the efficacy of interpersonal therapy for depressive disor-
    ders. Eur Arch Psychiatry Clin Neurosci 2005;255(2):75–82.
34. Markowitz JC. Psychotherapy of dysthymia. Am J Psychiatry 1994;151(8):
    1114–21.
35. Wilfley DE, Welch RR, Stein RI, et al. A randomized comparison of group cogni-
    tive behavior therapy and group interpersonal therapy for the treatment of over-
    weight individuals with binge-eating disorder. Arch Gen Psychiatry 2002;59(8):
    713–21.
36. Lipsitz JD, Markowitz JC, Cherry S, et al. Open trial of interpersonal psycho-
    therapy for the treatment of social phobia. Am J Psychiatry 1999;156(11):
    1814–6.
37. Lipsitz JD, Gur M, Vermes D, et al. A randomized trial of interpersonal therapy
    versus supportive therapy for social anxiety disorder. Depress Anxiety 2008;
    25(6):542–53.
38. Borge FM, Hoffart A, Sexton H, et al. Residential cognitive therapy versus resi-
    dential interpersonal therapy for social phobia: a randomized clinical trial.
    J Anxiety Disord 2008;22(6):991–1010.
39. Zerbe KJ. Unchartered waters: psychodynamic considerations in the diagnosis
    and treatment of social phobia. In: Menninger WW, editor. Fear of humiliation:
    integrated treatment of social phobia and comorbid conditions. Northvale
    (NJ): Jason Aronson; 1997. p. 1–19.
40. Gabbard GO. Psychodynamics of panic disorder and social phobia. Bull Men-
    ninger Clin 1992;56(2 Suppl A):A3–13.
41. Gabbard GO. Anxiety disorders in psychodynamic psychiatry in clinical prac-
    tice. Washington, DC: American Psychiatric Press; 2005.

42. Leichsenring F, Beutel M, Leibing E. Psychodynamic psychotherapy for social phobia: a treatment based on supportive-expressive therapy. Bull Menninger Clin 2007;71(1):56–83.
43. Gould RA, Buckminster S, Pollack MH, et al. Cognitive-behavioral and pharmacological treatment for social phobia: a meta-analysis. Clinical Psychology: Science and Practice 1997;4(4):291–306.
44. Fedoroff IC, Taylor S. Psychological and pharmacological treatments of social phobia: a meta-analysis. J Clin Psychopharmacol 2001;21(3):311–24.
45. Taylor S. Meta-analysis of cognitive-behavioral treatments for social phobia. J Behav Ther Exp Psychiatry 1996;27(1):1–9.
46. Heimberg RG, Liebowitz MR, Hope DA, et al. Cognitive behavioral group therapy vs. phenelzine therapy for social phobia. Arch Gen Psychiatry 1998; 55(12):1133–41.
47. Liebowitz MR, Heimberg RG, Schneier FR, et al. Cognitive-behavioral group therapy versus phenelzine in social phobia: long term outcome. Depress Anxiety 1999;10(3):89–98.
48. Blanco C, Heimberg RG, Schneier FR, et al. A placebo-controlled trial of phenelzine, cognitive behavioral group therapy and their combination for social anxiety disorder [Under review].
49. Blomhoff S, Haug TT, Hellström K, et al. Randomised controlled general practice trial of sertraline, exposure therapy and combined treatment in generalised social phobia. Br J Psychiatry 2001;179(1):23–30.
50. Haug TT, Blomhoff S, Hellström K, et al. Exposure therapy and sertraline in social phobia. 1 year follow up of a randomised controlled trial. Br J Psychiatry 2003; 182(4):312–8.
51. Guastella AJ, Richardson R, Lovibond PF, et al. A randomized controlled trial of D-cycloserine enhancement of exposure therapy for social anxiety disorder. Biol Psychiatry 2008;63(6):544–9.
52. Hofmann SG, Meuret AE, Smits JA, et al. Augmentation of exposure therapy with D-cycloserine for social anxiety disorder. Arch Gen Psychiatry 2006;63(6):298–304.
53. Westra HA, Dozois DJA. Preparing clients for cognitive behavioral therapy: a randomized pilot study of motivational interviewing for anxiety. Cognit Ther Res 2006;30(1):481–08.
54. Miller WR, Rollnick S. Motivational interviewing: preparing people for change. New York: Guilford; 2002.
55. Kabat-Zinn J. Mindfulness-based interventions in context: past, present, and future. Clinical Psychology: Science and Practice 2003;10(2):144–56.
56. Grossman P, Niemann L, Schmidt S, et al. Mindfulness-based stress reduction and health benefits: a meta-analysis. J Psychosom Res 2004;57(1):35–43.
57. Kabat-Zinn J, Massion AO, Kristeller J, et al. Effectiveness of a meditation-based stress reduction program in the treatment of anxiety disorders. Am J Psychiatry 1992;149(7):936–43.
58. Koszycki D, Benger M, Shlik J, et al. Randomized trial of a meditation-based stress reduction program and cognitive behavior therapy in generalized social anxiety disorder. Behav Res Ther 2007;45(10):2518–26.
59. Roemer L, Orsillo SM. An open trial of an acceptance-based behavior therapy for generalized anxiety disorder. Behav Ther 2007;38(1):72–85.
60. Dalrymple KL, Herbert JD. Acceptance and commitment therapy for generalized social anxiety disorder. Behav Modif 2007;31(5):543–68.
61. Ossman WA, Wilson KG, Storaasli RD, et al. A preliminary investigation of the use of acceptance and commitment therapy in a group treatment for social

phobia. International Journal of Pyschology and Pyschological Therapy 2006; 6(3):397–416.

62. Hayes SC, Wilson KG, Gifford EV, et al. Experiential avoidance and behavioral disorders: a functional dimensional approach to diagnosis and treatment. J Consult Clin Psychol 1996;64(6):1152–68.

63. Stein MB, Goldin PR, Sareen J, et al. Increased amygdala activation to angry and contemptuous faces in generalized social phobia. Arch Gen Psychiatry 2002;59(11):1027–34.

64. Furmark T, Tillfors M, Marteinsdottir I, et al. Common changes in cerebral blood flow in patients with social phobia treated with citalopram or cognitive-behavioral therapy. Arch Gen Psychiatry 2002;59(5):425–33.

65. Hofmann SG. Treatment of social phobia: potential mediators and moderators. Clinical Psychology: Science and Practice 2000;7(1):3–16.

66. Hofmann SG. Cognitive mediation of treatment change in social phobia. J Consult Clin Psychol 2004;72(3):392–9.

67. Moscovitch DA, Hofmann SG, Suvak MK, et al. Mediation of changes in anxiety and depression during treatment of social phobia. J Consult Clin Psychol 2005; 73(5):945–52.

68. Edelman RE, Chambless DL. Adherence during sessions and homework in cognitive-behavioral group treatment of social phobia. Behav Res Ther 1995; 33(5):573–7.

69. Leung AW, Heimberg RG. Homework compliance, perceptions of control, and outcome of cognitive-behavioral treatment of social phobia. Behav Res Ther 1996;34(5–6):423–32.

70. Woody SR, Adessky RS. Therapeutic alliance, group cohesion, and homework compliance during cognitive-behavioral group treatment of social phobia. Behav Ther 2002;33(1):5–27.

71. Hayes SA, Hope DA, VanDyke M, et al. Working alliance for clients with social anxiety disorder: relationship with session helpfulness and within-session habituation. Cogn Behav Ther 2007;36(1):34–42.

72. Safren SA, Heimberg RG, Juster HR. Clients' expectancies and their relationship to pretreatment symptomatology and outcome of cognitive-behavioral group treatment for social phobia. J Consult Clin Psychol 1997;65(4):694–8.

73. Chambless DL, Tran GQ, Glass CR. Predictors of response to cognitive-behavioral group therapy for social phobia. J Anxiety Disord 1997;11(3):221–40.

74. Taube-Schiff M, Suvak MK, Antony MM, et al. Group cohesion in cognitive-behavioral group therapy for social phobia. Behav Res Ther 2007;45(4): 687–98.

75. Stopa L, Clark DM. Cognitive processes in social phobia. Behav Res Ther 1993; 31(3):255–67.

76. Schultz LT, Heimberg RG. Attentional focus in social anxiety disorder: potential for interactive processes. Clin Psychol Rev 2008;28(7):1206–21.

77. Coles ME, Heimberg RG. Memory biases in the anxiety disorders: current status. Clin Psychol Rev 2002;22(4):587–627.

78. Brozovich F, Heimberg RG. An analysis of post-event processing in social anxiety disorder. Clin Psychol Rev 2008;28(6):891–903.

79. Papageorgiou C, Wells A. Nature, functions, and beliefs about depressive rumination. In: Papageorgiou C, Wells A, editors. Depressive rumination: nature, theory, and treatment. Hoboken (NJ): Wiley & Sons; 2003. p. 3–20.

80. Spasojevic J, Alloy LB, Abramson LY, et al. Reactive rumination: outcomes, mechanisms, and developmental antecedents. In: Papageorgiou C, Wells A,

editors. Depressive rumination: nature, theory, and treatment. Hoboken (NJ): Wiley & Sons; 2003. p. 43–58.

81. Brown EJ, Juster HR, Heimberg RG, et al. Stressful life events and personality styles: relation to impairment and treatment outcome in patients with social phobia. J Anxiety Disord 1998;12(3):233–51.

82. Watson D, Clark LA, Carey G. Positive and negative affectivity and their relation to anxiety and depressive disorders. J Abnorm Psychol 1988;97(3):346–53.

83. Hughes AA, Heimberg RG, Coles ME, et al. Relations of the factors of the tripartite model of anxiety and depression to types of social anxiety. Behav Res Ther 2006;44(11):1629–41.

84. Clark LA, Watson D. Mood and the mundane: relations between daily life events and self-reported mood. J Pers Soc Psychol 1988;54(2):296–308.

85. Kashdan T. Social anxiety spectrum and diminished positive experiences: theoretical synthesis and meta-analysis. Clin Psychol Rev 2007;27(3):348–65.

86. Grant DM, Beck JG. Attentional biases in social anxiety and dysphoria: does co-morbidity make a difference? J Anxiety Disord 2006;20(4):520–9.

87. Musa C, Lépine JP, Clark DM, et al. Selective attention in social phobia and the moderating effect of a concurrent depressive disorder. Behav Res Ther 2003; 41(9):1043–54.

88. Erwin BA, Heimberg RG, Juster H, et al. Comorbid anxiety and mood disorders among persons with social anxiety disorder. Behav Res Ther 2002;40(1):19–35.

89. Ledley DR, Huppert JD, Foa EB, et al. Impact of depressive symptoms on the treatment of generalized social anxiety disorder. Depress Anxiety 2005;22(4): 161–7.

90. Marom S, Gilboa-Schechtman E, Aderka IM, et al. Impact of depression on treatment effectiveness and gains maintenance in social phobia: a naturalistic study of cognitive behavior group therapy. Depress Anxiety 2009;26(3): 289–300.

91. Dimidjian S, Hollon SD, Dobson KS, et al. Randomized trial of behavioral activation, cognitive therapy, and antidepressant medication in the acute treatment of adults with major depression. J Consult Clin Psychol 2006;74(4):658–70.

92. Herbert JD, Hope DA, Bellack AS. Validity of the distinction between generalized social phobia and avoidant personality disorder. J Abnorm Psychol 1992;101(2): 332–9.

93. Holt CS, Heimberg RG, Hope DA. Avoidant personality disorder and the generalized subtype of social phobia. J Abnorm Psychol 1992;101(2):318–25.

94. Schneier FR, Spitzer RL, Gibbon D, et al. The relationship of social phobia subtypes and avoidant personality disorder. Compr Psychiatry 1991;32(6): 496–502.

95. Turner SM, Beidel DC, Townsley RM. Social phobia: a comparison of specific and generalized subtypes and avoidant personality disorder. J Abnorm Psychol 1992;101(2):326–31.

96. Heimberg RG. Social phobia, avoidant personality disorder, and the multiaxial conceptualization of interpersonal anxiety. In: Salkovskis PM, editor. Trends in cognitive and behavioural therapies. West Sussex: Wiley; 1996. p. 43–61.

97. Chambless DL, Fydrich T, Rodebaugh TL. Generalized social phobia and avoidant personality disorder: meaningful distinction or useless duplication? Depress Anxiety 2008;25(1):8–19.

98. Huppert JD, Strunk DR, Ledley DR, et al. Generalized social anxiety disorder and avoidant personality disorder: structural analysis and treatment outcome. Depress Anxiety 2008;25(5):441–8.

99. Brown EJ, Heimberg RG, Juster HR. Social phobia subtype and avoidant personality disorder: effect on severity of social phobia, impairment, and outcome of cognitive behavioral treatment. Behav Ther 1995;26(3):467–86.

100. Feske U, Perry KJ, Chambless DL, et al. Avoidant personality disorder as a predictor for treatment outcome among generalized social phobics. J Personal Disord 1996;10(2):174–84.

101. Taylor CT, Laposa JM, Alden LE. Is avoidant personality disorder more than just social avoidance? J Personal Disord 2004;18(6):571–94.

102. Barlow DH, Allen LB, Choate ML. Toward a unified treatment for emotional disorders. Behav Ther 2004;35(2):205–30.

103. Norton PJ, Philipp LM. Transdiagnostic approaches to the treatment of anxiety disorders: a quantitative review. psychotherapy theory, research, practice. Training 2008;45(2):214–26.

104. Morris EP, Stewart SH, Ham LS. The relationship between social anxiety disorder and alcohol use disorders: a critical review. Clin Psychol Rev 2005;25(6): 734–60.

105. Buckner JD, Ledley DR, Heimberg RG, et al. Treating comorbid social anxiety and alcohol use disorders: combining motivation enhancement therapy with cognitive-behavioral therapy. Clinical Case Studies 2008;7(3):208–23.

106. Jack MS, Heimberg RG, Mennin DS. Situational panic attacks: impact on social phobia with and without panic disorder. Depress Anxiety 1999;10(3):112–8.

107. Brozovich F, Jørstad-Stein EC, Heimberg R. Panic symptomatology among individuals with social anxiety disorder or generalized anxiety disorder [Poster session 3C: social anxiety, social phobia; abstract 5]. In: 42nd Annual Convention of the Association for Behavioral and Cognitive Therapies. Orlando: November 14–17, 2008.

108. Barrett PM, Rapee RM, Dadds MR, et al. Family enhancement of cognitive style in anxious and aggressive children. J Abnorm Child Psychol 1996;24(2): 187–203.

109. Beesdo K, Bittner A, Pine DS, et al. Incidence of social anxiety disorder and the consistent risk for secondary depression in the first three decades of life. Arch Gen Psychiatry 2007;64(8):903–12.

110. Barrett P, Turner C. Prevention of anxiety symptoms in primary school children: preliminary results from a universal school-based trial. Br J Clin Psychol 2001; 40(4):399–410.

111. Dadds MR, Holland DE, Laurens KR, et al. Early intervention and prevention of anxiety disorders in children: results at 2-year follow-up. J Consult Clin Psychol 1999;67(1):145–50.

112. Liebowitz MR, Heimberg RG, Fresco DM, et al. Social phobia or social anxiety disorder: what's in a name? Arch Gen Psychiatry 2000;57(2):191–2.

113. Schneier FR, Liebowitz MR, Beidel DC, et al. MacArthur data reanalysis for DSM-IV: social phobia. In: Widiger TA, Frances AH, Pincus HA, et al, editors, DSM-IV source book, vol. 4. Washington, DC: American Psychiatric Press; 1998. p. 307–28.

114. Stein MB, Chartier MJ, Hazen AL, et al. A direct interview family study of generalized social phobia. Am J Psychiatry 1998;155(1):90–7.

115. Vriends N, Becker ES, Meyer A, et al. Subtypes of social phobia: are they of any use? J Anxiety Disord 2007;21(1):59–75.

116. Butler G. Exposure as treatment for social phobia: some instructive difficulties. Behav Res Ther 1985;23(6):651–7.

117. Butler G. Issues in the application of cognitive and behavioral strategies to the treatment of social phobia. Clin Psychol Rev 1989;9(1):91–106.
118. Hope DA, Heimberg RG, Juster H, et al. Managing social anxiety: a cognitive-behavioral therapy approach (Client Workbook). New York: Oxford University Press; 2000.
119. Hope DA, Heimberg RG, Turk CL. Therapist guide for managing social anxiety: a cognitive-behavioral therapy approach. New York: Oxford University Press; 2006.
120. Lincoln TM, Rief W, Hahlweg K, et al. Effectiveness of an empirically supported treatment for social phobia in the field. Behav Res Ther 2003;41(11):1251–69.
121. Barlow DH, Levitt JT, Bufka LF. The dissemination of empirically supported treatments: a view to the future. Behav Res Ther 1999;37(S1):S147–62.
122. Gaston JE, Abbott MJ, Rapee RM, et al. Do empirically supported treatments generalize to private practice? A benchmark study of a cognitive-behavioural group treatment programme for social phobia. Br J Clin Psychol 2006;45(1):33–48.
123. McEvoy PM. Effectiveness of cognitive behavioural group therapy for social phobia in a community clinic: a benchmarking study. Behav Res Ther 2007;45(12):3030–40.

Obsessive–compulsive Disorder: Diagnostic and Treatment Issues

Dan J. Stein, MD, PhD[a],*, Damiaan Denys, MD, PhD[b],
Andrew T. Gloster, PhD[c], Eric Hollander, MD[d], James F. Leckman, MD[e],
Scott L. Rauch, MD[f], Katharine A. Phillips, MD[g]

KEYWORDS

- Obsessive-compulsive disorder
- Obsessive-compulsive spectrum • Diagnosis
- Pharmacotherapy • Psychotherapy • Nosology • DSM-V

Obsessive–compulsive (OC) symptoms are common, and obsessive–compulsive disorder (OCD) is a particularly disabling disorder. In the National Comorbidity Study-Replication (NCS-R), lifetime prevalence of OCD was 2.3%.[1] Similar rates are found in several other countries.[2–4] OC symptoms are much more frequent, however; more than 25% of NCS-R respondents reported obsessions or compulsions at some time in their lives. Similar rates were reported recently in a population-based sample in New Zealand.[5] In the NCS-R, OCD was associated with substantial comorbidity with anxiety, mood, substance use, and impulse control disorders. Greater severity of OCD was associated with higher comorbidity and poorer insight and greater role impairment. Indeed, in the World Health Organization (WHO)'s Global Burden of Disease

Several of the authors serve on the DSM-V Workgroup on Anxiety, Obsessive–Compulsive Spectrum, Posttraumatic, and Dissociative Disorders or on the DSM-V Task Force. Nevertheless, the views here do not necessarily represent the views or conclusions of the Workgroup or Taskforce.

[a] Deparment of Psychiatry and Mental Health, University of Cape Town, Cape Town, South Africa
[b] Department of Psychiatry, Academic Medical Center, University of Amsterdam and the Institute for Neuroscience of the Royal Netherlands Academy of Arts and Sciences, Amsterdam, The Netherlands
[c] Institute of Clinical Psychology and Pyschotherapy, Department of Psychology, Technische Universität Dresden, Dresden, Germany
[d] Department of Pyschiatry, Montefiore Medical Center, University Hospital of Albert Einstein College of Medicine, Bronx, NY, USA
[e] Child Study Center, Yale University, New Haven, CT, USA
[f] Department of Psychiatry, Harvard Medical School and McLean Hospital, Belmont, MA, USA
[g] Department of Psychiatry and Human Behavior, Brown University, Providence, RI, USA
* Corresponding author.
E-mail address: dan.stein@uct.ac.za (D.J. Stein).

study, OCD was among the most disabling of all medical disorders.[6] Furthermore, there are substantial financial costs associated with OCD.[7,8]

At the same time, OCD remains underdiagnosed and undertreated. In a 1997 survey of members of the Obsessive–Compulsive Foundation, mean lag time to diagnosis was 17 years.[9] Data from a psychiatric practice research network in the United States found that few patients were treated with recommended psychotherapy.[10] Prescription of benzodiazepines or antipsychotics was common, often in the absence of a serotonin reuptake inhibitor (SRI). European data similarly emphasize that many OCD patients do not receive optimal treatment.[11] Thus, despite important advances in the pharmacologic and psychological treatments for OCD, psychiatric care of OCD remains an area with substantial opportunity for improvement in quality.

In the past 20 to 30 years, much has been learned about the underlying psychobiology of OCD.[12,13] Advances in imaging technology have contributed to understanding the neurocircuitry underlying OCD, and there is a growing appreciation of the way in which particular molecular mechanisms in this circuitry underpin OC symptoms. There is growing understanding of the mechanisms underpinning the pharmacotherapy and psychotherapy of OCD, and there is now also a foundation from which to develop novel approaches to diagnosing and treating this condition.

This article reviews current approaches to diagnosing and treating OCD and considers future developments in this area. It also addresses some issues concerning the relationship between OCD and other anxiety disorders.

TREATMENT OF OBSESSIVE–COMPULSIVE DISORDER
Pharmacotherapy

The anecdotal discovery several decades ago that some patients who had OCD responded to clomipramine, a relatively serotonergic tricyclic antidepressant, was a key step forward in the treatment of this disorder. Subsequent systematic trials demonstrated that clomipramine was more effective than desipramine, a relatively noradrenergic tricyclic antidepressant, and that its benefits were apparent not only in adults but also in children and adolescents with OCD. Selective serotonin reuptake inhibitors (SSRIs) have tolerability advantages compared with the older tricyclics, and when these became available, they soon were studied in OCD, and shown in rigorous randomized controlled trials to be effective and safe. Meta-analyses have confirmed the efficacy of the SSRIs, and current guidelines emphasize the use of this class of agents as a first-line pharmacotherapy.[14,15] For example, a recent meta-analysis found that effect size for SRIs in OCD was 0.91.[16]

The recommended daily dose of SRIs for OCD is perhaps somewhat higher than in depression (ie, clomipramine, 75 to 300 mg; fluvoxamine, 50 to 300 mg; paroxetine, 20 to 60 mg; sertraline, 50 to 200 mg; citalopram, 20 to 60 mg, escitalopram, 10 to 20 mg; and fluoxetine, 20 to 60 mg). Indeed, a recent meta-analysis has indicated that higher doses of SSRI pharmacotherapy are more effective than lower-dose treatments in adults who have OCD.[17] Response may be slow and may not occur for several weeks; a treatment period of at least 12 weeks is required to assess response. The optimal time to maintain an individual who has responded to pharmacotherapy on medication is unclear, but after a satisfactory response, patients should be maintained on anti-OCD medication for at least 12 to 18 months before attempting to discontinue medication.[15,18,19]

Despite the efficacy of the SRIs, many patients respond only partially,[20] or fail to reach remission.[21] Switching to a different SRI may be useful. Further, a range of different agents has been studied in the augmentation of SRIs. Dopamine receptor blockers are of particular interest for many reasons, including evidence of dopaminergic involvement in animal models of OCD, genetic overlap in susceptibility to OCD and Tourette's disorder (which responds to these agents), and other evidence from clinical research that the dopamine system mediates OC symptoms[22–24] Furthermore, although the total number of patients entered into augmentation trials is relatively low, the most promising data are those from trials of dopamine blockers, with number needed to treat around 5.5 [25,26]

Psychotherapy

The introduction of the behavioral techniques of exposure and response prevention (ERP), a variation of cognitive-behavioral therapy (CBT), was a key advance in the treatment of OCD.[27] ERP involves systematically exposing a patient to the thoughts, images, situations, or stimuli that elicit the obsessive fear (exposure), while simultaneously helping the patient learn to refrain from engaging in compulsive rituals (response prevention), so that the patient can experience that the anxiety dissipates without engaging in the compulsion. Although effective, ERP is sometimes difficult to implement given the subtle and dynamic nature of the rituals and avoidance. Covert rituals (eg, praying, telling oneself "this is just an exercise," repeatedly asking for/ giving clarification, and counting) are more difficult to detect than overt rituals (eg, washing one's hands, checking the door). To overcome this, therapists are encouraged to conduct a functional analysis to thoroughly understand the relationship between all of the patients' obsessions and compulsions, although this can be somewhat complicated by patient's difficulty reporting accurate symptom covariations.[28] ERP is considered a form of CBT, because the techniques focus on thoughts and behaviors as they occur in the here and now and aim to help the patient learn new behaviors and associations.

ERP has been established as an empirically supported treatment and is considered the first-line psychological treatment approach in OCD. Across 13 studies, the mean effect size for ERP compared with control groups was 1.13, with significantly greater effect sizes for more recent studies.[29] ERP's efficacy has been demonstrated in Western and Eastern settings[30,31] in both individual and group formats,[32] with improvements lasting over 2 years in approximately 75% of the patients.[33] The efficacy of ERP also is supported in children and adolescents, although the literature is smaller than in adults.[34] Early work demonstrating that ERP, like pharmacotherapy with SRIs, reversed functional neuroanatomical abnormalities in OCD,[35] strengthened the hypothesis that it had significant psychobiological effects.

Despite the unequivocal efficacy of ERP when properly executed, room for progress remains. Improvement is needed especially with respect to residual symptoms, patient noncompliance and drop out, and a significant lack of access to professionals trained in ERP. Although such problems are germane to all exposure treatments,[36,37] they can be amplified in OCD. Additional work is needed on approaches to treatment-refractory patients. Preliminary work in this area suggests that some improvements can be made with these patients by further specifying the functionality of the symptoms with subsequent matching to treatment and intensification of some parameters.[38]

Cognitive therapy (CT) also has been shown to influence positively OCD symptoms. The aim of CT is to alter dysfunctional beliefs that maintain the symptomatology.[39] Examples of maintaining beliefs include exaggerated sense of responsibility and self-blame. The evidence base for CT[40] is much smaller than that of ERP, however, and CT trials have been criticized for incorporating exposure elements. As exposure is considered by many to be the necessary active ingredient for successful outcome, questions arise as to whether the cognitive techniques add anything above and beyond ERP. What is clear is that OCD patients suffer from a range of cognitive–affective dysfunctions, all of which can be targeted for psychotherapeutic intervention.

At a very basic level, psychoeducation is an important component of CBT; many patients are relieved to learn that OCD is a common disorder, with relatively well-investigated psychobiology, and often responsive to both psychotherapy and pharmacotherapy. There is also evidence of the value of using self-help platforms (eg, bibliotherapy, Internet-based therapy) to access behavioral therapy.[41]

Combined Treatment

Reviews of OCD management yield the tentative proposal that pharmacotherapy may be more likely than psychotherapy to yield an early response to treatment, while psychotherapy may be more likely than pharmacotherapy to lead to maintained effects even after discontinuation. There are some data to support the role of psychotherapy in maintained response,[42] and expert guidelines sometimes have suggested that the two modalities of treatment be combined, with psychotherapy particularly important before discontinuation of medication.

Relatively few studies however, have compared pharmacotherapy, psychotherapy, and combined treatment in adults with OCD systematically.[30] Most of the studies have been characterized by relatively small samples and short durations, and they have used different designs that limit direct comparisons. Take together, they have not demonstrated clearly that combined treatment is more effective than any single modality.[43] A few studies, nevertheless, have suggested that CBT may be effective in patients refractory to pharmacotherapy.[44,45] In pediatric OCD, there is some evidence that combined pharmacotherapy and CBT are more effective than either treatment alone.[46]

NEW TREATMENT DEVELOPMENTS

A range of pharmacological agents is receiving ongoing attention. Certain serotonergic receptors such as $5\text{-HT}_{1B/D}$ may play a particularly important role in OCD symptoms, and agents that act at multiple monoamine receptors, including different serotonin subreceptors, may prove useful.[47] The glutamate system likely is involved in mediation of OCD symptoms, and there are preliminary data that riluzole, which acts as a glutamate antagonist, is effective in some patients who have treatment-refractory OCD.[48,49] To date, there have been no controlled studies of riluzole, and the potential hepatoxicity of this agent is a concern. There is also growing interest in the use of nonmedication somatic treatments, such as transcranial magnetic stimulation and deep brain stimulation for treatment-refractory OCD.[50–52] Of note, while still experimental, substantial encouraging data have accrued,[53] leading to a humanitarian device exemption from the FDA with regard to deep brain stimulation for OCD.

Acceptance and commitment therapy (ACT), a variation of CBT, recently has been applied to OCD. ACT aims to help patients learn to distance themselves from their thoughts and not to treat them as literal, while decreasing experiential avoidance in the service of simultaneously increasing contact with their personal values. As applied to OCD, patients increase their willingness to experience obsessions while letting go of the struggle with their compulsions. A study of four patients using a multiple baseline across participants research design achieved clinically significant change in all four patients that were maintained at 3-month follow-up.[54] Although promising, these results must be interpreted cautiously until larger studies replicate the findings.

Within CBT, techniques have also been refined to target OCD subtypes and spectrum disorders. The introduction of adapted CBT treatments for hoarding and rigorous attention to the value of habit reversal for the management of tics in Tourette's disorder are particularly promising developments.[55,56] The development of motivational interventions for patients who are reluctant to try pharmacotherapy or CBT is promising.[57]

There is an exciting emerging set of studies on the combined use of D-cycloserine, a partial n-methyl-d-aspartate (NMDA) agonist, and CBT. Animal studies have indicated that D-cycloserine is able to facilitate extinction of fear conditioning, and clinical studies in simple and social phobia have found that D-cycloserine significantly enhances the effects of CBT in these populations.[58,59] Though there have been some encouraging findings using this strategy for OCD,[60] the results have been inconsistent overall, and the approach remains experimental, requiring further research.

UNDERLYING MECHANISMS

Research on the management of OCD has given impetus to, and intersected closely with, research on the underlying mechanisms of OCD. A good deal has been learned about the underlying neurocircuitry of OCD, and about the relevant molecular mechanisms that operate in those neurocircuits. Furthermore, there long has been interest in exploring how pharmacotherapy and psychotherapy are able to normalize the relevant functional neuroanatomy and molecular mechanisms.[61]

Evidence that OCD is mediated by specific neuronal circuits dates back to early case reports of OC symptoms in patients with particular neurological lesions.[62] Conversely, a range of neuropsychiatric and neuropsychological clinical research has documented such phenomena as increased neurological soft signs, and particular disruptions on neuropsychological tasks, pointing to the involvement of discrete circuitry in the mediation of the disorder.[63] The introduction of modern imaging technologies has played a particularly key role in demonstrating that OCD is mediated by orbitofrontal–striatal neurocircuitry.[64–70]

Evidence that particular molecular systems within the orbitofrontal–striatal circuitry are important in OCD dates back to early work demonstrating that clomipramine, a tricyclic antidepressant that acts predominantly on the SRI, was more effective than desipramine, a tricyclic antidepressant that acts predominantly on the norepinephrine reuptake inhibitor. Subsequent work has explored concentrations of monoamine and other neurotransmitter systems, behavioral and endocrine responses to pharmacological challenges, and a range of pharmacotherapeutic interventions. Molecular imaging techniques have provided further insight into the role of a range of different systems in the pathophysiology of OCD.[71] Studies of gene variants have indicated that several candidates may contribute to OCD symptoms,[72] and there is growing interest in particular endophenotypes as susceptibility factors for OCD.[73]

A growing animal literature provides a basis for a translational approach to understanding the psychobiology of OCD. Early work by MacLean indicated that habits were underpinned by the striatum.[74] Subsequent work has explored the neurobiology of behavioral, pharmacological, and genetic models of OCD. Behavioral models include naturally occurring stereotypy and innate motor behaviors (such as grooming) that occur after stress or after a behavioral manipulation. Pharmacologically induced stereotypy includes the quinpirole model, while genetic models include the D1CT-7 transgenic model of comorbid OCD and Tourette's Syndrome (TS), the Hoxb8 model, the SAP90/SAPAP3 model, the 5-HT$_{2C}$ receptor knockout model, and the DAT knock-down model.[47,75]

At a psychological level of analysis, debate continues as to the processes and mechanisms that maintain symptoms in OCD patients and what differentiates them from the many individuals who have OC symptoms without OCD.[76,77] Extensive experimental studies have attempted to identify the relevant psychological processes, including thought suppression,[78] inhibition and facilitation,[79,80] focused information processing,[81] and implicit and explicit appraisals.[82] Ideally, these theories are informed by and inform treatment.[83]

It should be emphasized that advances in OCD management often have relied on clinical intuitions and discoveries, rather than on basic knowledge of underlying mechanisms. Nevertheless, a growing understanding of the underlying psychobiology of OCD heterogeneity,[84–86] of differential effects of therapies on underlying mechanisms,[35,87] and of predictors of response to treatment,[88–90] may contribute to new approaches to treatment in the future. In the interim, some of these data may be useful in considering the optimal classification of OCD.

SIMILARITY TO OTHER ANXIETY DISORDERS

The question of whether OCD is conceptualized best as an anxiety disorder has generated debate.[91–93] The tenth edition of the *International Classification of Disorders* (ICD-10) emphasizes the distinctive nature of OCD, classifying it separately from other anxiety disorders, and some have argued that future iterations of the *Diagnostic and Statistical Manual of Mental Disorders (DSM)* should take a similar approach. On the other hand, there are also strong arguments for the opposing view. A survey asking experts on OCD about contentious issues in the classification of OCD found that 60% agreed that OCD should be removed from the current supraordinate category of anxiety disorders, while 40% disagreed.[94]

From a phenomenological perspective, it can be argued that obsessions increase anxiety, while compulsions are performed to reduce such anxiety. At the same time, there are patients for whom anxiety does not appear to be the main feature of their subjective experience. For example, patients who have symmetry concerns and compulsions may focus instead on the need to feel that things are "just right." Although the characteristic features of such OC symptoms may be distinctive, from a functional perspective it can be argued there may be some similarities with anxiety disorders (insofar as distress may emerge when things are not "just right").

There is also ongoing interest in clarifying the relationship of disorders to one another and in improving diagnostic validity by using neuroscience research.[95] An immediate question is whether findings on the neurocircuitry and neurochemistry of OCD are sufficiently specific and sensitive to differentiate this disorder from others. Although any particular study often is not able to include a broad range of disorders, there does seem to be some specificity to the psychobiology of OCD.[92,96]

One hypothesis is that OCD may be particularly closely related to a range of putative OCD spectrum disorders, such as Tourette's disorder and body dsymorphic disorder.[97–99] Certainly there long has been persuasive evidence of genetic overlap between OCD and Tourette's disorder.[100] At the same time, many of the other putative obsessive-compulsive spectrum disorders (OCSDs) have received relatively little study from an imaging or neurogenetic perspective, and few studies have compared these disorders directly.[99,101]

Questions about how groups should be grouped together in diagnostic classifications should be supplemented by considerations about clinical utility. The construct of an OC spectrum of disorders arguably has been useful in encouraging clinical awareness of a range of underdiagnosed conditions that have notable phenomenological overlap with OCD, and which may respond to pharmacotherapies or psychotherapies, that are useful in the treatment of OCD. From a clinical perspective, it also may be useful to consider the overlaps between the more cognitive OCSDs (eg, BDD, hypochondriasis, hoarding) and those between the more motoric OCSDs (eg, Tourette's, trichotillomania, skin picking).

One potential compromise between the proposal that OCD remain classified with the anxiety disorders versus classified instead in a category of OCSDs, would be to include both OCD and OCSDs within an umbrella of anxiety and OCDs. A potential weakness of this suggestion is that certain OCSDs (eg, Tourette's disorder) do not appear closely related to non-OCD anxiety disorders. On the other hand, such a compromise potentially encourages awareness of both those features of OCD, which overlap with anxiety disorders, and of the construct of a spectrum of OCDs that share features with OCD. Arguably, given the current data, many current nosological debates do not have a perfect solution, one only can aim for more and less optimal ones.[93]

IMPROVING DIAGNOSIS AND DISSEMINATION
Diagnostic Criteria

The diagnostic criteria for OCD have remained relatively unchanged since the publication of the *DSM-III* more than 25 years ago. Obsessions were defined there as intrusive thoughts, images, or impulses that led to an increase in anxiety or distress. In contrast, compulsions were described as repetitive behaviors that were performed in response to an obsession or according to rigidly applied rules, and which aimed to prevent or reduce distress.

The *DSM-IV* field trials examined three issues:[102]

First, the requirement that symptoms be viewed as excessive or unreasonable
Second, the presence of mental compulsions
Third, the *ICD-10* subcategories (eg, predominantly obsessive versus predominantly compulsive)

The field trial indicated that most patients were uncertain whether their symptoms were excessive or unreasonable, and the authors therefore argued that the requirement for insight should be de-emphasized. The field trial also found that most patients had both behavioral and mental compulsions, and the authors therefore proposed that mental rituals should be included in the definition of compulsions. The results on the *ICD-10* subcategories were equivocal, and so no recommendation was made to include these in *DSM-IV*.

There remain several concerns about the *DSM-IV* definitions of obsessions and compulsions (**Box 1**). First, the term impulse in the criteria is possibly confusing, insofar as impulsive symptoms are characteristic of the impulse control disorders. It might be useful to replace the term impulse with urge. Second, although it is certainly important to differentiate OCD obsessions from worries about real-life problems, this component of the definition is confusing, insofar as it is also important to differentiate obsessions from a whole range of other symptoms. It might be useful to instead include this concept in the criterion referring to other axis I disorders, noting that the content of the obsessions or compulsions is not restricted to worries in the presence of generalized anxiety disorder (GAD).

Another issue is that the definition of compulsion, unlike that of obsession, does not refer to or specify different forms of avoidance. It might complement the definition of

---

Box 1
DSM-IV-TR diagnostic criteria for 300.3 obsessive–compulsive disorder

Either obsessions or compulsions

Obsessions as defined by:

> Recurrent and persistent thoughts, impulses, or images that are experienced, at some time during the disturbance, as intrusive and inappropriate and that cause marked anxiety or distress

> The thoughts, impulses, or images are not simply excessive worries about real-life problems

> The person attempts to ignore or suppress such thoughts, impulses, or images, or to neutralize them with some other thought or action

> The person recognizes that the obsessional thoughts, impulses, or images are a product of his or her own mind (not imposed from without as in thought insertion)

Compulsions as defined by:

> Repetitive behaviors (eg, hand washing, ordering, checking) or mental acts (eg, praying, counting, repeating words silently) that the person feels driven to perform in response to an obsession, or according to rules that must be applied rigidly

> The behaviors or mental acts are aimed at preventing or reducing distress or preventing some dreaded event or situation; however, these behaviors or mental acts either are not connected in a realistic way with what they are designed to neutralize or prevent or are clearly excessive

At some point during the course of the disorder, the person has recognized that the obsessions or compulsions are excessive or unreasonable. This does not apply to children.

The obsessions or compulsions cause marked distress, are time-consuming (take more than 1 hour a day), or significantly interfere with the person 's normal routine, occupational (or academic) functioning, or usual social activities or relationships.

If another axis 1 disorder is present, the content of the obsessions or compulsions is not restricted to it (eg, preoccupation with food in the presence of an eating disorder; hair pulling in the presence of trichotillomania; concern with appearance in the presence of body dysmorphic disorder; preoccupation with drugs in the presence of a substance use disorder; preoccupation with having a serious illness in the presence of hypochondriasis; preoccupation with sexual urges or fantasies in the presence of a paraphilia; or guilty ruminations in the presence of major depressive disorder).

The disturbance is not caused by the direct physiological effects of a substance (eg, a drug of abuse, a medication) or a general medical condition.

Specify if:
With poor insight: if, for most of the time during the current episode, the person does not recognize that the obsessions and compulsions are excessive or unreasonable

International Classification of Disorders-10 diagnostic criteria for F42 obsessive–compulsive disorder

Either obsessions or compulsions (or both) present on most days for a period of at least 2 weeks

Obsessions (thoughts, ideas or images) and compulsions (acts) share the following features, all of which must be present:

> They are acknowledged as originating in the mind of the patient, and are not imposed by outside persons or influences.

> They are repetitive and unpleasant, and at least one obsession or compulsion must be present that is acknowledged as excessive or unreasonable.

> The subject tries to resist them (but if very long-standing, resistance to some obsessions or compulsions may be minimal). At least one obsession or compulsion must be present that is resisted unsuccessfully.

Performing the obsessive thought or compulsive act is not in itself pleasurable. This should be distinguished from the temporary relief of tension or anxiety.

The obsessions or compulsions cause distress or interfere with the subject's social or individual functioning, usually by wasting time.

Most commonly used exclusion criteria: not caused by other mental disorders, such as schizophrenia and related disorders (F2), or mood (affective) disorders (F3).

The diagnosis may be specified by the following four character codes:

F42.0—predominantly obsessional thoughts and ruminations

F42.1—predominantly compulsive acts

F42.2—mixed obsessional thoughts and acts

F42.8—other obsessive compulsive disorders

F42.9—obsessive–compulsive disorder, unspecified

compulsion if a note were added that, "the person actively avoids certain persons, places, or objects, because they fear that these situations will prompt the obsessive thoughts to occur." Although *DSM-IV* criteria emphasize that obsessions lead to anxiety, while compulsions act to neutralize distress, compulsions can result in increased anxiety and distress.

There is also a question as to whether the criterion that pertains to the person's recognition that the obsessions or compulsions are excessive or unreasonable should be deleted. These terms are not defined or operationalized, and it is unclear how clinicians and researchers interpret them. Presumably this criterion pertains to insight—that patients recognize that they spend too much time on their obsessions or compulsions (ie, they are excessive), or recognizes that their underlying beliefs are not actually true, or both. Studies have shown, however, that some patients with OCD have poor insight, and about 2% completely lack insight, in the sense that the belief underlying their obsession is delusional (eg, having complete conviction that if they do not check the stove over and over again, the house truly will burn down).[103,104] Technically speaking, according to *DSM-IV*, such delusional patients would receive a diagnosis of delusional disorder, not OCD. It is likely, however, that OCD is characterized by a spectrum of insight, including delusional beliefs, and that patients who have delusional disorder do not have a disorder that is distinct from OCD.[99] Thus, a consideration for *DSM-V* is whether criterion B should be deleted from OCD and OCD's delusional variant eliminated from the psychosis section of *DSM*. If this change is made, OCD's poor insight specifier could be expanded to include not only poor insight but a broader range of insight options, such as good, poor, and absent insight (ie, delusional thinking). Alternatively, if *DSM-V* adopts a dimensional approach to assessing delusionality/insight, such a dimension could be applied to OCD, replacing these categorical specifiers.

The clinical significance criterion[105] is under active debate across a range of different disorders. The current criterion refers to distress, to a duration of 1 hour or more a day spent on obsessions or compulsions, and to impairment in functioning in different domains. A first objection is that in medical disorders, a disease entity can and should be defined in terms of its core symptomatology or underlying pathophysiology, rather than in terms of its functional consequences. A cancer can and should be diagnosed, even if it is so early in its course that it is not yet causing distress and impairment. Many of the characteristic symptoms of psychiatric disorders (eg, the sadness of depression, the worries of GAD), however, are present in the same form, as part of everyday life, in many in the general population. Conversely, associated distress (or other similar emotions) is a characteristic feature of many psychiatric disorders, and so should be included in diagnostic criteria where appropriate. Furthermore, the etiology and psychophysiology of most psychiatric disorders are understood insufficiently to be useful for diagnostic purposes. Thus, the clinical significance criterion serves as a clinically useful cut point, one that although not able to cut nature at her joints, is helpful in differentiating disorder from normalcy, and in considering intervention.

A second objection to the clinical criterion might be that different individuals may have different thresholds for experiencing subjective distress and for displaying objective impairment in functioning. Thus, a more emotionally demonstrative person may voice distress in response to milder symptoms. A more resilient person may not display impairment in functioning despite suffering from severe symptoms. The functional impact of a particular level of symptoms also may differ depending upon the level of demand required by the person's occupation, or the amount of available social or financial support. Clinical judgment is therefore crucial in delineating the cut points of clinically relevant distress and impairment.

A 1-hour cut point for the time taken by OC symptoms seems somewhat arbitrary. At the same time, the authors are not aware of data that indicate that a lower or higher level allows greater diagnostic validity, or has higher clinical utility. The authors, however, would suggest that in assessing the time consumed by OCD symptomatology, the clinician also includes an assessment of avoidance (eg, a person who is obsessed about contamination may avoid important activities so he/she does not come into contact with contaminated objects).

It is important to note, however, that even patients who have subclinical OCD may have significant impairment in functioning. In a recent study, Denys and colleagues compared subjects with obsessions and compulsions, who did not meet all criteria for OCD (subthreshold disorders) with subjects who had full-blown OCD and with subjects without obsessions or compulsions. Data were derived from the Netherlands Mental Health Survey and Incidence Study (NEMESIS), a large representative sample of the general Dutch population (N=7076). Using the Composite International Diagnostic Interview (CIDI 1.1), three groups were distinguished: subjects without lifetime obsessions or compulsions (94.2%), subjects who had subthreshold OCD (4.9%) and subjects who had full-blown OCD according to *DSM-III-R* (0.9%). These three groups were compared on various items, such as psychological vulnerability, health and functional status, psychiatric comorbidity, and seeking treatment. Subthreshold subjects scored equally to OCD subjects on most items measured. Thus, there was little difference between subthreshold cases and OCD subjects in health, functional status, psychological vulnerability, and psychiatric comorbidity. OCD subjects and subthreshold subjects scored worse on most of these items when compared with controls without obsessions or compulsions. Similar results have been reported recently in New Zealand.[5]

Symptom Dimensions

Clinicians long have noted that although the form of obsessions and compulsions in OCD may be similar, the content can vary. Early work contrasted washers and checkers, with some findings of subtle clinical differences, but no clear evidence that these comprised two separate subtypes of OCD. Baer undertook a factor analysis of OCD symptoms and found that there were three symptom factors: symmetry/

hoarding, contamination/cleaning, and pure obsessions.[106] Of note, only the first factor was related to a lifetime history of tics, suggesting that this particular factor was associated with unique clinical and perhaps psychobiological features.

Many subsequent factor and cluster analyses subsequently have been published. In a recent meta-analysis, Bloch and colleagues included 21 studies with over 5000 participants.[107] They generated four factors:

1. symmetry obsessions and repeating, ordering, and counting compulsions
2. forbidden thoughts: aggression, sexual, religious, and somatic obsessions and checking compulsions
3. cleaning: cleaning and contamination
4. hoarding: hoarding obsessions and compulsions

Such symptom dimensions can be assessed with the Dimensional Yale-Brown Obsessive-Compulsive Scale (Y-BOCS).[108]

It has been suggested that a dimensional approach is particularly valuable for genetic studies.[109] An early family study suggested that symmetry and ordering symptoms had a significant genetic component.[110] In the OCD Collaborative Genetics Study, significant sibling–sibling associations were found for four of five factors, with hoarding and taboo thoughts the most robustly familial.[111] At the same time, heritability for OC symptoms in general may be greater than that for any particular symptom dimensions. In multigenerational families with OCD and hoarding, OC symptoms had higher heritability than hoarding.[112] In a population-based twin study, all symptom dimensions shared variation with a latent common factor (ie, OC behavior). Variation in this common factor was explained by both genes (36%) and environmental factors (64%), and only the contamination dimension was influenced by specific genes and seemed relatively independent.[113] Several genetic studies have found links between candidate genes or chromosomal regions and symptom dimensions, particularly hoarding, although again data have not always been consistent.[114–117] Taken together, these various studies support the potential value of assessing symptom dimensions, but also call for work to replicate and elucidate fully the findings.

There is some additional evidence that different symptom dimensions have a somewhat different psychobiology. Functional imaging studies suggest, for example, that exposure of OCD patients to symptoms from different dimensions results in the engagement of different neural circuits.[118] It may argued, however, that this simply reflects the fact that different parts of the brain are responsible for processing different kinds of material, rather than a difference in the underlying pathogenesis of OCD. Indeed, although larger samples are needed, structural imaging findings show a larger relationship of anatomical changes to OCD severity than to particular symptom dimensions.[119] Nevertheless, treatment studies suggest that OCD patients who have certain symptoms dimensions, such as hoarding/symmetry, may not respond as robustly to treatment with SSRIs.[120,121] This is consistent with a range of basic research, suggesting that hoarding is mediated by distinct (perhaps more dopaminergic) neurocircuitry.[122,123]

Given these data, there is an argument that it may be appropriate to document the presence of prominent symptom dimensions through the use of specifiers (eg, OCD with prominent contamination and cleaning compulsions). If a decision is made to use OC symptom dimension specifiers in DSM-V, then it will be crucial to decide which ones should be included. Leading candidates are contamination/cleaning, exactness/symmetry and ordering, harm and forbidden thoughts/related compulsions, and hoarding. In addition, if these specifiers are used, then several practical issues will need to be addressed, including addition of text to describe precisely each of the symptom dimensions, and whether to include a severity rating scale.

The question has been raised of whether hoarding should, in addition to being a dimensional specifier for OCD, also be considered as a separate diagnosis. First, hoarding may not be performed in response to an obsessional thought or be done in a compulsive way. A recent population-based study found that nearly 5% of the population had prominent hoarding symptoms, but none of these individuals met criteria for OCD.[124] When hoarders with and without OCD are compared, those with comorbid OCD may have a unique clinical profile, with a more severe and disabling form of the disorder.[125] Second, although not all data are consistent, hoarding may be associated with specific neurocircuitry[126–128] and neurogenetic correlates. Furthermore, hoarding may have specific treatment implications, perhaps responding less well to SSRIs and dropping out earlier during CBT.[129] At the same time, the literature on patients with hoarding who do not meet OCD criteria is sparse, and neurobiological and treatment research is an early stage.

Dimensions other than symptom dimensions also may be relevant to the nosology of OCD. The severity of anxiety and of mood symptoms certainly forms an important part of patient evaluation. Across the anxiety disorders, it is also relevant to consider the extent to which there are avoidant symptoms; some of the disability associated with OCD is because of avoidant behaviors, rather than obsessions and compulsions per se.

Other Subtyping

The heterogeneity of OCD may be useful in explaining variations between individuals in clinical research studies (eg, of imaging) and in treatment trials. In addition to symptom dimensions, several other subtypes of OCD have received significant attention[130] and may contribute to enhancing diagnostic validity and clinical utility when assessing and treating patients who have OCD.

Obsessive–compulsive disorder with tics

Although the exact rate of tics varies from study to study, it is clear that subjects who have OCD, and their first degree relatives, have an increased vulnerability to tic disorders. There is a growing literature on the psychobiology of tics, and there is some evidence that within particular families, similar neurocircuitry is involved in the production of either OCD or tics in different individuals.[131] There is ongoing investigation of the relevant genes that contribute to comorbid tics in OCD.[132,133] In the interim, there is some evidence of a differential response to treatment with SRIs in both adult and pediatric OCD patients with and without tics.[24,134]

Obsessive–compulsive disorder with early onset

Several studies have indicated that OCD patients with early onset have particular characteristics, including a greater preponderance among males, greater symptom severity, and greater familiality.[135] There is some overlap with the category of OCD with tics, as early onset OCD also is more likely to be characterized by comorbid tics. Imaging studies again have found that OCD with early onset is characterized by distinctive features.[136] Studies use somewhat different criteria to determine the cut point of early onset OCD. Notably, long-term outcome in early onset OCD is not necessarily poor.[137]

Obsessive–compulsive disorder with poor insight

As discussed previously, *DSM-IV* allows the diagnosis of an OCD subtype with poor insight. Nevertheless, there are relatively few studies demonstrating that such patients have differentiating clinical or psychobiological characteristics,[138,139] and those data that do exist suggest that they may not respond any differently to treatment.[140] Nevertheless, it is possible that insight is conceptualized best as a dimensional rather than categorical characteristic of OCD, and that more rigorous description of this dimension would enhance diagnostic validity and clinical utility.

Obsessive–compulsive disorder with evidence of streptococcal infection

Seminal studies by Swedo and colleagues suggested that in at least some patients, infection with *Streptococcus* is followed by acute onset of OC symptoms or tics.[141] This subgroup of patients may have specific neurobiological characteristics (eg, increased striatal volume) and may respond to immunological therapies.[142] There is also preliminary evidence of an association between *Streptococcus* and some putative OC spectrum disorders.[143] Much of the relevant research, however, has been done by only a few groups.

In summary, currently, there is perhaps most evidence for the diagnostic validity and clinical utility of identifying several subtypes of OCD: with/without tics (this may be especially useful because of treatment implications) and perhaps with/without early onset. There is, however, some overlap between these particular subtypes. Awareness of their existence would encourage clinicians to assess comorbid tics, and to include a developmental perspective in their evaluation.

Other Issues

As noted at the start of this article, there is significant room for improving awareness of OCD and appropriate treatment. Given that many patients have onset in childhood, there is a particular need to encourage awareness of OCD in youth. SSRIs have proven to be an important advance in the treatment of OCD, but further work is needed for managing treatment-refractory patients. CBT also has been a key development, but access to well-trained practitioners remains a problem in many areas. There have been ongoing advances in the understanding of the psychobiology of OCD, and it is timely to consider the implications of these data for the optimal diagnostic criteria and subtyping of OCD. An improved nosology also may be useful in encouraging appropriate diagnosis and treatment of OCD and OC spectrum disorders.

REFERENCES

1. Ruscio AM, Stein DJ, Chiu WT, et al. The epidemiology of obsessive–compulsive disorder in the National Comorbidity Survey replication. Mol Psychiatry 2008 Aug 26 [Epub ahead of print].
2. Weissman MM, Bland RC, Canino GJ, et al. The cross-national epidemiology of obsessive– compulsive disorder. J Clin Psychiatry 1994;55:5–10.
3. Fontenelle LF, Mendlowicz MV, Versiani M. The descriptive epidemiology of obsessive-compulsive disorder. Prog Neuropsychopharmacol Biol Psychiatry 2006;30:327–37.
4. Wittchen HU, Jacobi F. Size and burden of mental disorders in Europe—a critical review and appraisal of 27 studies. Eur Neuropsychopharmacol 2005;15: 357–76.

5. Fullana MA, Mataix-Cols D, Caspi A, et al. Obsessions and compulsions in the community: prevalence, interference, help-seeking, developmental stability, and co-occurring psychiatric conditions. Am J Psychiatry 2009;166:329–36.

6. Murray CJL, Lopez AD. In: Global burden of disease: a comprehensive assessment of mortality and morbidity from diseases, injuries, and risk factors in 1990 and projected to 2020, vol 1. Harvard (MA): World Health Organization; 1996.

7. Dupont RL, Rice DP, Shiraki S, et al. Economic costs of obsessive–compulsive disorder. Med Interface 1995;8:102–9.

8. Leon AC, Portera L, Weissman MM. The social costs of anxiety disorders. Br J Psychiatry 1995;166:19–22.

9. Hollander E, Stein DJ, Broatch J, et al. A pharmacoeconomic and quality-of-life study of obsessive–compulsive disorder. CNS Spectr 1997;2:16–25.

10. Blanco C, Olfson M, Stein DJ, et al. Treatment of obsessive–compulsive disorder by US psychiatrists. J Clin Psychiatry 2006;67:946–51.

11. Denys D, Van Megen H, Westenberg H. The adequacy of pharmacotherapy in outpatients with obsessive–compulsive disorder. Int Clin Psychopharmacol 2002;17(3):109–14.

12. Graybiel AM, Rauch SL. Toward a neurobiology of obsessive–compulsive disorder. Neuron 2000;28:343–7.

13. Stein DJ, Fineberg N. Obsessive–compulsive disorder. Oxford (UK): Oxford University Press; 2007.

14. Stein DJ, Ipser JC, Baldwin DS, et al. Treatment of obsessive–compulsive disorder. CNS Spectr 2007;12:28–35.

15. Koran LM, Hanna GL, Hollander E, et al. Practice guideline for the treatment of patients with obsessive–compulsive disorder. Am J Psychiatry 2007;164:5–53.

16. Eddy KT, Dutra L, Bradley R, et al. A multidimensional meta-analysis of psychotherapy and pharmacotherapy for obsessive–compulsive disorder. Clin Psychol Rev 2004;24:1011–30.

17. Bloch MH, McGuire JEA. Meta-analysis of the dose–response relationship of SSRI in obsessive–compulsive disorder. Mol Psychiatry 2009 May 26 [Epub ahead of print].

18. Baldwin DS, Anderson IM, Nutt DJ, et al. Evidence-based guidelines for the pharmacological treatment of anxiety disorders: recommendations from the British Association for Psychopharmacology. J Psychopharmacol 2005;19:567–96.

19. Zohar J, Hollander E, Stein DJ, et al. Consensus statement. CNS Spectr 2007;12(2 Suppl 3):59–63.

20. Tolin DE, Abramowitz JS, Diefenbach GJ. Defining response in clinical trials for obsessive-compulsive disorder: a signal detection analysis of the Yale-Brown obsessive–compulsive scale. J Clin Psychiatry 2005;66:1549–57.

21. Simpson HB, Huppert JD, Petkova E, et al. Response versus remission in obsessive–compulsive disorder. J Clin Psychiatry 2006;67:269–76.

22. Stein DJ. Seminar on obsessive–compulsive disorder. Lancet 2002;360:397–405.

23. Denys D, Zohar J, Westenberg HG. The role of dopamine in obsessive–compulsive disorder: preclinical and clinical evidence. J Clin Psychiatry 2004; 65:11–7.

24. March JS, Franklin ME, Leonard H, et al. Tics moderate treatment outcome with sertraline but not cognitive–behavior therapy in pediatric obsessive–compulsive disorder. Biol Psychiatry 2007;61:344–7.

25. Ipser JC, Carey P, Dhansay Y, et al. Pharmacotherapy augmentation strategies in treatment-resistant anxiety disorders. Cochrane Database Syst Rev 2006: CD005473.

26. Bloch MH, Landeros-Weisenberger A, Kelmendi B, et al. A systematic review: antipsychotic augmentation with treatment refractory obsessive–compulsive disorder. Mol Psychiatry 2006;11:622–32.
27. Meyer V, Levy R. Modification of behavior in obsessive–compulsive disorders. In: Adams IHE, Unikel P, editors. Issues and trends in behavior therapy. Springfield (IL): Charles C Thomas; 1973.
28. Gloster AT, Richard DC, Himle J, et al. Accuracy of retrospective memory and covariation estimation in patients with obsessive-compulsive disorder. Behav Res Ther 2008;46:642–55.
29. Rosa-Alcázar AI, Sánchez-Meca J, Gómez-Conesa A, et al. Psychological treatment of obsessive–compulsive disorder: a meta-analysis. Clin Psychol Rev 2008;28:1310–25.
30. Foa EB, Liebowitz MR, Kozak MJ, et al. Randomized, placebo-controlled trial of exposure and ritual prevention, clomipramine, and their combination in the treatment of obsessive–compulsive disorder. Am J Psychiatry 2005;162:151–61.
31. Nakatani E, Nakagawa A, Nakao T, et al. A randomized controlled trial of Japanese patients with obsessive–compulsive disorder: effectiveness of behavior therapy and fluvoxamine. Psychother Psychosom 2005;74:269–76.
32. McLean PD, Whittal ML, Söchting I, et al. Cognitive versus behavior therapy in the group treatment of obsessive–compulsive disorder. J Consult Clin Psychol 2001;69:205–14.
33. Foa EB, Kozak MJ. Psychological treatments for obsessive compulsive disorder. In: Mavissakalian MR, Prien RP, editors. Long-term treatments of anxiety disorders. Washington, DC: American Psychiatric Press; 1996.
34. March JS, Franklin ME, Nelson A, et al. Cognitive–behavioral psychotherapy for pediatric obsessive–compulsive disorder. J Clin Child Psychol 2001;30: 8–18.
35. Brody AL, Saxena S, Schwartz JM, et al. FDG-PET predictors of response to behavioral therapy and pharmacotherapy in obsessive–compulsive disorder. Psychiatry Res 1998;84:1–6.
36. Hembree EA, Cahill SP. Obstacles to successful implementation of exposure therapy. In: Richard DCS, Lauterbach D, editors. Handbook of exposure therapies. Burlington (MA): Academic Press; 2007.
37. Richard DCS, Gloster AT. Exposure therapy has a public relations problem: a dearth of litigation amid a wealth of concern. In: Richard DCS, Lauterbach D, editors. Handbook of exposure therapies. Burlington (MA): Academic Press; 2007.
38. VanDyke MM, Pollard CA. Treatment of refractory obsessive–compulsive disorder: the St. Louis model. Cogn Behav Pract 2005;12:30–9.
39. Salkovskis PM. Obsessional compulsive problems: a cognitive–behavioral analysis. Behav Res Ther 1985;23:571–83.
40. Wilson KA, Chambless DL. Cognitive therapy for obsessive–compulsive disorder. Behav Res Ther 2005;43:1645–54.
41. Tolin DF, Hannan S, Maltby N, et al. A randomized controlled trial of self-directed versus therapist-directed cognitive–behavioral therapy for obsessive–compulsive disorder patients with prior medication trials. Behav Ther 2007;38:179–91.
42. Simpson HB, Liebowitz MR, Foa EB, et al. Post-treatment effects of exposure therapy and clomipramine in obsessive-compulsive disorder. Depress Anxiety 2004;19:225–33.
43. Kuzma JM, Black DW. Integrating pharmacotherapy and psychotherapy in the management of anxiety disorders. Curr Psychiatry Rep 2004;6:268–73.

44. Simpson HB, Foa EB, Liebowitz MR, et al. A randomized, controlled trial of cognitive–behavioral therapy for augmenting pharmacotherapy in obsessive–compulsive disorder. Am J Psychiatry 2008;165:621–30.

45. Tolin DF, Maltby N, Diefenbach GJ, et al. Cognitive–behavioral therapy for medication nonresponders with obsessive–compulsive disorder: a wait list-controlled open trial. J Clin Psychiatry 2004;65:922–31.

46. March JS, Foa E, Gammon P, et al. Cognitive–behavior therapy, sertraline, and their combination for children and adolescents with obsessive–compulsive disorder—the Pediatric OCD Treatment Study (POTS) randomized controlled trial. JAMA 2004;292:1969–76.

47. Joel D, Stein J, Schreiber R. Animal models of obsessive–compulsive disorder: from bench to bedside via endophenotypes and biomarkers. In: Robert AM, Franco B, editors. Animal and translational models for CNS drug discovery. San Diego (CA): Academic Press; 2008. p. 133–64.

48. Pittenger C, Kelmendi B, Wasylink S, et al. Riluzole augmentation in treatment-refractory obsessive–compulsive disorder—a series of 13 cases, with long-term follow-up. J Clin Psychopharmacol 2008;28:363–7.

49. Grant P, Lougee L, Hirschtritt M, et al. An open-label trial of riluzole, a glutamate antagonist, in children with treatment-resistant obsessive–compulsive disorder. J Child Adolesc Psychopharmacol 2007;17:761–7.

50. Cosgrove GR. Deep brain stimulation and psychosurgery. J Neurosurg 2004; 101:574–5.

51. Burdick A, Goodman WK, Foote KD. Deep brain stimulation for refractory obsessive–compulsive disorder. Front Biosci 2009;14:1880–90.

52. Mantovani A, Lisanby SH, Pieraccini F, et al. Repetitive transcranial magnetic stimulation (rTMS) in the treatment of obsessive–compulsive disorder (OCD) and Tourette 's syndrome (TS). Int J Neuropsychopharmacol 2006;9:95–100.

53. Greenberg BD, Gabriels LA, Malone DA Jr, et al. Deep brain stimulation of the ventral internal capsule/ventral striatum for obsessive-compulsive disorder: worldwide experience. Mol Psychiatry, in press.

54. Twohig MP, Hayes SC, Masuda A. Increasing willingness to experience obsessions: acceptance and commitment therapy as a treatment for obsessive-compulsive disorder. Behav Ther 2006;37:3–13.

55. Himle MB, Woods DW, Piacentini JC, et al. Brief review of habit reversal training for Tourette syndrome. J Child Neurol 2006;21:719–25.

56. Tolin DF, Frost RO, Steketee G. An open trial of cognitive–behavioral therapy for compulsive hoarding. Behav Res Ther 2007a;45:1461–70.

57. Maltby N, Tolin DF. A brief motivational intervention for treatment-refusing OCD patients. Cogn Behav Ther 2005;34:176–84.

58. Davis M, Ressler K, Rothbaum BO, et al. Effects of D-cycloserine on extinction: translation from preclinical to clinical work. Biol Psychiatry 2006;60: 369–75.

59. Hofmann SG, Meuret AE, Smits JA, et al. Augmentation of exposure therapy with D-cycloserine for social anxiety disorder. Arch Gen Psychiatry 2006;63(3): 298–304.

60. Wilhelm S, Buhlmann U, Tolin DF, et al. Augmentation of behavior therapy with D-cycloserine for obsessive-compulsive disorder. Am J Psychiatry 2008;165(3): 335–41.

61. Baxter LR, Schwartz JM, Bergman KS, et al. Caudate glucose metabolic rate changes with both drug and behavior therapy for OCD. Arch Gen Psychiatry 1992;49:681–9.

62. Cheyette SR, Cummings JL. Encephalitis lethargica: lessons for contemporary neuropsychiatry. J Neuropsychiatry Clin Neurosci 1995;7:125–35.
63. Purcell R, Maruff P, Kyrios M, et al. Cognitive deficits in obsessive–compulsive disorder on tests of frontal–striatal function. Biol Psychiatry 1998;43:348–57.
64. Whiteside SP, Port JD, Abramowitz JS. A meta-analysis of functional neuroimaging in obsessive–compulsive disorder. Psychiatr Res 2004;132:69–79.
65. Menzies L, Chamberlain SR, Laird AR, et al. Integrating evidence from neuroimaging and neuropsychological studies of obsessive–compulsive disorder: the orbitofronto–striatal model revisited. Neurosci Biobehav Rev 2008;32:525–49.
66. Rotge JY, Guehl D, Dilharreguy B, et al. Provocation of obsessive–compulsive symptoms: a quantitative voxel-based meta-analysis of functional neuroimaging studies. J Psychiatry Neurosci 2008;33:405–12.
67. Rotge JY, Guehl D, Dilharreguy B, et al. Meta-analysis of brain volume changes in obsessive–compulsive disorder. Biol Psychiatry 2009;65:75–83.
68. Baxter LR Jr, Schwartz JM, Bergman KS, et al. Caudate glucose metabolic rate changes with both drug and behavior therapy for obsessive-compulsive disorder. Arch Gen Psychiatry 1992;49(9):001–0.
69. Rauch SL, Jenike MA, Alpert NM, et al. Regional cerebral blood flow measured during symptom provocation in obsessive-compulsive disorder using oxygen 15-labeled carbon dioxide and positron emission tomography. Arch Gen Psychiatry 1994;51:62–70.
70. Saxena S, Rauch SL. Functional neuroimaging and the neuroanatomy of obsessive-compulsive disorder. Psychiatr Clin North Am 2000;23(3):563 86.
71. Talbot PS. The molecular neuroimaging of anxiety disorders. Curr Psychiatry Rep 2004;6:274–9.
72. Hemmings SM, Stein DJ. The current status of association studies in obsessive–compulsive disorder. Psychiatr Clin North Am 2006;29:411–44.
73. Chamberlain SR, Menzies L, Hampshire A, et al. Orbitofrontal dysfunction in patients with obsessive–compulsive disorder and their unaffected relatives. Science 2008;321:421–2.
74. MacLean PD. A triune concept of the brain and behavior. Toronto: University of Toronto Press; 1973.
75. Korff S, Harvey BH. Animal models of obsessive–compulsive disorder: rationale to understanding psychobiology and pharmacology. Psychiatr Clin North Am 2006;29:371–90.
76. Rachman S, De Silva P. Abnormal and normal obsessions. Behav Res Ther 1978;16:233–48.
77. Salkovskis PM, Harrison J. Abnormal and normal obsessions—a replication. Behav Res Ther 1984;22:549–52.
78. Purdon C. Empirical investigations of thought supression in OCD. J Behav Ther Exp Psychiatry 2004;35:121–36.
79. Bannon S, Gonsalvez CJ, Croft RJ. Processing impairments in OCD: it is more than inhibition! Behav Res Ther 2008;46:689–700.
80. Moritz S, von Mühlenen A. Inhibition of return in patients with obsessive–compulsive disorder. J Anxiety Disord 2005;19:117–26.
81. Soref A, Dar R, Argov G, et al. Obsessive–compulsive tendencies are associated with a focused information processing strategy. Behav Res Ther 2008;46:1295–9.
82. Teachman BA, Woody SR, Magee JC. Implicit and explicit appraisals of the importance of intrusive thoughts. Behav Res Ther 2006;44:785–805.

83. Franklin ME, Foa EB. Obsessive–compulsive disorder. In: Barlow D, editor. Clinical handbook of psychological disorders. New York: Guilford; 2008.
84. Mataix-Cols D, Rosario-Campos MC, Leckman JF. A multidimensional model of obsessive-compulsive disorder. Am J Psychiatry 2005;162:228–38.
85. Rauch SL, Dougherty DD, Shin LM, et al. Neural correlates of factor-analyzed OCD symptom dimensions: a PET study. CNS Spectrums 1998;3:37–43.
86. Saxena S, Brody AL, Maidment KM, et al. Cerebral glucose metabolism in obsessive-compulsive hoarding. Am J Psychiatry 2004;161(6):1038–48.
87. Schwartz JM, Stoessel PW, Baxter LR Jr, et al. Systematic changes in cerebral glucose metabolic rate after successful behavior modification treatment of obsessive-compulsive disorder. Arch Gen Psychiatry 1996;53(2):109–13.
88. Denys D, de Geus F. Predictors of pharmacotherapy response in anxiety disorders. Curr Psychiatry Rep 2005;7:252–7.
89. Saxena S, Brody AL, Maidment KM, et al. Localized orbitofrontal and subcortical metabolic changes and predictors of response to paroxetine treatment in obsessive-compulsive disorder. Neuropsychopharmacology 1999;21(6):683–93.
90. Rauch SL, Dougherty DD, Cosgrove GR, et al. Cerebral metabolic correlates as potential predictors of response to anterior cingulotomy for obsessive compulsive disorder. Biol Psychiatry 2001;50(9):659–67.
91. Storch EA, Abramowitz J, Goodman WK. Where does obsessive–compulsive disorder belong in DSM-V? Depress Anxiety 2008;25:336–47.
92. Hollander E, Braun A, Simeon D. Should OCD leave the anxiety disorders in DSM-V? The case for obsessive–compulsive-related disorders. Depress Anxiety 2008;25:317–29.
93. Stein DJ. Is disorder x in category or spectrum y? General considerations and application to the relationship between obsessive–compulsive disorder and anxiety disorders. Depress Anxiety 2008;25:330–5.
94. Mataix-Cols D, Pertusa A, Leckman JF. Issues for DSM-V: how should obsessive–compulsive and related disorders be classified? Am J Psychiatry 2007; 164:1313–4.
95. Hyman SE. Can neuroscience be integrated into the DSM-V? Nat Rev Neurosci 2007;8:725–32.
96. Stein DJ. Psychobiology of anxiety disorders and obsessive–compulsive spectrums disorders. CNS Spectr 2008;13(Suppl 14):23–8.
97. Hollander E, Kwon JH, Stein DJ, et al. Obsessive–compulsive and spectrum disorders: overview and quality-of-life issues. J Clin Psychiatry 1996; 57:3–6.
98. Lochner C, Stein DJ. Does work on obsessive–compulsive spectrum disorders contribute to understanding the heterogeneity of obsessive–compulsive disorder? Prog Neuropsychopharmacol Biol Psychiatry 2006;30:353–61.
99. Phillips KA, Price LH, Greenberg BD, et al. Should the DSM diagnostic groupings be changed? In: Phillips KA, First MB, Pincus HA, editors. Advancing DSM: dilemmas in psychiatric diagnosis. Washington, DC: American Psychiatric Association; 2003.
100. Pauls DL, Towbin KE, Leckman JF, et al. Gilles de la Tourette 's syndrome and obsessive– compulsive disorder: evidence supporting a genetic relationship. Arch Gen Psychiatry 1986;43:1180–2.
101. Stein DJ. Neurobiology of the obsessive–compulsive spectrum disorders. Biol Psychiatry 2000;47:296–304.
102. Foa EB, Kozak MJ. DSM-IV field trial—obsessive–compulsive disorder. Am J Psychiatry 1995;152:90–6.

103. Eisen JL, Phillips KA, Coles ME, et al. Insight in obsessive–compulsive disorder and body dysmorphic disorder. Compr Psychiatry 2004;45:10–5.
104. Phillips KA, Pinto A, Menard W, et al. Obsessive-compulsive disorder versus body dysmorphic disorder: a comparison study of two possibly related disorders. Depress Anxiety 2007;24:399–409.
105. Spitzer RL, Wakefield JC. DSM-IV diagnostic criterion for clinical significance: does it help solve the false-positive problem? Am J Psychiatry 1999;156: 1856–64.
106. Baer L. Factor analysis of symptom subtypes of obsessive–compulsive disorder and their relation to personality and tic disorders. J Clin Psychiatry 1994;55: 18–23.
107. Bloch MH, Landeros-Weisenberger A, Rosario MC, et al. Meta-analysis of the symptom structure of obsessive–compulsive disorder. Am J Psychiatry 2008; 165:1532–42.
108. Rosario-Campos MC, Miguel EC, Quatrano S, et al. The Dimensional Yale-Brown Obsessive-Compulsive Scale (DY-BOCS): an instrument for assessing obsessive–compulsive symptom dimensions. Mol Psychiatry 2006;11:495–504.
109. Miguel EC, Leckman JF, Rauch S, et al. Obsessive–compulsive disorder phenotypes: implications for genetic studies. Mol Psychiatry 2005;10:258–75.
110. Alsobrook JP, Leckman JF, Goodman WK, et al. Segregation analysis of obsessive compulsive disorder using symptom-based factor scores. Am J Med Genet 1999;88:669–75.
111. Pinto A, Greenberg BD, Grados MA, et al. Further development of YBOCS dimensions in the OCD Collaborative Genetics Study: symptoms versus categories. Psychiatr Res 2008;160:83–93.
112. Mathews CA, Nievergelt CM, Azzam A, et al. Heritability and clinical features of multigenerational families with obsessive–compulsive disorder and hoarding. Am J Med Genet B Neuropsychiatr Genet 2007;144B:174–82.
113. van Grootheest DS, Boomsma DI, Hettema JM, et al. Heritability of obsessive–compulsive symptom dimensions. Am J Med Genet B Neuropsychiatr Genet 2008;147B:473–8.
114. Lochner C, Kinnear CJ, Hemmings SM, et al. Hoarding in obsessive–compulsive disorder: clinical and genetic correlates. J Clin Psychiatry 2005;66:1155–60.
115. Samuels J, Shugart YY, Grados MA, et al. Significant linkage to compulsive hoarding on chromosome 14 in families with obsessive–compulsive disorder: results from the OCD collaborative genetics study. Am J Psychiatry 2007;164: 493–9.
116. Alonso P, Gratacos M, Menchon JM, et al. Genetic susceptibility to obsessive–compulsive hoarding: the contribution of neurotrophic tyrosine kinase receptor type 3 gene. Genes Brain Behav 2008;7:778–85.
117. Zhang H, Leckman JF, Pauls DL, et al. Genome-wide scan of hoarding in sib pairs in which both sibs have Gilles de la Tourette syndrome. Am J Hum Genet 2002;70:896–904.
118. Phillips ML, Mataix-Cols D. Patterns of neural response to emotive stimuli distinguish the different symptom dimensions of obsessive–compulsive disorder. CNS Spectr 2004;9:275–83.
119. Gilbert AR, Mataix-Cols D, Lawrence N, et al. Brain structure and symptom dimension relationships in obsessive–compulsive disorder (OCD): a voxel-based morphometry (VBM) study. Neuropsychopharmacology 2006;31:83.
120. Mataix-Cols D, Rauch SL, Manzo PA, et al. Use of factor-analyzed symptom dimensions to predict outcome with serotonin reuptake inhibitors and placebo

in the treatment of obsessive–compulsive disorder. Am J Psychiatry 1999;156: 1409–16.

121. Stein DJ, Carey PD, Lochner C, et al. Escitalopram in obsessive–compulsive disorder: response of symptom dimensions to pharmacotherapy. CNS Spectr 2008;13:492–8.

122. Stein DJ, Seedat S, Potocnik F. Hoarding: a review. Isr J Psychiatry Relat Sci 1999;36:35–46.

123. Saxena S. Recent advances in compulsive hoarding. Curr Psychiatry Rep 2008; 10:297–303.

124. Samuels JF, Bienvenu OJ, Grados MA, et al. Prevalence and correlates of hoarding behavior in a community-based sample. Behav Res Ther 2008;46: 836–44.

125. Pertusa A, Fullana MA, Singh S, et al. Compulsive hoarding: OCD symptom, distinct clinical syndrome, or both? Am J Psychiatry 2008;165:1289–98.

126. Anderson SW, Damasio H, Damasio AR. A neural basis for collecting behaviour in humans. Brain 2005;128:201–12.

127. Saxena S, Brody AL, Maidment KM, et al. Cerebral glucose metabolism in obsessive–compulsive hoarding. Am J Psychiatry 2004;161:1038–48.

128. An SK, Mataix-Cols D, Lawrence NS, et al. To discard or not to discard: the neural basis of hoarding symptoms in obsessive–compulsive disorder. Mol Psychiatry 2009;14:318–31.

129. Mataix-Cols D, Marks IM, Greist JH, et al. Obsessive-compulsive symptom dimensions as predictors of compliance with and response to behaviour therapy: results from a controlled trial. Psychother Psychosom 2002;71: 255–62.

130. Lochner C, Stein DJ. Heterogeneity of obsessive–compulsive disorder: a literature review. Harv Rev Psychiatry 2003;11:113–32.

131. Moriarty J, Eapen V, Costa DC, et al. HMPAO SPET does not distinguish obsessive–compulsive and tic syndromes in families multiply affected with Gilles de la Tourette 's syndrome. Psychol Med 1997;27:737–40.

132. Nicolini H, Cruz C, Paez F, et al. Dopamine D2 and D4 receptor genes distinguish the clinical presence of tics in obsessive–compulsive disorder. Gac Med Mex 1998;134:521–7.

133. Urraca N, Camarena B, Gomez-Caudillo L, et al. Mu opioid receptor gene as a candidate for the study of obsessive–compulsive disorder with and without tics. Am J Med Genet B Neuropsychiatr Genet 2004;127:94–6.

134. McDougle CJ, Goodman WK, Leckman JF. Haloperidol addition in fluvoxamine-refractory obsessive–compulsive disorder: a double-blind placebo-controlled study in patients with and without tics. Arch Gen Psychiatry 1994;51:302–8.

135. Geller D, Biederman J, Jones J, et al. Is juvenile obsessive–compulsive disorder a developmental subtype of the disorder? A review of the pediatric literature. J Am Acad Child Adolesc Psychiatry 1998;37:420–7.

136. Busatto GF, Buchpiguel CA, Zamignani DR, et al. Regional cerebral blood flow abnormalities in early onset obsessive–compulsive disorder: an exploratory SPECT study. J Am Acad Child Adolesc Psychiatry 2001;40:347–54.

137. Stewart SE, Geller DA, Jenike M, et al. Long-term outcome of pediatric obsessive–compulsive disorder: a meta-analysis and qualitative review of the literature. Acta Psychiatr Scand 2004;110:4–13.

138. Aigner M, Zitterl W, Prayer D, et al. Magnetic resonance imaging in patients with obsessive–compulsive disorder with good versus poor insight. Psychiatr Res 2005;140:173–9.

139. Matsunaga H, Kiriike N, Matsui T, et al. Obsessive–compulsive disorder with poor insight. Compr Psychiatry 2002;43:150–7.
140. Eisen JL, Rasmussen SA, Phillips KA, et al. Insight and treatment outcome in obsessive–compulsive disorder. Compr Psychiatry 2001;42:494–7.
141. Swedo SE, Leonard HL, Garvey M, et al. Pediatric autoimmune neuropsychiatric disorders associated with streptococcal infections: clinical description of the first 50 cases. Am J Psychiatry 1998;155:264–71.
142. Snider LA, Swedo SE. PANDAS: current status and directions for research. Mol Psychiatry 2004;9:900–7.
143. Hounie AG, Pauls DL, Mercadante MT, et al. Obsessive–compulsive spectrum disorders in rheumatic fever with and without Sydenham's chorea. J Clin Psychiatry 2004;65:994–9.

Posttraumatic Stress Disorder and Stress-Related Disorders

Arieh Y. Shalev, MD

KEYWORDS

- Stress-disorder posttraumatic • Anxiety disorders • DSM-V
- Therapy (pharmacological) • Therapy (psychological)

Numerous studies have established the frequent occurrence of posttraumatic stress disorder (PTSD) among individuals exposed to traumas including wars, disasters, terrorist attacks, road traffic accidents, and interpersonal violence.[1-5] The estimated lifetime prevalence of PTSD in the US population is about 10%.[6,7] Lower prevalence rates are found in Europe, along with a lower frequency of trauma exposure.[8,9] The conditional probability of developing PTSD is more stable across continents but varies between types of traumatic events and genders. The lifetime prevalence of PTSD is higher in women, although it remains unclear whether this can be explained by the more frequent occurrence of gender-related incidents (eg, rape, assault).[9,10]

The validity of the diagnosis of PTSD has been challenged, with particularly critical emphasis on the implied etiological role of the traumatic event.[10-13] Nevertheless, a re-evaluation of the prevalence of PTSD among Vietnam veterans with an independent corroboration of combat exposure[1] yielded a somewhat smaller but still impressive lifetime (18.7%) and point prevalence (11.1%) of the disorder in this population.

Studies that have examined the construct validity of the syndrome, as defined in the Diagnostic and Statistical Manual of Mental Disorders, 4th edition (DSM-IV), have generally confirmed its current latent structure, with some suggestions for the possible separation of the DSM-IV Avoidance/Numbing diagnostic criterion into "effortful avoidance" and "emotional numbing" components.[14-16] The latter components (ie, diminished interest in significant activities, feeling of detachment or estrangement from others, restricted range of affect, and sense of a foreshortened future) resemble symptoms of depression and might explain part of the observed comorbidity of the

This work was supported by US Public Health Service Grant No. MH71651 to Dr. Shalev. Department of Psychiatry, Hadassah University Hospital, Ein Kerem Campus, P.O. Box 12000, 91120 Jerusalem, Israel
E-mail address: ashalev@cc.huji.ac.il

Psychiatr Clin N Am 32 (2009) 687–704
doi:10.1016/j.psc.2009.06.001
0193-953X/09/$ – see front matter © 2009 Elsevier Inc. All rights reserved.

two conditions; however, unlike other anxiety disorders in which the onset of depression tends to follow that of anxiety, the co-occurrence of PTSD and depression exists from the very beginning of the disorder.[17]

The high prevalence of PTSD among deployed servicemen of current wars (eg, 24% of US reservists of the Iraq and Afghanistan campaigns 1 year after homecoming[4,18]) continues to be worrisome. The degree of functional disability and quality of life impairments in patients with PTSD are comparable with and, in many instances, greater than that in other anxiety and mood disorders.[19,20]

Longitudinal studies (reviewed in[21]) indicate that PTSD symptoms appear shortly after the traumatic event, subside in many survivors, and persist in others in the form of chronic PTSD. Accordingly, PTSD might be seen as a "disorder of recovery" from the early responses to psychologically traumatic events.[22] In an epidemiological study,[6] about 40% of survivors with early PTSD had diagnosable PTSD 6 years later.[6] Importantly, 95% of those who recover do so within the year that follows the traumatic event. On the basis of the extant therapies, Kessler and colleagues[6] questioned the advantage of administering treatment with the purpose of reducing the long-term prevalence of PTSD.

Chronic PTSD usually co-occurs with mood, anxiety, and substance use disorders. It is highly reactive to environmental reminders of the traumatic event and to renewed life stressors; therefore, it may have a fluctuating course.[23]

The implications for treatment of these particularities are important. The saliency of the traumatic event and the early expression of typical symptoms create an opportunity for preventive interventions. Treatment of chronic PTSD, on the other hand, should set realistic goals (eg, stabilization versus remission) and evaluate the relative merit of properly therapeutic efforts versus rehabilitation. Similarities between PTSD and emotional learning have led to novel therapeutic attempts to affect the acquisition, the extinction, and the reconsolidation of fear responses in this disorder.

This article separately addresses treatment of the early forms of PTSD (acute stress disorder [ASD] and acute PTSD) and that of chronic PTSD. Psychopharmacology and psychotherapy are addressed in each section. Each section starts by pointing to relevant treatment targets and ends by discussing novel therapies and future directions.

The treatment of PTSD has been the object of recent meta-analyses and critical reviews.[24–33] Treatment guidelines have been published by several professional and national agencies (eg, the US Institute of Medicine,[34] the American Psychiatric Association,[35] the UK National Institute of Clinical Excellence,[36] the World Federation of Societies of Biological Psychiatry,[37] the Australian National Center for PTSD,[38] and the British Association for Psychopharmacology[39]). This article is informed by these publications, as well as by the re-evaluation of PTSD within the revision of the DSM (DSM-V).

ACUTE STRESS DISORDER AND ACUTE POSTTRAUMATIC STRESS DISORDER

Converging evidence from basic and clinical studies suggests that there is a window of opportunity to help those persons who are vulnerable to develop chronic PTSD in the early aftermath of trauma.[40–45] There is also convincing evidence that preventing chronic PTSD is imperative, because chronic PTSD can be pernicious and disabling for many across the lifespan.[1,6,46] Even more alarming, when individuals with chronic PTSD overcome various personal, familial, cultural, economic, and logistical barriers and obtain care, they may still not get the care they need,[4,47] their problems may be so entrenched that they fail to benefit from formal treatment,[48] or they may drop out of treatment prematurely.[49,50] Finding early interventions that effectively prevent chronic PTSD is perceived as a critical public health mandate.[34,51]

The meta-analysis by Brewin and colleagues[52] of risk factors for PTSD suggests that adversity and lack of social support after the traumatic event contribute significantly to the maintenance of PTSD symptoms. The duration of expressing early PTSD symptoms may have an independent pathogenic effect in that it repeats and strengthens the association between reminders of the traumatic event and alarm responses. This idea is subsumed under Antelman's "time-dependent sensitization" model,[53] Post's kindling model,[54] and McEwen'sallostatic stress model.[55,56] These models predict the occurrence of irreversible changes to the central nervous system within a critical period, during which a triggering event is followed by repeated reinforcements. The persistence of external stressors, but also the continuation of inner states of hypervigilence,[57] or repeated and distressing recall of the traumatic event can be seen as such reinforcements. This view predicts that early interventions could have an inherent advantage to the degree that they prevent the repeated reinforcements of the responses to the traumatic event.

Targets for Early Intervention

The main target of early intervention is the prevention of chronic PTSD. Effective prevention requires accurate case identification, accessible services, acceptance of care by survivors at risk, and efficacious interventions.

Defining candidates for early intervention is the first challenge. Historically, the most popular preventive intervention for PTSD has been psychological debriefing provided to groups of exposed survivors regardless of initial symptoms; however, systematic reviews and meta-analyses[58-60] have failed to confirm the efficacy of this technique. Moreover, Mayou and colleagues[61] reported adverse long-term effects of debriefing. A review of other "interventions for all," such as education,[62] collaborative care,[63,64] and trauma-focused counseling,[65] similarly concluded that those methods are unlikely to have a clinically important effect on subsequent PTSD.[33,36] The collapse of the scientific basis for using trauma exposure as a risk indicator underscores the need to better identify the factors that put an individual at high risk to selectively offer services to survivors at high risk before offering therapies.

ASD is one potential identifier. The essential feature of ASD is the expression of PTSD and dissociation symptoms within a month of trauma exposure. As many as 80% of ASD patients develop chronic PTSD;[66] however, the majority of those who develop PTSD do not have diagnosable ASD. Consequently, ASD cannot be used to exclusively define the risk group in need of treatment. Acute PTSD (ie, PTSD developing between 1 and 3 months of the traumatic event) can supplement ASD in defining high-risk survivors.

Pharmacotherapy for Acute Stress Disorder or Acute Posttraumatic Stress Disorder

Because medications can be easily dispensed and delivered (eg, in disaster-prone areas or war zones), developing pharmacological prevention of PTSD is of particular interest; however, currently, there is no good evidence that pharmacological interventions can prevent the development of PTSD. Furthermore, the number and quality of current studies are limited.

Selective serotonin reuptake inhibitors (SSRIs) have been recommended for use in chronic PTSD, but their effect on ASD is virtually unexplored. A randomized controlled study of escitalopram for acute PTSD[67] found no positive effect of that drug over placebo or wait list control; however, the small study sample (22 in each arm) calls for larger replications.

Minor tranquilizers are often used to abate anxious responses to life stressors; however, studies of benzodiazepines in recent trauma survivors showed either no beneficial effect[68] or a higher likelihood of subsequent PTSD.[69] Again, these studies are limited by their sample size and design and require large-scale replications.

A retrospective chart review of the antipsychotic risperidone given 5 days after a traumatic event[70] suggests that this agent can reduce sleep disturbances, nightmares, and hyperarousal; however, these results should be interpreted with caution given the lack of randomized studies.

Several theory-driven, exploratory studies of early interventions have been published. Theory suggests that blocking the adrenergic responses to a traumatic event might prevent its long-term encoding as a fear response. In a randomized, double-blind controlled study, Pitman and colleagues[42] administered the beta-adrenergic blocking agent propranolol to trauma survivors who had an elevated initial heart rate within hours of a traumatic event. The treatment failed to decrease the intensity of PTSD symptoms 3 months later. Similarly, Stein and colleagues[71] found that neither propranolol nor the anticonvulsive agent gabapentin could reduce PTSD symptoms when administered within 48 hours of a traumatic injury.

Promising yet preliminary results were obtained in a study by Schelling and colleagues[72] in which injured trauma survivors who received stress doses of cortisol showed lower levels of PTSD symptoms at follow-up. Although other small studies and case series have been published, the most pertinent observation is that the pharmacological prevention of PTSD is for the most part unexplored.

Psychological Interventions for Acute Stress Disorder or Acute Posttraumatic Stress Disorder

Systematic reviews and meta-analyses have established the efficacy of early, trauma-focused, exposure-based cognitive behavioral therapy (CBT) in preventing chronic PTSD;[33,73–76] however, there is significant heterogeneity among studies.

Several studies have found a beneficial effect of exposure-based CBT. Foa and colleagues[77] compared four CBT sessions (n = 10) with repeated assessments of trauma-related psychopathology (n = 10). Active treatment significantly reduced the prevalence of PTSD (10% versus 70%) and the intensity of PTSD symptoms. Echeburua and colleagues[78] compared five 1-hour sessions of cognitive therapy (CT) and coping skills training (n = 12) with progressive muscle relaxation (n = 12) in treatment-seeking sexual assault survivors within 3 months of the assault. Survivors in the CT arm had a lower level of PTSD symptoms 1 year later. A series of studies by Bryant and colleagues[73–76] showed a relative advantage of early exposure-based CBT relative to supportive counseling at 6-month and 4-year intervals from the traumatic event. The addition of anxiety management techniques to exposure-based CBT did not increase its efficacy. The effects were maintained at 3-year follow-up. Ehlers and colleagues[79] compared twelve weekly sessions of CT with a self-help booklet and repeated assessments in motor vehicle accident survivors. The treatment started approximately 4 months after the traumatic event. CT was superior to both control conditions.

Bryant and colleagues[80] compared CBT, CBT plus hypnosis, and supportive counseling. Both active treatment modalities were better than the comparator. Hypnosis did not add to the already substantial effect of CBT. Bryant and colleagues[75] found that exposure-based CBT was superior to cognitive restructuring in reducing PTSD symptoms among survivors with ASD. Shalev and colleagues[67] compared exposure-based CBT with CT and wait list control and found that the two active treatments were similarly effective in reducing the prevalence of PTSD (20% and 22%, respectively, versus 56% in the control group) and the intensity of PTSD and symptoms.

Other studies have failed to show a beneficial effect of early CBT. Bisson and colleagues[81] compared four 1-hour CBT sessions with no intervention in individuals endorsing at least moderate PTSD symptoms 1 to 3 weeks after mild-to-moderate physical injury. There were no statistical differences between the treatment groups. van Emmerik and colleagues[82] failed to find a difference between five 1.5-hour sessions of CBT and structured writing therapy among trauma survivors with ASD. Foa and colleagues[83] compared four weekly 2-hour sessions of CBT with social counseling and repeated assessments in female survivors of sexual and physical aggression within 4 weeks of the assault. The results did not differentiate the CBT group from the assessment only group. The investigators suggested that downplaying the necessity of in vivo exposure and homework-based imaginal exposure in this trial may have attenuated the effects of the CBT. Sijbrandij and colleagues[84] evaluated the effect of four sessions of brief CBT (n = 79) relative to wait list control (n = 64) provided within 3 months of a traumatic event and found a transient beneficial effect in the active treatment group (1 week following treatment completion), which was not evident any more 4 months later.

Despite the heterogeneity between studies, the weighted evidence[25,35,36,38] seems to suggest that exposure-based, trauma-focused CBT is efficacious in the early aftermath of a traumatic event. The effect of CT without exposure is still uncertain. The number of treatment sessions needed to achieve an effect is unknown. Indeed, rather than specifying the number of sessions, one could use treatment outcome in each case as an indication to either stop or continue treatment. Patients may differ in their ability to learn and practice CBT. There is no knowledge about "booster sessions" and other means to enhance or maintain the effect of an initial intervention. Most importantly, the effectiveness of preventive CBT in large groups has not been explored.

Challenges to Early Interventions

Challenges to early interventions include the lack of accurate threshold criteria for selecting survivors for treatment and the time lag between the traumatic event and the beginning of therapy. With regard to threshold criteria, a recent review of early psychological interventions[33] suggests that survivors who do not meet the full diagnostic criteria for acute PTSD recover with or without treatment and thus may not need treatment. Similarly, Shalev and colleagues[67] performed a randomized controlled study of CBT, CT, and an SSRI and found that survivors with partial PTSD fared as well with or without treatment at 5 and 8 months after the traumatic event.

The time lag between the traumatic event and the onset of treatment has been examined in a study by Shalev and colleagues[67] in which participants of the wait list control group (n = 60) started exposure-based CBT upon completion of the early phase of the study. At the study's completion (8 months), there was no difference between the early and late treatment group in the prevalence of PTSD (19% versus 22%) and in the severity of PTSD symptoms. One can conclude that early treatment should start within the first 5 months after exposure, include survivors with full PTSD, and consist of trauma-focused CBT.

Additionally, there are significant barriers to receiving early care among trauma-exposed civilians and military personnel.[3,85–87] In the study by Shalev and colleagues,[67] 49% of 1501 civilian survivors who were assessed by telephone interviews and found to have distressing ASD symptoms declined an offer to see a clinician, and 27% of those seen by clinicians and diagnosed as having acute PTSD declined an offer to begin treatment.

Recent studies of combat veterans from the Iraq and Afghanistan wars[4,18] have shown an increase in the prevalence of PTSD in the years following their homecoming. Although the true incidence of delayed-onset PTSD is considered to be rare,[88] the saliency of early symptoms might be limited by the survivors' need to cope with ongoing stressors (eg, injury) or to continue to perform under stress (eg, in a war zone) or otherwise dampen their emotionality. The presence of a "delayed onset" or a "mute" form of early PTSD reduces the number of survivors who will seek or accept early care.

Even if the previous barriers were overcome, early psychological interventions would be frustrated by the availability of adequate resources and the dissemination of treatment skills. Skilled cognitive behavioral therapists are rare in developed countries and virtually inexistent in the developing world. Even when they exist, the demand for such services will often exceed the supply (eg, in mass casualty events). Disseminating CBT skills to professionals and nonspecialists and possibly modifying face-to-face techniques are major future challenges.[89,90] On a positive note, the recent implementation of a very short CBT protocol in earthquake survivors in Turkey[91] significantly reduced the prevalence and the severity of PTSD. Efforts to simplify, test, and disseminate CBT deserve further attention.

CHRONIC POSTTRAUMATIC STRESS DISORDER

Formally defined as having more than 3 months duration, chronic PTSD is often much longer. Epidemiological studies have shown that the average duration of a PTSD episode is more than 7 years.[19] This longer form of PTSD is often comorbid with other disorders and difficult to treat. The US Institute of Medicine[34] found that the scientific evidence on treatment modalities for PTSD was "below the level of certainty that would be desired for such a common and serious disorder." The Institute of Medicine has identified but one treatment component of CBT, exposure therapy, to have convincing evidence behind it. The evidence for other treatment modalities including pharmacological therapies has been found to be inadequate.

Other practice guidelines[35,92,93] recommend the use of exposure-based, trauma-focused CBT as well as SSRIs. The British National Institute for Clinical Excellence practice guidelines[36] found the evidence on pharmacotherapy to be tentative, and recommended that medication be offered if psychological treatments are not effective or in the case of comorbid depression or severe hyperarousal that interferes with psychotherapy.

Pharmacotherapy

Many PTSD patients receive pharmacological treatment. For example, 80% of PTSD patients treated by the US Veteran's Administration received psychotropic medication during the year 2004 (a total of 274,297 prescriptions); 89% of the patients were prescribed antidepressants, 61% received anxiolytics/sedative-hypnotics, and 34% received antipsychotics.[94] Although some of these compounds might have been prescribed for comorbid conditions, the numbers are still in sharp contrast with the empirical evidence of drug efficacy in PTSD.

Early pharmacological studies focused on the tricyclic antidepressants and monoamine oxidase inhibitors. More recent work has addressed SSRIs and newly introduced antidepressants (nefazodone, venlafaxine, mirtazapine). Fewer studies have evaluated the role of anticonvulsive agents, atypical neuroleptics, and prazosin, an adrenergic-inhibiting agent.

Large-scale randomized controlled trials have found that SSRIs are effective in reducing PTSD and associated symptoms.[95–98] Research support to date is particularly strong for paroxetine,[97,98] sertraline,[95,96] and fluoxetine,[99] but a negative study has also been reported.[100] Consequently, SSRIs have been considered to be a first-line pharmacological treatment for the disorder.[101] As noted by Friedman and colleagues,[101] SSRIs also have a potential use for co-occurring conditions such as depression, other anxiety disorders, and impulsivity. Several SSRIs have been approved by the FDA (sertraline, paroxetine) and the European Medical Agency (sertraline) for the treatment for PTSD.

A systematic review of pharmacotherapy for PTSD[32] concluded that SSRIs were effective in treating PTSD on a short- (14 weeks) and long-term (eg, 1 year) basis. More cautiously, Zhang and Davidson's review[102] proposes that the "Existing pharmacologic agents produce meaningful results and bear the advantage of treating depression and other comorbid disorders, yet still fall short of being ideal due to limited response and remission rates and tolerability issues." This statement truly summarizes the state of facts, that is, SSRIs may produce clinically meaningful alleviation of suffering, but the magnitude of the response leaves many patients with partial PTSD. Specifically, the response rates of SSRIs rarely exceed 60%, and less than 20% to 30% of the patients achieve remission.[103]

Non-SSRI antidepressants (venlafaxine, nefazodone, trazodone, and mirtazapine) have been evaluated in open-label trials and case studies and cannot be recommended for systematic use in PTSD. Several of the older antidepressants and monamine oxidase inhibitors have inconsistent effects, and most of them have been abandoned with the advent of SSRIs.[104]

The atypical antipsychotic olanzapine has been evaluated as single agent or adjunct to SSRIs with positive yet preliminary results.[29,105] Pae and colleagues[29] recommend caution in interpreting the current evidence given the quality and availability of the data.

One single-blind study and three case reports have evaluated the effect of the antiepileptic compound valproate in PTSD symptoms and showed statistically significant reduction of some PTSD symptoms.[106] Preliminary studies have also evaluated the effect of other anticonvulsant drugs (lamotrigine, carbamazepine, clonidine) in PTSD, but the evidence does not amount to clear clinical recommendations.[35] Prazosin, an adrenergic-inhibiting agent, has been evaluated for its effects on nightmares and insomnia and seems to produce a beneficial effect.[107,108]

One way to understand the gap between prescribing routines and the empirical evidence of efficacy in PTSD is by recognizing the discrepancy between the criteria used in clinical trials (mainly, symptom reduction) and what patients and treating psychiatrists may try to achieve in real world practice (eg, stabilization, better sleep, better controllability of emotional reactions, reduction of self-medication with alcohol or substances of abuse). Many PTSD patients continue to receive medication despite their limited effect. Furthermore, the lack of accepted criteria of "success" and "remission"[34] leaves clinicians without clear indications about stopping medication, switching to other compounds, or using augmentation techniques. For many practitioners, the pharmacological treatment of the chronic PTSD patient is experienced as a long struggle within the boundaries of their professional ability to help. Reliable information about the patients' perspective is lacking, yet it is likely that even small effects of medication would be viewed as helpful.

Psychotherapies

Trauma-focused CBT has the largest research base of well-designed randomized controlled studies, systematic reviews,[27] and meta-analyses.[25,33] The latter has addressed 25 randomized controlled studies and found (1) a significant reduction of clinician-rated symptoms (14 studies with 649 subjects; standardized mean difference [SMD], 1.4; 95% CI, −1.89 to −0.91); (2) a significant reduction in patient self-rated PTSD symptoms (9 studies with 428 subjects; SMD, −1.7; 95% CI, −2.1 to −1.24); and (3) a significant decrease in PTSD diagnoses (relative risk, 0.44; 95% CI, 0.37 to 0.57). Withdrawal rates were higher in the wait list group.

The components of CBT that have been associated with the largest effects in the treatment of PTSD are CT and prolonged exposure. CT mainly addresses trauma-related cognitive distortions regarding the dangerousness of the world, the imminence of harm, and the limitations of one's own resources. Prolonged exposure relies on exposing patients during sessions and in homework practices to inner (psychological) and external reminders of the traumatic event in ways that reduce their avoidance and the associated fearfulness (fear structure).

Marks and colleagues[109] found equivalent reductions in PTSD symptoms with CT alone, prolonged exposure alone, and CT with prolonged exposure combined. Similarly, Tarrier and colleagues[49] found equivalent reductions in PTSD symptoms with imaginal exposure and CT. Resick and colleagues[110] found equivalent reductions in PTSD symptoms with cognitive processing therapy and prolonged exposure. Foa and colleagues[111] compared prolonged exposure with stress inoculation training (containing CT) and found no difference between the treatments in the reduction of PTSD severity.

Treatment guidelines have consistently recommended trauma-focused CBT for chronic PTSD. Several treatment protocols have been published[112,113] and are available to clinicians. Several studies have examined the effect of a variant of trauma-focused CBT, the eye movement desensitization and reprocessing treatment (EMDR), which is a technique that combines imaginal exposure to trauma reminders with repeated lateral eye movements.[114–117] Critics of this procedure cite evidence suggesting that the procedural components that purportedly differentiate it from exposure (ie, the guided eye movement) are inactive. Nevertheless, as a treatment package (ie, eye movement and exposure), EMDR has been effective in several well-controlled studies.

A systematic review and meta-analysis by Bisson and colleagues[25] evaluated 12 studies of EMDR, seven studies of stress management techniques, and six studies of other therapies. EMDR was better than a wait list in reducing PTSD symptoms, and there was some evidence that both CBT and EMDR were better than supportive/nondirective therapies. These investigators have noted the absence of data on side effects and early withdrawal from treatment (intent-to-treat analyses).

New Approaches

New approaches include theory-driven and enhanced therapies. The disorder's fear-conditioning theory postulates that PTSD has, at its core, an acquired (conditioned) fear response in which the traumatic event serves as a conditioning stimulus and the immediate reaction to the event is an unconditioned response, and suggests that the disorder consists of an abnormal conservation of a strong associative link between reminders of the conditioning stimulus and fear responses (conditioned responses). The determining event in PTSD is, accordingly, the conservation and the subsequent generalization of fear (or alarm) responses over time as opposed to their expected decline via extinction. Much of the current research in PTSD concerns the conditions that interfere with the extinction of traumatic memories. Hypothesis-driven therapies of PTSD are based on hypotheses driven from this model.

Attempts to manipulate the strength of the initial learning by modifying the endocrine modulators of emotional learning (cortisol and norepinephrine) led to the previously mentioned studies of propranolol and cortisol.[22,71,72] An attempt to enhance glutamatergic transmission by D-cycloserine, which, in theory, could enhance a cortical (predominantly glutamatergic) control over midbrain fear circuits,[118] is another theory-driven trial. This particular study did not separate active treatment from placebo. Unpublished studies are evaluating the ability of D-cycloserine to enhance the effect of CBT with the same rationale.

Other attempts to enhance the effect of therapies refer to the ability of virtual reality to enhance the patient's engagement in reliving and exploring previously traumatic experiences.[119] Recently, a "Virtual Iraq" has been designed as an aid to exposure therapy of war veterans.[120] Germain and colleagues[121] compared the efficacy of CBT via video conference with that of face-to-face sessions and found that the two methods produced a similar reduction in PTSD symptoms.

Recent animal research[45] has shown that an experimental reactivation of conditioned fear responses is followed by their forgetfulness when protein synthesis is inhibited. The process that enables retention after recall has been referred to as reconsolidation. The requirement of such rewriting of memories after recall is at the origin of novel and experimental research in which drugs that interfere with reconsolidation are administered during deliberate recall of traumatic memories with the hope of somehow dissolving them.[122,123] This line of experiments is worth following.

Current efforts are directed toward circumventing the problem of service delivery by using Web-based CBT.[124] The results of these efforts should be followed with great interest.

Active Ingredients of Therapies: Explaining How They Work

Current evidence consistently supports the efficiency of CBT and less consistently that of pharmacological treatment. There are many ways to interpret the relative success of CBT and the limited performance of medication in PTSD. With regard to medication, it might be true that the nature of PTSD—a learned fear response—can be particularly resistant to pharmacological manipulations. PTSD patients show uncontrollable emotional and physiological responses to reminders of the trauma.[125] These responses specifically involve an activation of the amygdala, the locus of fear-driven learning. The parsimonious interpretation of the relatively limited effect of medications, most of which affect the brain's distributed modulatory systems (eg, the serotonin, dopamine, norepinephrine, and GABA-ergic systems), is that these modulatory systems cannot affectively modify this type of learned responses or cannot affect them to the extent that they do in disorders driven by emotionality (eg, depression, anxiety disorders). Because emotional learning is a natural, normal, and absolutely necessary process in all humans, it is robust and resistant to change[126] and may only be marginally affected by modifying its serotonergic or adrenergic environment. Implicit learning, such as that of skills, habits, and conditioned responses, defies forgetting and age. Instead, its alteration essentially requires corrective learning. In that sense, PTSD may resemble several other disorders that involve over-learning or overreinforcement of an initially normal response (eg, dieting in anorexia, drinking or using substances for pleasure in the various addictions, and many of the anxiety disorders). Indeed, the extent to which PTSD resists current pharmacological manipulation resembles the relative resistance of eating or addictive disorders to pharmacological therapies when used as single agents.

It might be true that pharmacotherapy should be used to create conditions that enable psychological changes in PTSD (as is the case with some anorectic patients, in which SSRIs reduce some of the craving for thinness and the redundant rumination about weight and calories). Unfortunately, there are currently no controlled studies of combined pharmacotherapy and psychotherapy in PTSD.

More mundane explanations of the relative poor performance of pharmacological agents in PTSD suggest that, with the exception of SSRIs, nothing has been tried systematically and on a large enough scale. Moreover, most SSRIs have been tried for short periods of time, and there is no systematic study of pharmacological augmentation techniques, combination of medication, or other means of modulating central nervous system responses.

Current pharmacological therapies, despite their imperfections, have major stabilizing effects on the patient's life. Stabilizing a chronic PTSD patient is a valuable treatment goal that should not be overlooked.

Toward the DSM-V

Reactive disorders

Currently classified among the anxiety disorders, PTSD differs by virtue of the fact that it is linked with a triggering event. The latter is both the point of onset of symptoms and their essential reference (eg, it even appears in the content of nightmares and intrusive recollections, and places and situations are avoided that resemble the event). PTSD is at the same time similar to other anxiety disorders because of the clear presence of anxiety within the disorder, which is also the disorder-defining feature of other anxiety disorders (eg, obsessions, phobias, panic attacks); however, the association of the syndrome with a triggering external event and the continuous reactivity to environmental stimuli which exist in PTSD might argue for the inclusion of this disorder in a wider category of stress-reactive disorders. Along with PTSD, one could see dissociative identity disorders, reactive psychoses, and adjustment disorders as possible members of this group. The extent to which creating a new category will better inform the study of each disorder is currently unclear. Moreover, the existence of common pathogenic and pathophysiological mechanisms behind the reactive disorders remains hypothetical.

Place of criterion A (the traumatic event)

The diagnosis of PTSD requires an exposure to a traumatic event (DSM-IV PTSD criterion A). Several studies have shown that persons in whom PTSD develops are significantly more likely to report intense levels of fear, helplessness, or horror during the traumatic event than persons who do not.[17,44,66] Other studies have shown that PTSD more likely follows an initial bodily and emotional response.[66,127,128] Other initial emotions such as guilt or anger have also been linked with the development of PTSD;[129] however, in a large epidemiological study, the conditional probability of developing PTSD following a traumatic event was not substantially affected by the inclusion or the omission of criterion A2 among survivors who were exposed to a traumatic event.[130] This finding might be explained by the small proportion of survivors who experience fear, helplessness, or horror that subsequently develop PTSD.[66] The epidemiological perspective differs here from that of clinicians, for whom the existence of a traumatic event clearly marks the onset of an often chronic condition.

From a clinical point of view, the discussion concerning the appropriateness of criterion A has two weaknesses. The first concerns the place of the traumatic event in the complex causation of PTSD. The second has to do with the wish to identify specific events as "traumatic."

Like many other disorders, the etiology of PTSD is complex and involves vulnerability, triggering, and maintaining factors.[131] In such complex causation, any single contributing factor can only account for a small portion of the total causation. This observation does not mean that one or several critical factors cannot have a decisive role, in which case they become necessary but not sufficient to explain the occurrence of the disorder. The traumatic event is such a critical factor. Moreover, this critical factor will only trigger PTSD in the presence of other contributing conditions and pre-disposing factors, such as biographical vulnerability factors (eg, prior mental illness, child abuse/neglect, or prior trauma), psychological factors (eg, co-occurring loss or loneliness), biological factors (eg, inherited vulnerability), appraisal of the traumatic event (including appraisal by the group, scapegoating), and the quality of the recovery environment. Consequently, even the most dramatic events are only potentially trau-matic in that they will lead to PTSD only under specific conditions. Much of the current debate concerning criterion A reflects confusion between the traumatic event's critical role in the etiology of PTSD with its relative contribution to the total causation of the disorder.

The second problem stems from DSM-IV preferential use of descriptive criteria, which forces a focus on well-defined events behind PTSD. It is possible that psycho-logical dimensions within specific events (eg, perceived intensity, controllability, escape, or self-efficacy) determine their potential to generate PTSD. For example, the presence during an event of grotesqueness or an incongruous incomprehensible novelty may trigger a redundant cycle of ruminative elaboration that is typical of PTSD, even in the absence of threat (eg, among body handlers or rescue workers). An attempt to define specifically traumatic events should be replaced by delineating specific traumatic elements of events and their aftermath.

SUMMARY

The study of PTSD has made major progress during the last decade. The disorder's defining symptoms have been re-evaluated and found to be robust and consistent across populations and traumatic events. The disorder's natural course is better known, fostering attempts at early prevention. Many of the neurobiological mecha-nisms of PTSD (eg, fear conditioning, memory consolidation, reconsolidation) have been explored in animal studies, and several of these investigations have been trans-lated into preliminary human studies. Despite criticism, PTSD has gained increasing acceptance and recognition by clinicians and researchers. Knowledge about the disorder's therapies has converged into a few well-studied interventions.

Progress made in understanding the therapy of PTSD has already shown a ceiling effect of pharmacotherapy and psychological therapies. At present, many PTSD patients continue to suffer despite treatment. Moreover, effective psychotherapies for PTSD require resources that are not available in most places. Studies of more sophisticated pharmacotherapies (eg, via augmentation of association with psycho-logical therapies) are badly missing. There is currently no efficient way to prevent the disorder under its naturally occurring circumstances.

Despite advances in knowledge, PTSD remains prevalent, chronic, disabling, and costly. Nonetheless, the emergence of theory-driven biological therapies designed to alter the longitudinal course of the disorder is encouraging, particularly when such therapies are applied during the disorder's critical first few months.

REFERENCES

1. Dohrenwend BP, Turner JB, Turse NA, et al. The psychological risks of Vietnam for US veterans: a revisit with new data and methods. Science 2006;313(5789): 979–82.

2. Hoge CW, Auchterlonie JL, Milliken CS. Mental health problems, use of mental health services, and attrition from military service after returning from deployment to Iraq or Afghanistan. JAMA 2006;295(9):1023–32.

3. Hoge CW, Castro CA, Messer SC, et al. Combat duty in Iraq and Afghanistan, mental health problems, and barriers to care. N Engl J Med 2004;351(1):13–22.

4. Milliken CS, Auchterlonie JL, Hoge CW. Longitudinal assessment of mental health problems among active and reserve component soldiers returning from the Iraq war. JAMA 2007;298(18):2141–8.

5. Mills MA, Edmondson D, Park CL. Trauma and stress response among Hurricane Katrina evacuees. Am J Public Health 2007;97(Suppl 1):S116–23.

6. Kessler RC, Sonnega A, Bromet E, et al. Posttraumatic stress disorder in the National Comorbidity Survey. Arch Gen Psychiatry 1995;52(12):1048–60.

7. Breslau N, Kessler RC, Chilcoat HD, et al. Trauma and posttraumatic stress disorder in the community: the 1996 Detroit Area Survey of Trauma. Arch Gen Psychiatry 1998;55(7):626–32.

8. Perkonigg A, Kessler RC, Storz S, et al. Traumatic events and post-traumatic stress disorder in the community: prevalence, risk factors and comorbidity. Acta Psychiatr Scand 2000;101(1):46–59.

9. Wittchen HU, Gloster A, Beesdo K, et al. PTSD: diagnostic and epidemiological perspectives. CNS Spectr 2009;14(1):5–12.

10. Freedman SA, Gluck N, Tuval-Mashiach R, et al. Gender differences in responses to traumatic events: a prospective study. J Trauma Stress 2002; 15(5):407–13.

11. McNally RJ. Psychology: psychiatric casualties of war. Science 2006;313(5789): 923–4.

12. Young A, Breslau N. Troublesome memories: reflections on the future. J Anxiety Disord 2007;21(2):230–2.

13. Heir T, Piatigorsky A, Weisaeth L. Longitudinal changes in recalled perceived life threat after a natural disaster. Br J Psychiatry 2009;194(6):510–4.

14. Elhai JD, Ford JD, Ruggiero KJ, et al. Diagnostic alterations for post-traumatic stress disorder: examining data from the National Comorbidity Survey Replication and National Survey of Adolescents. Psychol Med 2009 Apr 20:1–10 [Epub ahead of print].

15. King DW, Leskin GA, King LA, et al. Confirmatory factor analysis of the Clinician-Administered PTSD Scale: evidence for the dimensionality of posttraumatic stress disorder. Psychol Assess 1998;10:90–6.

16. Simms LJ, Watson D, Doebbeling BN. Confirmatory factor analyses of posttraumatic stress symptoms in deployed and nondeployed veterans of the Gulf War. J Abnorm Psychol 2002;111(4):637–47.

17. Shalev AY, Freedman S, Peri T, et al. Prospective study of posttraumatic stress disorder and depression following trauma. Am J Psychiatry 1998; 155(5):630–7.

18. Grieger TA, Cozza SJ, Ursano RJ, et al. Posttraumatic stress disorder and depression in battle-injured soldiers. Am J Psychiatry 2006;163(10):1777–83 [quiz: 1860].

19. Kessler RC. Posttraumatic stress disorder: the burden to the individual and to society. J Clin Psychiatry 2000;61(Suppl 5):4–12 [discussion: 13–4].

20. Seedat S, Lochner C, Vythilingum B, et al. Disability and quality of life in post-traumatic stress disorder: impact of drug treatment. Pharmacoeconomics 2006;24(10):989–98.

21. Peleg T, Shalev AY. Longitudinal studies of PTSD: overview of findings and methods. CNS Spectr 2006;11(8):589–602.

22. Shalev AY. PTSD: a disorder of recovery? In: Kirmayer L, Lemelson R, Barad M, editors. Understanding trauma: integrating biological clinical and cultural perspectives. Cambridge (UK): Cambridge University Press; 2007. p. 207–23.
23. Niles BL, Newman E, Fisher LM. Obstacles to assessment of PTSD in longitudinal research. In: Shalev AY, Yehuda R, McFarlane AC, editors. International handbook of human response to trauma. New York: Kluwer Academic/Plenum Publishers; 2000. p. 213–22.
24. Bisson JI, Ehlers A, Matthews R, et al. Psychological treatments for chronic posttraumatic stress disorder: systematic review and meta-analysis. Br J Psychiatry 2007;190:97–104.
25. Bisson J, Andrew M. Psychological treatment of post-traumatic stress disorder (PTSD). Cochrane Database Syst Rev 2007;(3):CD003388.
26. Bisson J, Andrew M. Psychological treatment of post-traumatic stress disorder (PTSD). Cochrane Database Syst Rev 2005,(2).CD003388.
27. Bradley R, Greene J, Russ E, et al. A multidimensional meta-analysis of psychotherapy for PTSD. Am J Psychiatry 2005;162(2).214–27.
28. Hofmann SG, Smits JA. Cognitive-behavioral therapy for adult anxiety disorders: a meta-analysis of randomized placebo-controlled trials. J Clin Psychiatry 2008; 69(4):621–32.
29. Pae CU, Lim HK, Peindl K, et al. The atypical antipsychotics olanzapine and risperidone in the treatment of posttraumatic stress disorder: a meta-analysis of randomized, double-blind, placebo-controlled clinical trials. Int Clin Psychopharmacol 2008;23(1):1–8.
30. Seidler GH, Wagner FE. Comparing the efficacy of EMDR and trauma-focused cognitive-behavioral therapy in the treatment of PTSD: a meta-analytic study. Psychol Med 2006;36:1515–22.
31. Stein DJ, Zohar J. The Cape town consensus on posttraumatic stress disorder: introduction. CNS Spectr 2009;14(1 Suppl 1).
32. Stein DJ, Ipser JC, Seedat S. Pharmacotherapy for posttraumatic stress disorder (PTSD). Cochrane Database Syst Rev 2006;(1):CD002795.
33. Roberts NP, Kitchiner NJ, Kenardy J, et al. Systematic review and meta-analysis of multiple-session early interventions following traumatic events. Am J Psychiatry 2009;166(3):293–301.
34. IOM, Committee on Treatment of Posttraumatic Stress Disorder. Treatment of posttraumatic stress disorder: an assessment of the evidence. Washington, (DC): The National Academies Press; 2008.
35. Ursano RJ, et al. Practice guideline for the treatment of patients with acute stress disorder and posttraumatic stress disorder. Am J Psychiatry 2004;161(11 Suppl):3–31.
36. NICE, National Collaborating Centre for Mental Health. The management of posttraumatic stress disorder in primary and secondary care. London: National Institute for Clinical Excellence; 2005.
37. Bandelow B, et al. World Federation of Societies of Biological Psychiatry (WFSBP) guidelines for the pharmacological treatment of anxiety, obsessive-compulsive and post-traumatic stress disorders–first revision. World J Biol Psychiatry 2008;9(4):248–312.
38. Forbes D, et al. Australian guidelines for the treatment of adults with acute stress disorder and post-traumatic stress disorder. Aust N Z J Psychiatry 2007;41(8):637–48.
39. Baldwin DS, Anderson IM, Nutt DJ, et al. Evidence-based guidelines for the pharmacological treatment of anxiety disorders: recommendations from the British Association for Psychopharmacology. J Psychopharmacol 2005;19:567–96.

40. Rothbaum BO, Foa EB, Riggs DS, et al. Prospective examination of post-traumatic stress disorder in rape victims. J Trauma Stress 1992;5:455–75.
41. Shalev AY, Peri T, Brandes D, et al. Auditory startle response in trauma survivors with posttraumatic stress disorder: a prospective study. Am J Psychiatry 2000; 157(2):255–61.
42. Pitman RK, Sanders KM, Zusman RM, et al. Pilot study of secondary prevention of posttraumatic stress disorder with propranolol. Biol Psychiatry 2002;51(2): 189–92.
43. Orr SP, Metzger LJ, Lasko NB, et al. Physiologic responses to sudden, loud tones in monozygotic twins discordant for combat exposure: association with posttraumatic stress disorder. Arch Gen Psychiatry 2003;60(3):283–8.
44. Zatzick DF, Russo J, Pitman RK, et al. Reevaluating the association between emergency department heart rate and the development of posttraumatic stress disorder: a public health approach. Biol Psychiatry 2005;57(1):91–5.
45. Milad MR, Rauch SL, Pitman RK, et al. Fear extinction in rats: implications for development of posttraumatic stress disorder. Biol Psychol 2006;73(1):61–71.
46. Kulka RA, Schlenger WE, Fairbank JA. Trauma and the Vietnam War generation: report of findings from the National Vietnam Veterans Readjustment Study. Philadelphia: Brunner/Mazel; 1990.
47. Becker CB, Zayfert C, Anderson E. A survey of psychologists' attitudes towards and utilization of exposure therapy for PTSD. Behav Res Ther 2004;42:277–92.
48. Schnurr PP, Friedman MJ, Foy DW. Randomized trial of trauma-focused group therapy for posttraumatic stress disorder: results from a Department of Veterans Affairs Cooperative Study. Arch Gen Psychiatry 2003;60:481–9.
49. Tarrier N, Pilgrim H, Sommerfield C, et al. A randomized trial of cognitive therapy and imaginal exposure in the treatment of chronic posttraumatic stress disorder. J Consult Clin Psychol 1999;67:13–8.
50. Van Minnen A, Arntz A, Keijsers GPJ. Prolonged exposure in patients with chronic PTSD: predictors of treatment outcome and dropout. Behav Res Ther 2002;40:439–57.
51. Litz BT, Gray MJ. Early intervention for trauma in adults: a framework for first aid and secondary prevention. In: Litz BT, editor. Early intervention for trauma and traumatic loss. New York: Guilford Press; 2004. p. 87–111.
52. Brewin C, Andrews B, Valentine J. Meta-analysis of risk factors for posttraumatic stress disorder in trauma exposed adults. J Consult Clin Psychol 2000;68: 748–66.
53. Antelman SM. Time-dependent sensitization as the cornerstone for a new approach to pharmacotherapy: drugs as foreign/stressful stimuli. Drug Dev Res 1988;14:1–30.
54. Post RM, Weiss SRB, Smith M. Sensitization and kindling: implications for the evolving neural substrates of post-traumatic stress disorder. In: Friedman JM, Charney DS, Deutch AY, editors. Neurobiological and clinical consequences of stress. Philadelphia: Lipincott-Raven; 1995. p. 203–24.
55. McEwen BS. Stressful experience, brain, and emotions: developmental, genetic, and hormonal influences. In: Gazzaniga MS, editor. editor. The cognitive neurosciences. Cambridge (MA): MIT Press; 1995. p. 1117–35.
56. McEwen BS. Allostasis and allostatic load: implications for neuropsychopharmacology. Neuropsychopharmacology 2000;22(2):108–24.
57. Schell TL, Marshall GN, Jaycox LH. All symptoms are not created equal: the prominent role of hyperarousal in the natural course of posttraumatic psychological distress. J Abnorm Psychol 2004;113(2):189–97.

58. Suzanna RO, Jonathan BI, Simon WE. Psychological debriefing for preventing post traumatic stress disorder (PTSD). Cochrane Database Syst Rev 2002;(2): CD000560.

59. Rose S, Bisson B, Wessely S. A systematic review of brief psychological interventions ("debriefing") for the treatment of immediate trauma related symptoms and the prevention of post-traumatic stress disorder. The Cochrane Collaboration (database on-line) Wiley; 2005. Updated issue 3.

60. Van Emmerick AA, Kamphuis JH, Hulsbosch AM, et al. Single session debriefing after psychological trauma: a meta-analysis. Lancet 2002;360:766–71.

61. Mayou RA, Ehlers A, Hobbs M. Psychological debriefing for road traffic accident victims: three-year follow-up of a randomised controlled trial. Br J Psychiatry 2000;176:589–93.

62. Rose S, Brewin CR, Andrews B, et al. A randomized controlled trial of individual psychological debriefing for victims of violent crime. Psychol Med 1999;29: 793–9.

63. Zatzick DF, Roy-Byrne P, Russo JE, et al. Collaborative interventions for physically injured trauma survivors: a pilot randomized effectiveness trial. Gen Hosp Psychiatry 2001;23(3):114–23.

64. Zatzick D, Roy-Byrne P, Russo J, et-al. A randomized effectiveness trial of stepped collaborative care for acutely injured trauma survivors. Arch Gen Psychiatry 61(5):498–506.

65. Brom D, Kleber RJ, Hofman MC. Victims of traffic accidents: incidence and prevention of post-traumatic stress disorder. J Clin Psychol 1993;49:131–40.

66. Bryant R. Early predictors of posttraumatic stress disorder. Biol Psychiatry 2003; 53(9):789–95.

67. Shalev AY, Peleg T, Ankri Y, et al. Prevention of PTSD by early treatment: results from the Jerusalem Trauma Outreach and Prevention (J-TOPS) study. in press.

68. Mellman T, Clark R, Peacock W. Prescribing patterns for patients with posttraumatic stress disorder. Psychiatr Serv 2003;54:1618–21.

69. Gelpin E, Bonne O, Peri T, et al. Treatment of recent trauma survivors with benzodiazepines: a prospective study. J Clin Psychiatry 1996;57(9):390–4.

70. Stanovic JK, James KA, VanDevere CA. The effectiveness of risperidone on acute stress symptoms in adult burn patients. a preliminary retrospective pilot study. Journal of Burn Care & Rehabilitation 2001;22:210–3.

71. Stein MB, Kerridge C, Dimsdale JE, et al. Pharmacotherapy to prevent PTSD: results from a randomized controlled proof-of-concept trial in physically injured patients. J Trauma Stress 2007;20(6):923–32.

72. Schelling G, Kilger E, Roozendaal B, et al. Stress doses of hydrocortisone, traumatic memories, and symptoms of posttraumatic stress disorder in patients after cardiac surgery: a randomized study. Biol Psychiatry 2004;55(6):627–33.

73. Bryant A, Sackville T, Dang ST, et al. Treating acute stress disorder: an evaluation of cognitive behavior therapy and supportive counseling techniques. Am J Psychiatry 1999;156(11):1780–6.

74. Bryant RA, Harvey AG, Dang ST, et al. Treatment of acute stress disorder: a comparison of cognitive-behavioral therapy and supportive counseling. J Consult Clin Psychol 1998;66:862–6.

75. Bryant RA, Mastrodomenico J, Felmingham KL, et al. Treatment of acute stress disorder: a randomized controlled trial. Arch Gen Psychiatry 2008;65(6): 659–67.

76. Bryant RA, Moulds ML, Nixon RV. Cognitive behaviour therapy of acute stress disorder: a four-year follow-up. Behav Res Ther 2003;41(4):489–94.

77. Foa EB, Hearst-Ikeda DE, Perry KJ. Evaluation of a brief cognitive-behavioral program for the prevention of chronic PTSD in recent assault victims. J Consult Clin Psychol 1995;63:948–55.

78. Echeburua E, de Corral P, Sarasua B, et al. Treatment of acute posttraumatic stress disorder in rape victims: an experimental study. J Anxiety Disord 1996; 10:185–99.

79. Ehlers A, Clark DM, Hackman A, et al. A randomized controlled trial of cognitive therapy, a self-help booklet, and repeated assessments as early interventions for posttraumatic stress disorder. Arch Gen Psychiatry 2003;60(10): 1024–32.

80. Bryant R, Moulds M, Guthrie R, et al. The additive benefit of hypnosis and cognitive-behavioural therapy in treating acute stress disorder. J Consult Clin Psychol 2005;73(2):334–40.

81. Bisson JI, Shepherd JP, et al. Early cognitive-behavioural therapy for post-traumatic stress symptoms after physical injury: randomised controlled trial. Br J Psychiatry 2004;184:63–9.

82. van Emmerik AA, Kamphuis JH, Emmelkamp PM. Treating acute stress disorder and posttraumatic stress disorder with cognitive behavioural therapy or structured writing therapy: a randomized controlled trial. Psychother Psychosom 2008;77(2):93–100.

83. Foa EB, Zoellner LA, Feeny NC. An evaluation of three brief programs for facilitating recovery after assault. J Trauma Stress 2006;19(1):29–43.

84. Sijbrandij M, Olff M, Reitsma J, et al. Treatment of acute posttraumatic stress disorder with brief cognitive behavioural therapy: a randomized controlled trial. Am J Psychiatry 2007;164:82–90.

85. Weisaeth L. Acute posttraumatic stress: nonacceptance of early intervention. J Clin Psychiatry 2001;62(Suppl 17):35–40.

86. Stuber J, Galea S, Boscarino JA, et al. Was there unmet mental health need after the September 11, 2001 terrorist attacks? Soc Psychiatry Psychiatr Epidemiol 2006;41(3):230–40.

87. Brewin CR, Scragg P, Robertson M, et al. Promoting mental health following the London bombings: a screen and treat approach. J Trauma Stress 2008;21(1): 3–8.

88. Frueh BC, Grubaugh AL, Yeager DE, et al. Delayed-onset post-traumatic stress disorder among war veterans in primary care clinics. Br J Psychiatry 2009;194: 515–52.

89. Cahill SP, Foa EB, et al. Dissemination of exposure therapy in the treatment of posttraumatic stress disorder. J Trauma Stress 2006;19(5):597–610.

90. Foa EB. Psychosocial therapy for posttraumatic stress disorder. J Clin Psychiatry 2006;67(Suppl 2):40–5.

91. Basoglu M, Salcioglu E, et al. A randomized controlled study of single-session behavioural treatment of earthquake-related post-traumatic stress disorder using an earthquake simulator. Psychol Med 2007;37(2):203–13.

92. US Department of Veterans Affairs. Diagnostic- and symptom-guided drug selection. J Clin Psychiatry 2008;69(6):959–65.

93. Foa EB, Keane TM, Friedman MJ, editors. Effective treatments for PTSD: practice guidelines from the International Society for Traumatic Stress Studies. New York: Guilford Press; 2000.

94. Mohamed S, Rosenheck RA. Pharmacotherapy of PTSD in the US Department of Veterans Affairs: diagnostic- and symptom-guided drug selection. J Clin Psychiatry 2008;69(6):959–65.

95. Brady K, Pearlstein T, Asnis GM, et al. Efficacy and safety of sertraline treatment of posttraumatic stress disorder: a randomized controlled trial. JAMA 2000; 283(14):1837–44.

96. Davidson JR, Rothbaum BO, van der Kolk BA, et al. Multicenter, double-blind comparison of sertraline and placebo in the treatment of posttraumatic stress disorder. Arch Gen Psychiatry 2001;58(5):485–92.

97. Marshall RD, Beebe KL, Oldham M, et al. Efficacy and safety of paroxetine treatment for chronic PTSD: a fixed-dose, placebo-controlled study. Am J Psychiatry 2001;158(12):1982–8.

98. Tucker P, Zaninelli R, Yehuda R, et al. Paroxetine in the treatment of chronic posttraumatic stress disorder: results of a placebo-controlled, flexible-dosage trial. J Clin Psychiatry 2001;62(11):860–8.

99. Martenyi F, Brown EB, Zhang II, et al. Fluoxetine versus placebo in prevention of relapse in post-traumatic stress disorder. Br J Psychiatry 2002;181: 315–20.

100. Martenyi F, Brown EB, Caldwell CD. Failed efficacy of fluoxetine in the treatment of posttraumatic stress disorder: results of a fixed-dose, placebo-controlled study. J Clin Psychopharmacol 2007;27(2):166–70.

101. Friedman MJ, Donnelly CL, Mellman TA. Pharmacotherapy for PTSD. Psychiatr Ann 2003;33(1):57–62.

102. Zhang W, Davidson JR. Post-traumatic stress disorder: an evaluation of existing pharmacotherapies and new strategies. Expert Opin Pharmacother 2007;8(12): 1861–70.

103. Berger W, Mendlowicz MV, et al. Pharmacologic alternatives to antidepressants in posttraumatic stress disorder: a systematic review. Prog Neuropsychopharmacol Biol Psychiatry 2009;33(2):169–80.

104. Asnis GM, Kohn SR, et al. SSRIs versus non-SSRIs in post-traumatic stress disorder: an update with recommendations. Drugs 2004;64(4):383–404.

105. Stein MB, Kline NA, et al. Adjunctive olanzapine for SSRI-resistant combat-related PTSD: a double-blind, placebo-controlled study. Am J Psychiatry 2002;159(10):1777–9.

106. Adamou M, Puchalska S, et al. Valproate in the treatment of PTSD: systematic review and meta-analysis. Curr Med Res Opin 2007;23(6):1285–91.

107. Raskind MA, Peskind ER, et al. A parallel group placebo controlled study of prazosin for trauma nightmares and sleep disturbance in combat veterans with post-traumatic stress disorder. Biol Psychiatry 2007;61(8):928–34.

108. Taylor HR, Freeman MK, et al. Prazosin for treatment of nightmares related to posttraumatic stress disorder. Am J Health Syst Pharm 2008;65(8):716–22.

109. Marks I, Lovell K, Noshirvani H, et al. Treatment of posttraumatic stress disorder by exposure and/or cognitive restructuring: a controlled study. Arch Gen Psychiatry 1998;55:317–25.

110. Resick PA, Nishith P, Weaver TL, et al. A comparison of cognitive-processing therapy with prolonged exposure and a waiting condition for the treatment of chronic posttraumatic stress disorder in female rape victims. J Consult Clin Psychol 2002;70:867–79.

111. Foa EB, Dancu CV, Hembree EA, et al. A comparison of exposure therapy, stress inoculation training, and their combination for reducing posttraumatic stress disorder in female assault victims. J Consult Clin Psychol 1999;67: 194–200.

112. Resick PA, Schnicke MK. Cognitive processing therapy for rape victims: a treatment manual. Newbury Park (CA): Sage; 1993.

113. Foa EB, Hembree EA, Rothbaum BO. Prolonged exposure therapy for PTSD: emotional process of traumatic experiences–therapist guide. Oxford (UK): Oxford University Press; 2007.

114. Devilly GJ, Spence SH. The relative efficacy and treatment distress of EMDR and a cognitive behavior trauma treatment protocol in the amelioration of post-traumatic stress disorder. J Anxiety Disord 1999;13:131–57.

115. Ironson GI, Freund B, Strauss JL, et al. Comparison of two treatments for traumatic stress: a community-based study of EMDR and prolonged exposure. J Clin Psychol 2002;58:113–28.

116. Rothbaum BO, Astin MC, Marsteller F. Prolonged exposure versus EMDR for PTSD rape victims. J Trauma Stress 2005;18:607–16.

117. Taylor S, Thordarson DS, Maxfield L, et al. Comparative efficacy, speed, and adverse effects of three PTSD treatments: exposure therapy, EMDR and relaxation training 2003.

118. Heresco-Levy U, Kremer I, et al. Pilot-controlled trial of D-cycloserine for the treatment of post-traumatic stress disorder. Int J Neuropsychopharmacol 2002;5(4):301–7.

119. Rothbaum BO, Hodges LF, et al. Virtual reality exposure therapy for Vietnam veterans with posttraumatic stress disorder. J Clin Psychiatry 2001;62(8):617–22.

120. Rizzo AA, Difede J, et al. VR PTSD exposure therapy results with active duty OIF/OEF combatants. Stud Health Technol Inform 2009;142:277–82.

121. Germain V, Marchand A, Bouchard S, et al. Effectiveness of cognitive behavioural therapy administered by videoconference for posttraumatic stress disorder. Cogn Behav Ther 2009;38(1):42–53.

122. Taubenfeld S, Riceberg JS, et al. Preclinical assessment for selectively disrupting a traumatic memory via postretrieval inhibition of glucocorticoid receptors. Biol Psychiatry 2009;65(3):249–57.

123. Yehuda R, Flory JD, et al. Developing an agenda for translational studies of resilience and vulnerability following trauma exposure. Ann N Y Acad Sci 2006; 1071:379–96.

124. Litz BT, Engel CC, et al. A randomized, controlled proof-of-concept trial of an Internet-based, therapist-assisted, self-management treatment for posttraumatic stress disorder. Am J Psychiatry 2007;164(11):1676–83.

125. Pitman RK, Orr SP, Forgue DF, et al. Psychophysiology of PTSD imagery in Vietnam combat veterans. Arch Gen Psychiatry 1987;44:970–5.

126. LeDoux JE, Romanski L, Xagoraris A. Indelibility of subcortical emotional networks. J Cogn Neurosci 1989;1:238–43.

127. Shalev AY, Sahar T, Freedman S, et al. A prospective study of heart rate responses following trauma and the subsequent development of PTSD. Arch Gen Psychiatry 1998;55:553–9.

128. Freedman SA, Peri T, Brandes D, et al. Predictors of chronic PTSD: a prospective study. Br J Psychiatry 1999;174:353–9.

129. Hathaway LM, Boals A, et al. "PTSD symptoms and dominant emotional response to a traumatic event: an examination of DSM-IV criterion A2." Anxiety Stress Coping 2009 Apr 20:1–8 [Epub ahead of print].

130. Weathers FW, Keane TM. The criterion a problem revisited: controversies and challenges in defining and measuring psychological trauma. J Trauma Stress 2007;20(2):107–21.

131. Yehuda R, McFarlane AC. Conflict between current knowledge about posttraumatic stress disorder and its original conceptual basis. Am J Psychiatry 1995; 152:1705–13.

Index

Note: Page numbers of article titles are in **boldface** type.

A

Acceptance and commitment therapy (ACT), for generalized anxiety disorder, 633–634
    for obsessive-compulsive disorder, 668
    for social phobia, 647
    in CBT, 529–530, 537–538
        unified treatment protocol for, 539
Acute stress disorder (ASD), comparison of CBT and CBT with adjunctive therapy for, 690–691
    critical period for irreversible CNS changes in, 688–689
    pharmacotherapy for, 689–690
    psychological interventions for, exposure-based, trauma-focused CBT, 690–691
Agomelatine, for generalized anxiety disorder, 615
Agoraphobia, in children and adolescents, course of, 505
        prevalence of, 496–499
Amino acid neurotransmitters, in generalized anxiety disorder, 564
    in panic disorder, 554–555
    in social anxiety disorder, 561
Amygdala, in anxiety disorders, 510–511
    in fear response, 550–551
    in generalized anxiety disorder, 617
    in social anxiety disorder, 561
Anterior cerebral cortex (ACC), in social anxiety disorder, 561
Anticonvulsants, for panic disorder, 594
Antidepressants, for PTSD, 692
    for specific phobias, 582
Antiepileptics, for PTSD, 693
Antipsychotics, for PTSD, 690
Anxiety, and depression, models for, 511
    criteria for, child-specific, 485
    description of, 483–484
    developmental issues and implications for DSM-V, **483–524**
    in children, assessment of, features in, 484
    in children and adolescents, assessment instruments for, 492
        assessment of, 488–491
        categorical inventories of, 493–494
        developmental issues in, 485
        epidemiology of, 487, 495
        normative, 484, 486
        onset of, 487, 495–496
        prevalence of, 487, 495–496

Psychiatr Clin N Am 32 (2009) 705–718
doi:10.1016/S0193-953X(09)00067-7
0193-953X/09/$ – see front matter © 2009 Elsevier Inc. All rights reserved.

Moving?

Make sure your subscription moves with you!

To notify us of your new address, find your **Clinics Account Number** (located on your mailing label above your name), and contact customer service at:

Email: journalscustomerservice-usa@elsevier.com

800-654-2452 (subscribers in the U.S. & Canada)
314-447-8871 (subscribers outside of the U.S. & Canada)

Fax number: 314-447-8029

Elsevier Health Sciences Division
Subscription Customer Service
3251 Riverport Lane
Maryland Heights, MO 63043

*To ensure uninterrupted delivery of your subscription, please notify us at least 4 weeks in advance of move.